Advanced
Early Years
Care and Education

For levels 4 and 5

lai

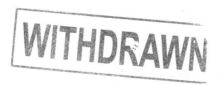

www.heinemann.co.uk
✓ Free online support
✓ Useful weblinks
✓ 24 hour online ordering

01865 888058

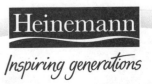

Heinemann

Inspiring generations

Heinemann Educational Publishers
Halley Court, Jordan Hill, Oxford OX2 8EJ
Part of Harcourt Education

Heinemann is the registered trademark of Harcourt Education Limited

© Iain MacLeod-Brudenell, Vicky Cortvriend, Elaine Hallet, Janet Kay, Vivienne Walkup, 2004

First published 2004

09 08 07
10 9 8 7 6

British Library Cataloguing in Publication Data is available
from the British Library on request.

978 0 435401 78 8

Designed by Kamae Design
Typeset by 🅣 Tek-Art, Croydon, Surrey
Original illustrations © Harcourt Education Limited, 2004
Cover design by The Wooden Ark Studio
Cover photo: © Alamy Images

Printed in the UK by CPI Bath

Acknowledgements
Every effort has been made to contact copyright holders of material
reproduced in this book. Any omissions will be rectified in subsequent
printings if notice is given to the publishers.

Tel: 01865 888058 www.heinemann.co.uk

Contents

About the authors

Iain MacLeod-Brudenell has taught in all phases of education and has had teaching, advisory, inspection and teacher training experience in early years education. He has provided nursery and early years teachers with their initial training. He has also developed a multi-disciplinary BA (Hons) degree in Early Childhood Studies (extended and developed by Janet Kay), an HND in Early Childhood Studies (with Vicky Cortvriend) and, more recently, a sector and non-sector endorsed foundation degree in Educare (with Elaine Hallet), which addresses all four routes of the sector endorsed Foundation Degree.

Vicky Cortvriend holds a degree in Nursing Management and Education. She worked as a midwife, then as a psychiatric nurse involved in student and client education. She has been a lecturer in early childhood studies since 1994. Vicky holds an early years qualification and is involved in teaching health and early years; at present, she is working with HND an BA students. She is also conducting her own research towards a Masters degree in professional development, focussing on four-year-olds in reception classes.

Elaine Hallet has wide early years experience, having taught in nursery and infant settings. She has a particular interest in the professional development of early years practitioners. She has delivered curriculum professional development courses in early literacy and has taught initial training childcare programmes. As senior lecturer at the University of Derby, she has taught on the BA Early Childhood Studies course. She was involved in writing the DFES Surestart Early Years sector endorsed approved Foundation Degree in Educare and Early Childhood and is its programme leader. Her research interests include early literacy development and reflective practice.

Janet Kay trained as a social worker specialising in child protection. After gaining a PGCE in Further Education, she became a lecturer in social care at North Derbyshire Tertiary College and went on to become the programme leader of the Early Childhood Studies BA at the University of Derby. She is the author of several publications on child protection and other early years subjects and is currently a senior lecturer in Early Childhood Studies at Sheffield Hallam University.

Vivienne Walkup is team leader in Education Studies at the University of Derby. She was previously a teacher and lecturer in English before becoming a lecturer in psychology. She is a practising counsellor and has a particular interest in child psychology. She is the mother of five children.

Acknowledgements

Iain MacLeod-Brudenell wishes to thank:
Joy Foster, University of Central Lancashire, for her support and encouragement.
Iain's grandchildren Patrick and Eleanore, George and Flora for providing him with a constant flow of source material for vignettes
… and Tamsin who was left out last time!

Vicky Cortvriend wishes to thank her husband and children.

Janet Kay wishes to thank:
Viv and Iain and all the team at Derby for your support and friendship during my time there – may it long continue!
My children Amie, Laura and Dan for spending their early childhood under surveillance and for wanting to be in the book.

Vivienne Walkup wishes to thank:
Her sons and daughters, who have provided her with constant inspiration.

Photo acknowledgements

Gareth Boden: 24, 28, 101, 177, 217, 291, 427, 433
Haddon Davies: 52
Gerald Sunderland: 88 and 89
Getty Images UK / Digital Vision: 162
Trevor Clifford: 192
Mark Thomas: 473

Introduction

This book will be of interest to all those who are taking courses in early childhood studies at levels 4 and 5 but particularly those who are foundation degree students. The book interest other practitioners in early years care and education who are not, as yet, following a formal course of study. A foundation degree in early years aims to equip students with a combination of the technical abilities, academic knowledge and transferable skills that employers in the early years sector are increasingly demanding. Many practitioners on Foundation Degrees and other courses will already have a range of rich and varied experiences of working with children and families, although students may be beginning academic study from different starting points. This book will focus on aiding you to fully recognise your existing academic and practice skills, to further develop these skills, and to extend your knowledge and understanding the many issues within early years care and education.

Students on Foundation Degrees may also be considering further study on completion. Although the foundation degree is a valuable higher education qualification in its own right, it is also seen by the government as making a valuable contribution to the 'ladder of lifelong learning', providing opportunities for students to progress to an honours degree and further professional qualifications.

Early Years Foundation Degrees aim to integrate study and work in order to enhance practice, often through work-based modules and projects, but also through assessment by means of reflecting on practice-based application of theory. This book will help you to become more aware of developmental approaches to learning and to reflect upon practice, which will extend your professional competence and effectiveness in supporting the well-being of children.

Encouraging equity

Effective communication between adults and children involves critical analysis of one's own interpersonal interactions with adults as well as children. This should include the ability to evaluate the effect of one's actions on other people in the environment in which you work. A central theme within this book is reflection on factors that contribute to effective communication with others including children, parents and other professionals. The practitioner's awareness of equity, anti-discriminatory practice and equality of opportunity should permeate every area of practice.

In line with current practice in educare documentation and practice, we use the term 'equity' throughout this book in preference to the broad and less defined term 'equal opportunities'. Equity is a proactive approach, concerning 'doing' rather than 'offering'. In order to provide equality of opportunity, individual children may require different and often unequal treatment so that they have complete access to opportunities offered to other children. For example, a child who has difficulty developing social skills may require additional support. A child who is learning to use English when it is not his or her first language will also require support in order to access the curriculum. Equitable approaches will therefore reflect developmentally appropriate early years practice.

About this book

The term 'educare' is used throughout this book. It is indicative of the increasingly close link between the two aspects – care and education (early learning) – that are present in government initiatives in the early years. Although this term may be of recent origin, the combination of these two aspects of early childhood support has a long history. This is explored in Chapter 1 and provides a rationale for the integrated approach to early childhood studies taken within this book.

Reflection on workplace issues, as well as theoretical educare issues, will aid you in your growth as a reflective practitioner with a commitment to lifelong learning. Reflective evaluation and analysis of practice is introduced in Chapter 2 and forms a strand throughout this book.

Understanding the physical development of children and issues related to health and physical safety are important and often neglected aspects of courses within higher education. Early years foundation degrees seek to redress this imbalance within their curricula and we reflect this aim in Chapter 3 (physical development) and Chapter 14 (health).

Similarly, not all practitioners have had an opportunity to study aspects of cognitive, emotional and social development. We address these issues in Chapters 4 and 5 at a level that provides a stimulus both for novices and for more experienced students.

Reflection upon your own personal and professional growth will require consideration of your own attitudes to teaching and learning. As discussed in Chapter 8, a considered approach to planning, which takes account of a child's individual needs, encourages the provision of richer learning experiences.

Evaluation of practice often involves the practitioner in research. In this book, Chapter 9 covers observation and research, and Chapter 10 focuses on undertaking a small-scale research project. Practitioners may be feel that research is a luxury confined to those with more time on their hands. In fact, practitioners often conduct informal but essential research in their daily work, such as by using different types of observation in the assessment of emotional, social or cognitive development of children. Data gathered may be used to inform planning. In many. This book encourages practitioners to extend their forms of research, in order to enable more considered and focused reflection of a single issue.

An understanding of the regulatory and legislative framework for early years is essential for all practitioners. The developing climate of collaboration between childcare and education services for young children is, in many ways, a response to failures in protecting and supporting children. A context of multi-agency co-operation requires all those who work with children to be better informed of their responsibilities and those of others. Chapter 11 provides a background discussion and some starting points to direct you to further detailed study of legislation in care and education.

The physical and emotional safety of children is a dynamic issue in legislation. A full discussion of the results of shortcomings in policy and practice relating to child protection and the actions taken in response is presented as a critical issue in Chapter 12 and, more specifically, in Chapter 15.

Working with parents and those with parental responsibility raises many issues of 'partnership' (Chapter 13). Professional practice must respond to the needs of children and their families, and requires that practitioners are competent in a broad range of communication and interpersonal skills in order to achieve effective collaboration.

Features of this book

Most early years foundation degree students will be undertaking their course through part-time study and will find that their academic studies complement and inform skills in their current jobs. Other students who have little practice-based experience will undertake this as part of their course. A variety of learning modes are provided within the book because you need to progress at your own pace, using methods that are best suited to you.

The learning that takes place during work experience is invaluable, not simply for improving and enhancing practice, but also for the place it has in contextualising the taught elements of the programme of study. In this book, vignettes and case studies provide examples from practice that illustrate key teaching points. The place of work experience is supported within each chapter in order to aid you in your ability to draw together taught elements of your course with practice-based learning. Both elements will be recognised in the formal assessment of your course.

By posing questions for your consideration and by presenting contentious issues for you to address, we aim to prepare you for progression to further qualifications. You are also encouraged, through the use of discussion points, activities and suggested further reading, to evaluate and monitor your developing skills.

Given the limited space that any book allows, it would be impossible to tackle every area in the depth that we would wish. Therefore, each chapter provides ideas for practice-based activities and a list of further references.

These will to help you understand, explain and evaluate the theoretical issues in the field of early childhood studies and to apply your critical understanding to a variety of issues in the workplace.

It is strongly recommended that you keep a log or a reflective diary during your programme of study. This is where you can record all your new learning, such as your developing skills in time management, your thoughts and reflections on practice, and the links you are making between theory and practice. Each chapter in this book will encourage you to consider the importance of becoming aware of an important issue in educare. As such, we will provide you with some ideas for developing platforms for self-knowledge and devising a programme of personal development.

Finally...

... we hope that you will find this book a valuable support in your studies. Good luck with your course!

Traditions and trends in early years care and education

1

Iain MacLeod-Brudenell

This chapter is designed to encourage you to extend your knowledge of the work of some of those who have made significant contributions to the study of young children. Following through key ideas from their original conception to the present day will enable you to gain insights into current practice. This chapter introduces the term educare, which is used throughout this book. It is widely used to describe an approach to working with young children that is more than its constituent parts: education and care. Educare approaches are not new but have enjoyed a revival and been given greater prominence over the past decade in the government agenda for combined early childhood support and provision. Increased emphasis has been placed on the integrated approach to early learning and the care of young children in England within recent years in both theory and practice: for example, in the Sure Start (2003) publication *Birth to Three Matters* and in the Curriculum Guidance for the Foundation Stage (QCA/DfEE (2001)). In other countries, formal documentation for the very early years is not provided but is embedded in practice.

There is a strong tradition of combining early learning and care in an holistic approach to working with young children. 'Education' may not be the most appropriate term to apply to younger children in the home and pre-school as the word has associations for many people with more formal, planned approaches to learning.

This chapter addresses the following areas:

⊃ why we should be aware of historical traditions in care and education
⊃ major theorists and their influence
⊃ the traditions today
⊃ traditions becoming trends
⊃ the work of Robert Owen
⊃ the work of Margaret McMillan

By undertaking the suggested study within this chapter it is hoped that you will be able to:

1 recognise the origins of some of the philosophical foundations of current methods and practices in early years education and care

2 identify the influence of key figures in the history of early childhood philosophy on present-day practice in educare

3 make informed reflections upon recent issues in educare provision.

Introduction

This chapter does not attempt to look at each and every person who has influenced early years practice. Instead it begins by focusing on a few aspects of the work of some leading theorists in early childhood studies – in particular Froebel, Montessori and Steiner. Emphasis is then given to the theories and work of two key practitioners – Robert Owen and Margaret McMillan; the focus on these two people is not because they are the most important theorists but rather because they are examples of practitioners who use an approach that draws on the combined provision of care and early learning.

Why we should be aware of historical traditions in care and education

Degree courses in the study of early childhood may vary in the focus they place upon the study of early learning, education and care. A common feature, however, is the emphasis placed upon a combined holistic approach to children's care and educational needs. This appears to be a model that is favoured by current legislation in England (DfES, 2002) and has been promoted in Scotland and in Wales. All courses in early childhood studies seek to:

- encourage students to explain and evaluate theoretical issues in the field of early childhood studies
- apply their critical understanding of such issues in appropriate practice settings.

Thus, there are two key strands in studying for a degree in early childhood studies: theory and practice. In order to better understand early childhood education and care (educare) theory we believe that students should be encouraged to reflect upon practice as well as engage in practice: to think as well as 'do'. This chapter presents ideas that were promoted by key thinkers in the study of early childhood, which have shaped the provision of educare today, and are present in many of the issues that appear in current legislation and practice.

As practitioners in early years settings we take many of our practice methods for granted. We have generally agreed ways of working that are defined by national criteria (Ofsted for example); curriculum guidance (as seen in documentation such as *Birth to Three Matters* (Sure Start, 2003); Curriculum Guidance for the Foundation Stage (QCA, 2000); and the National Curriculum. Statutory requirements as defined by the Children Act (1989) will also affect methods of working and these are usually well established. For some, the approach to early learning and care may also be offered using a particular approach such as High/Scope, or it may follow a particular philosophy such as is found in Steiner or Montessori nurseries and schools. In our expectations of children there may be close links to their performance in achieving the tasks outlined in such curricula.

We may also take for granted such ideas as 'parents as partners' and 'child-centred approaches'. Familiarity with such terms, or frequency of use, sometimes blurs the power of such statements. But where do these ideas originate? In your previous studies you may have looked at some of the main sources of early years curriculum and care theory; you may also be aware of such thinkers as Piaget and Vygotsky, of practitioners such as the McMillan sisters and Steiner. It may not be clear to you where the linkage between the theories expounded by these thinkers and present-day practice lies. This chapter aims to demonstrate some of these links.

Major theorists and their influence

Many seminal thinkers have influenced contemporary early childhood education and care. We regard these thinkers as important today, but they may have been seen very differently in their own time. For some of their contemporaries, these theorists appeared to reflect the values of a few people, but with hindsight we can see that they all functioned within the context of the values of the time. Their influence has not only been long lasting but has also influenced early years curricula throughout the world.

A starting point for any recent study of traditions in early education must be to acknowledge the work of Bruce (1987) in her comparison of the work of three leaders in the field of early childhood studies: Froebel, Montessori and Steiner. (Bruce further develops her discussion by comparing their work with that of more recent thinkers: Piaget, Vygotsky, Bruner and Mia Kelmer Pringle.)

Brief details of the work of Froebel, Montessori and Steiner are provided in this section. To discuss all aspects of the work of each theorist would detract from the key message that you should take from this discussion and, therefore, the aim is to illustrate some of the key aspects of their work only to enable you to compare and contrast ideas. You should refer to websites listed at the end of this chapter for more detailed information.

Friedrich Wilhelm Froebel
(1782–1852)

Froebel developed the concept of focused early learning experiences, based on the idea of 'natural unfolding'. Through close observation of children, adults – both parents and teachers – could determine the child's readiness to learn and thus provide appropriate activities. The role of the mother in recognising the capacity for learning in their children and for nurturing this learning was an important underpinning feature of Froebel's vision. The role of the teacher was as a guide and support in developing children's inherent capacity for learning.

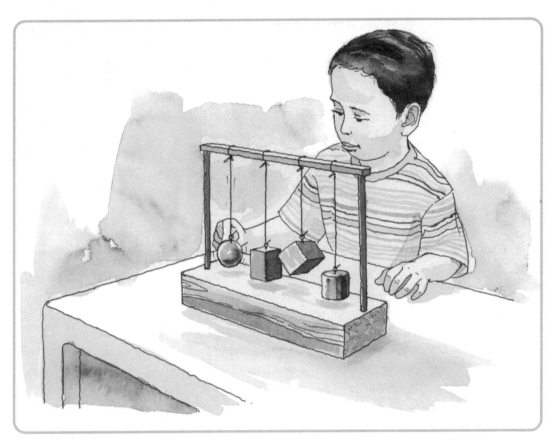

Froebel's gifts are intended to develop complex skills of perception, manipulation and combination

Froebel formulated the idea of the kindergarten as a means of educating young children. The term **Kindergarten** ('children's garden') reflects the metaphors he used to describe and explain his educational theory. In Froebel's view of early childhood, a child was likened to a seed, the process of learning 'unfolding' to the flower emerging from a bud, and the educator likened to a gardener nurturing the plant.

To Froebel, both the child's own nature and the more universal aspect of nature were in close harmony. To enable the child to develop his/her inherent capacity for learning, the supportive adult had to be trained in this particular method. Froebel's curriculum was carefully planned. Children were encouraged to learn through playful activity and songs. Froebel's 'gifts' were an essential aspect of his structure for learning. Gifts included balls of different colour and size, cubes, cylinders and spheres. The kindergarten teacher supported the child in using these objects, to handle and consider them in order to acquire an understanding of shape, size and colour, of concepts such as contrasting, counting and measuring. Occupations comprised materials for developing psychomotor skills: for example, cutting, folding, modelling, stringing beads and sewing.

Key points of Froebel's approach

Froebel's approach emphasised the following:

- ⮑ children are able to develop their unique capacity for learning 'unfolding' through play. Active learning is essential, as is the use of concrete manipulative materials in the learning process
- ⮑ the importance of mothers in the education of young children
- ⮑ children learn through carefully structured play, matched to their readiness, with guidance, appropriate direction and an organised and prepared learning environment
- ⮑ the importance of training for early childhood (kindergarten) teachers. The first kindergarten was established in England in 1851 and the first specific training establishment – the Froebel Training College – was opened in 1876.

Influence of Froebel's work on current practice

These points are as contentious today as they were in the early 19th century. The emphasis on active learning is well established within early years settings, but there is emphasis placed upon meeting targets within current guidance from central government (QCA, 2000; 2003). It may be argued that those targets are indicative of 'normal' expectations of children's development; however, there appears to be widespread misunderstanding and misinterpretation of the guidance in practice. Worksheets are regularly used in some pre-school settings, and yet there is no requirement or expectation for their use; it is a misunderstanding of the curriculum guidance. Supportive materials provided in the Curriculum Guidance for the Foundation Stage (QCA, 2000) emphasise the need to be aware of the differences in individual developmental rates, and yet in practice, play appears to be subservient to the taught curriculum. Documents will allow, some may say encourage, play-based activity. Evidence provided by interpretation of the inspection of early years settings would indicate that play-based learning is not a priority.

The role of mothers

The role of mothers in child rearing continues to be an issue for debate. Froebel believed that mothers should be encouraged to devote their time to caring for and educating their children. In today's society, in the United Kingdom, it may be argued that there is subtle pressure from government and the media to encourage mothers of young children to work rather than to remain at home. Teaching and nurturing children in the home appears to be regarded as less effective or desirable than education in more formal, out-of-home settings.

Training of practitioners for work in early years settings

Froebel believed that the training of workers for early years settings was essential. Children are now being admitted to out-of-home settings at a progressively earlier age than was formerly the case. The training of practitioners in educare is, therefore, an area that has received some considerable attention in recent years. In effect, current practice is now trying to catch up with ideas that Froebel proposed many years ago. Courses leading to a wide range of specific childcare qualifications, at a variety of levels of academic and practice-based competence, are now available in the United Kingdom. Basic skills have been met in knowledge and understanding of childcare through, for example, the NVQ qualifications route. More rigorous study on BA Early Childhood Studies programmes has ensured that potentially a highly qualified workforce is available to work with young children. However, the government has not organised the range of qualifications within an appropriate framework effectively, either in matching qualifications to the needs of children and parents, or the students on such courses, and so has some way to go to meet Froebel's vision. Current developments through new childcare and education programmes, such as the emergent foundation degrees, enhance practitioner confidence and skills through a mixture of academic and work-related study. These may prove to be an effective short-term solution to meeting government targets by supplying greater numbers of more highly qualified staff for early years settings than is presently available. The initial training of teachers in early years settings remains largely focused on meeting government agendas or political imperatives (and is controlled by inspection) rather than focusing on those areas of child development that are prominent in the curricula of similar training schemes in other parts of the world. The syllabus of Froebel's Training College has been largely superseded in English teacher education by emphasis on a much narrower curriculum, despite valiant efforts by a number of universities and colleges.

> **Activity 1** **Varying practices in training practitioners for early years settings**
>
> Extend your awareness of different practice in the training of early years staff.
>
> Talk to colleagues about the content of their training course, for example:
>
> ⊃ nursery nurses
> ⊃ classroom teaching assistants
> ⊃ play workers
> ⊃ social workers working with young children
> ⊃ teachers.
>
> If you wish, you may combine this activity with some practice in using research methods (see Chapter 10), either now or at a later date.

Devise a questionnaire or a schedule for informal interviews

Devise a questionnaire, or a schedule, for informal interviews. Your questions may focus on the following or other similar issues:

- ⊃ similarities in the content of the courses, the curriculum
- ⊃ comparability between the length of the different courses and future roles and responsibilities
- ⊃ the monitoring of work practice or placement
- ⊃ assessment of practice-based study
- ⊃ the proportion of time allocated to child development as part of training.

Comment on research activity

If you undertake this research, either informally through conversation with colleagues, or through a more focused interview or questionnaire, it will illustrate just how much variation there is in early years training. This research should provide some very interesting comparisons between training in different locations. The period in which training was undertaken will also reveal different emphases in curriculum content.

Consistency of approach to training at different times and in different locations is more likely to occur in centres that follow a particular philosophy. Such training may now be undertaken in training centres, colleges and through distance learning. National and international organisations often advertise, or inform interested parties, through websites. This is the case with those following the Montessori method for training teachers.

The work of Maria Montessori (1870–1952)

Montessori's method draws on the ideas of Rousseau and Pestalozzi and the practical approaches to teaching devised by Froebel. Emphasis was placed on the child experiencing carefully organised preparatory activities, rather than repetition as a means of developing competence in skills.

first the education of the senses, then the education of the intellect.

Maria Montessori
(1870–1952)

The essential thing is for the task to arouse such an interest that it engages the child's whole personality.

Montessori (1967:206)

Montessori's first involvement with young children was as a medical practitioner and not an educationalist. In fact, she was the first woman in Italy to qualify as a physician.

Her work with those children who were regarded as difficult to educate, including those whom we would now classify as having special needs, prompted her initial interest in educational methodology.

Montessori method of training teachers

Montessori's method of teaching has been successful in a wide range of contexts. This is in part due to the emphasis placed on the training of teachers in the Montessori method. There is a particular emphasis on the need for good observational skills, in order to inform planning and support and guide children's learning. Montessori intended teacher intervention to be appropriately applied – children guided rather than over-directed. This approach has led to 'de-centring' of the teacher's role. Montessori settings strive to present a stimulating environment. They would also claim that they encourage children to participate more fully in taking responsibility for their own learning. (Such claims would also be made by those following a more mainstream curriculum and other methodological approaches such as High/Scope.) Montessori was one of the first to stress the importance of these aspects of early learning.

Rudolf Steiner

A third key person, who is very influential on present-day practice in many countries, is Rudolf Steiner. As well as having influenced approaches used within 'mainstream' nursery and early years education curricula, Steiner educational theory is used in its complete form in Steiner Waldorf schools in over 40 countries. There are currently more than 800 schools, and, although each school is independently managed they all conform to Steiner's principles. Often, these private schools provide an alternative to the national prescribed curricula present in mainstream education, within different cultural and social contexts.

Spiritual dimension to Steiner's approach

Steiner education, or Waldorf/Steiner education as it is often known, has its origins in a vision of education as a means of changing society. In this respect, there are many similarities between Steiner's intentions and those of Owen (see page 17) and McMillan (see page 21). Steiner differs markedly from the other two educational and social reformers in that the spiritual dimension was the key to his entire approach to life. His philosophy has at its core a view that the person is a threefold being of spirit, soul and body. These three aspects unfold in three developmental stages on the path to adulthood: early childhood, middle childhood and adolescence. In many ways, there are clear links to the perceptions of stages of childhood and adolescence that are reflected in the organisation of stages of teaching the curriculum: in England in the Key Stages, in nursery, first, middle and upper schools, or in nursery, primary and secondary schools. This staged approach has been reflected in curricula throughout the world and at different times.

The origins of Waldorf/Steiner schools have links with industry and philanthropy. In the period following the First World War, Europe was suffering from political instability, economic uncertainty and great social problems. In 1919, Rudolf Steiner was asked by Emil Molt, the owner of the Waldorf Astoria cigarette factory in Austria, to open a school for the children of his employees. This type of philanthropy was not uncommon: schools linked with factories, the most notable of which was Owen's ground-breaking venture at New Lanark in Scotland, were well established. The link with workplace nurseries today is obvious.

Conditions set by Steiner

Steiner's Waldorf School, *Die Freie Waldorfschule*, was free in more than name. The four conditions set by Steiner were:

- ⊃ that the school be open to all children
- ⊃ that it be co-educational
- ⊃ that it be a unified twelve-year school
- ⊃ that the teachers, those individuals actually in contact with the children, have primary control of the school, with minimum interference from the state or from economic sources.

These preconditions indicated a philosophical approach to teaching and learning that was very different from those employed in Austria at that time.

The Waldorf/Steiner curriculum aimed then, and continues, to develop an approach to learning which draws fully on three dimensions: the body, the mind and the spirit. Although much of the language used in Steiner's approach may appear to be exclusive and rooted in theological dogma, in essence there are many aspects of his theory which most early educators would strive to attain a balance between: sound skills in literacy, languages and numeracy, and confidence in aesthetic awareness and practice (in music, art, craft and physical development).

Steiner's approach to training teachers

Training of teachers is very well supported with a rigorous training programme in theoretical and practice-based child-centred education. There are 50 teacher training centres around the world. In Waldorf/Steiner teacher training, one course offers two years of college-based work, followed by one year in placement. A range of pre-service and in-service courses ensures that teaching methods are consistent and conform to the Waldorf/Steiner model.

Rudolf Steiner
(1861–1925)

Steiner's approach to the education and care of young children has a strong emphasis on the spiritual dimension. There is an attempt in the Waldorf/Steiner method to 'unfold', to develop the full potential of every child. Childhood is seen as a stage but within a much broader perspective than in other theoretical approaches. Steiner's philosophy, *Anthroposophy*, acknowledges existence before birth and after death.

Stages of Waldorf/Steiner education match children's developmental stages with a broad and child-focused curriculum. 'Rhythm' and 'balance' are frequently used terms in the curriculum. This is manifest in the respect given to seasons and times of the year, as well as times of life. The balance of skills and knowledge is fostered by equal emphasis on artistic, practical and intellectual work throughout the school curriculum. At the heart of this approach is the child and a recognition that, in order to promote the inner development of the child, it is necessary to provide appropriate experiences for each determined stage of development.

Values feature prominently in Waldorf/Steiner education: social awareness is fostered, and empathy and sensitivity to others are promoted.

Individual aptitudes and needs are nurtured by the sustained, ongoing and supportive relationship between a child and his or her teacher.

Key points of Steiner's approach

Steiner's approach emphasised the following:

⊃ a broad curriculum is offered. There is a balance of aesthetic, social, emotional, spiritual and cognitive development within the taught curriculum

⊃ the curriculum responds to developmental stages.

Activity 2) Research the contributions made by Froebel, Steiner and Montessori

1 Undertake a web search to find out more about Froebel, Steiner and Montessori.

2 Look at some of the websites of Montessori and Waldorf/Steiner schools.

3 Based on the very brief summaries offered here and your web-based research, what do you consider to be the most important contribution of each of these thinkers to current practice in your workplace?

The traditions today

Although Bruce's discussion (1987) is limited in range to only three 'leading theorists', these people are probably the most important in terms of influencing current educational thought and practice. Bruce has provided a valuable and influential framework.

The Early Years Curriculum Group (EYCG, 1992), who adapted Bruce's principles (Fisher, 1996:32), have in turn been very influential in curriculum development, the effects of which can be seen in the current documentation for the Foundation Stage (QCA, 2000). The child-centred approaches to early childhood education and care outlined by Rousseau and Pestalozzi can be seen clearly in the theories of other early childhood educators such as Owen (1771–1858) as well as later figures such as Margaret McMillan and Susan Isaacs. It is well to recognise their contributions, whilst not diminishing the roles of those whom Bruce has chosen to discuss.

The Ten Common Principles

The Ten Common Principles of early childhood education (Bruce 1987:10) are based on the philosophical approaches of the three figures that Bruce considers to be the most important influential pioneers in this field: Froebel, Montessori and Steiner (see Figure 1.1).

Childhood is a part of life, not simply a preparation for the future.

The whole child is considered to be important.

Learning is not compartmentalised, for everything links.

Intrinsic motivation, resulting in child-initiated, self-directed study, is valued.

Self-discipline is emphasised.

There are specially receptive periods for learning at different stages of development.

What children can do (rather than what they cannot do) is the starting point in the child's education.

There is an inner life in the child which emerges especially under favourable conditions.

The people (both adults and children) with whom the child interacts are of central importance.

The child's education is seen as an interaction between the child and the environment the child is in including, in particular, other people and knowledge itself.

(Bruce 1987:10)

Figure 1.1
Principles of early childhood education

The influences of Jean-Jacques Rousseau (1712–1778)

In your reading you will begin to identify how thinkers influence each other and how their ideas are modified to meet the needs of children in different social, historical and geographical contexts. One of the earliest and most influential thinkers was Jean-Jacques Rousseau, a man of many talents: a philosopher with an interest in social and political ideas, a musician, a botanist and, above all, an influential writer. In the sphere of early childhood study, his novel *Émile* (1762) introduced a new theory of education. This approach emphasised the nurturing of the child to encourage free expression rather than repression, a common response to children in his time.

Rousseau's theory of education can be viewed on numerous websites (information is provided at the end of this chapter). His psychologically orientated method of education led to new methods of education and care and his influence can be seen in the theories and practice of Johann Heinrich Pestalozzi, Robert Owen and Friedrich Froebel. Their influence continues to be felt in the present day through figures such as the McMillan sisters, Susan Isaacs, John Dewey and other pioneers of modern early childhood education and care. Rousseau was probably the first widely read writer to identify the link between emotional/physical care and education in the context of effective learning.

Starting points: traditions becoming trends

There are two main responses to early childhood education and both are recorded in Roman times. One view, recorded by Plato in *The Republic*, sees early childhood as a special stage in life and recommends that adults take particular care when educating the young, as 'in all things the beginning is the most important part'.

The second view, which sees children being in need of training by submission of the will is recorded by Seneca. This approach to education viewed the child as 'an empty vessel' to be filled with knowledge. The teacher instructed and the child would learn. If learning was not successful the problem lay with the child rather than the teacher.

These two traditions have run parallel through history and can be discerned in present-day practice, particularly in later primary education. Generally, most educators regard the earliest years of education as different from the later years in that practice is more child-focused in the earliest years. It may be argued that the drive to a narrower skills-based curriculum may eventually displace a child-focused one.

Child-centred learning

Johann Pestalozzi (1746–1827) advocated teaching through kindness and he was the first to apply Rousseau's ideas of child-centred learning approaches in practice. A child-centred curriculum was also fundamental to the teaching method of Robert Owen. (See page 17 for a discussion of Owen's work.)

In Owen's time it was not unusual for children to be exploited and maltreated; they were employed in mills and other industrial settings where mortality rates were high. The living conditions of the working poor were also appalling. The kindness with which the teachers at Owen's school at his factory complex at New Lanark treated the children was, therefore, in marked contrast to the usual life experiences of young children in the early 19th century. Another remarkable aspect of the teaching method at New Lanark was that children were not physically punished but were managed in their behaviour through kindness – a very unusual procedure in the 19th century.

Early years education as a means of combating child 'crime'

The converse of this attitude is demonstrated by Samuel Wilderspin, who was active in the 1840s. He advocated infant schools chiefly as a means of combating child 'crime' (Cusden, 1938:3).

This approach is not far removed from some more recent responses to socio-educational issues. The National Commission on Education report *Learning to Succeed* (1993) emphasised the importance of nursery education and the dangers of admitting children to formal schooling at too early an age. The report urged expansion of nursery education, with provision in priority areas being seen as the most urgent need. The argument proposed within the document, however, was that the cost of such expansion would be offset by reduction in the costs of remedial action in adolescence and by reduced social costs, which arise from youth unemployment and juvenile crime (National Commission on Education, 1993:137).

Divergence of opinion

One of the main reasons why there is such divergence in opinion on the methods of caring for and educating young children is the recognition that young children up to the age of 8 are impressionable and can be moulded to conform to particular social patterns.

McMillan considered that the natural end of early childhood was reached at the age of 7, which corresponds with the traditional end of infant education in England and Scotland. At this age, too, many other countries begin their formal education of children.

The claim by the Jesuits that the period from birth to 7 is of crucial importance to a child's education is well known. It has a basis in fact, as the rates of development and learning are at their most rapid during this stage of childhood.

It may be argued, therefore, that the young child needs to be encouraged and stimulated through the provision of a wide range of experiences.

Developmentally appropriate curriculum

Much has been written about a **developmentally appropriate curriculum**. Blenkin (1994) indicates the extent to which international research studies in early learning and early childhood education have been remarkable for the consistency of their recommendations and findings. This is demonstrated in, for example, the New Zealand ECCE Working Group, the work of the Canadian Ministry of Education in their early years papers and in policies and practices emerging in European countries (Mills and Mills, 1998). This research has helped to clarify what a developmentally appropriate curriculum for young children would look like and to identify the demands that such a curriculum would make on practitioners in early years settings, thereby clarifying their training needs (Blenkin, 1994).

There is very little current training at higher level for those working with very young children. The needs of those working with babies and toddlers are not well served by publications that often focus on the early years of childhood from 3 years and upwards. Until recently, little attention was paid to the age range from 3 to 5 years, where a developmentally appropriate curriculum may be seen as having the greatest potential impact. As Bruce's published works drew on the work of key early childhood thinkers and presented them for the 1980s, Hurst and Joseph (1998) have interpreted these theories for the turn of the 21st century. These Principles for a Developmental Curriculum are now widely recognised as an appropriate theoretical underpinning for early childhood curriculum programme development (see Figure 1.2).

(For articulate and compelling arguments, see Hurst and Joseph (1998) and Blenkin and Kelly (1994); and Siraj-Blatchford (1997:17) for some cautionary comments.) It can be seen that there are strong similarities between these principles and those outlined by Bruce (1997; see Figure 1.1 on page 11).

Guidance on supporting early childhood development

There are many different visions of what is required of the adult in supporting early childhood development and yet there are also some common themes. The following guidance documents all draw on the themes indicated within Figures 1.1 and 1.2:

- ⊃ Curriculum Guidance for the Foundation Stage (2000), which presents materials for use with children between 3 years of age and admission to Year 1 of infant education
- ⊃ the Foundation Stage Profile (2003), which assesses children before they proceed to Year 1 (usually in the term after their fifth birthday)

⊃ Each child is an individual and should be respected and treated as such.

⊃ The early years are a period of development in their own right, and education of young children should be seen as a specialism with its own valid criteria of appropriate practice.

⊃ The role of the educator of young children is to engage actively with what most concerns the child, and to support learning through these preoccupations.

⊃ The educator has a responsibility to foster positive attitudes in children to both self and others, and to counter negative messages which children may have received.

⊃ Each child's cultural and linguistic endowment is seen as the fundamental medium of learning.

⊃ An anti-discriminatory approach is the basis of all respect-worthy education, and is essential as a criterion for a developmentally appropriate curriculum (DAC).

⊃ All children should be offered equal opportunities to progress and develop, and should have equal access to good-quality provision. The concepts of multiculturalism and anti-racism are intrinsic to this whole educational approach.

⊃ Partnership with parents should be given priority as the most effective means of ensuring coherence and continuity in children's experiences, and in the curriculum offered to them.

⊃ A democratic perspective permeates education of good quality and is the basis of transactions between people.

(Hurst and Joseph 1998:xi)

Figure 1.2
Principles for a Developmental Curriculum

⊃ *Birth to Three Matters* (2003), which presents guidance for those working with children under 3 years of age,

However, the interpretation of such guidance by settings managers or teachers may result in very different experiences for children.

The curriculum method devised by Owen in 1816 indicates that he was conscious of the need to devise a programme that was appropriate to the needs he perceived young children to have. This appeared to work. But given enthusiastic practitioners, it may be argued that even more formal approaches to education may also work. Perhaps the key to success is the respect for children by those who care for and educate them.

The youngest, or infant class, under the age of five, ... (were under the) charge of a male and female superintendent, and whose principal office it is to encourage amongst them habits and feelings of good-will and affection towards each other.

Our party walked down to the village, and entered the children's play ground. God bless their little faces, I see them now. There were some bowling hoops, some drumming on two sticks – all engaged in some

infantine amusement or other. Not a tear – not a wrangle. Peaceful innocence pervaded the whole group. As soon as they saw us, curtsies and bows saluted us from all quarters.

(from a report by the Duke of Kent's personal physician in McNab (1819), quoted in Siraj-Blatchford (1997))

Anyone familiar with young children in nursery settings will recognise the responses of these children. A new face in the nursery is soon accosted and questioned; we may no longer have curtsies and bows, but the personal response is the same.

The theorists discussed in this chapter did not have a unified approach to every aspect of early childhood education and care; often their vision and their priorities differed markedly from one another. Four key aspects, however, are present in the educational ideology of every one of these thinkers. These are illustrated in Figure 1.3.

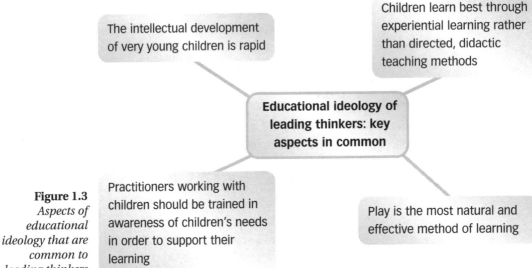

Figure 1.3
Aspects of educational ideology that are common to leading thinkers

Key aspects that are common to the theoretical approaches to the care of young children are shown in Figure 1.4:

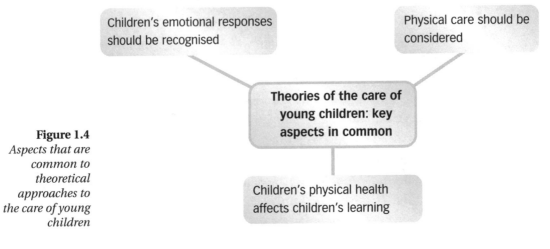

Figure 1.4
Aspects that are common to theoretical approaches to the care of young children

To illustrate the link between the aspects of education and care illustrated in Figures 1.3 and 1.4, the work of two important pioneers in the field of 'educare', Robert Owen and Margaret McMillan, is briefly examined.

The work of Robert Owen (1771–1858)

Owen lived in times of great change. This was a period of rapid industrial development, with the exploitation of the workforce of women and young children as well as men. It was time of great social and political unrest in Britain and revolution in Europe. His motives for developing an interest in early childhood education reflect his political values. A free thinker in an age when religious practice was the norm, Owen was a philanthropist and a political theorist who was not driven by religious imperatives. He was self-educated, a draper's assistant who had become a successful and very wealthy businessman as an owner of cotton mills.

In 1816, Robert Owen established the first school for infants in Britain, at New Lanark in Scotland, a fact that is often overlooked. The age range of the children is also of interest: 1 to10 years. The novelty of his approach was attractive to those who were interested in industrial productivity as well as education. He claimed that the substantial profits generated by his cotton mills were due to the type of education he provided for the children of his workers. The school had visitors from across the world, many of whom commented on the happiness of the children.

It was unusual at this time for employers to be concerned about the welfare of their employees. Owen's motives for establishing a school were to promote social improvement. He was appalled by the conditions of working people and particularly of children. He is credited as one of the founders of the co-operative and socialist movements in Britain.

Educational environment is key

In your previous studies you will doubtless have encountered the nature/nurture debate, that is, the extent to which children are influenced by genetic inheritance or by the environment. Robert Owen firmly believed that the educational environment was a main contributing factor in shaping the ways in which children responded to educative experiences, social behaviour and value systems. Owen was scathing about any influence that heredity might have on a child's development.

He believed that by the use of good role models and appropriate educative and social experiences, children's individual characters could be shaped at a very early age. To this end, he employed male and female teachers who were required to have 'a great love for and unlimited patience with infants'.

A stimulating curriculum

Owen's emphasis was on a stimulating curriculum that offered freedom for the child from the pressures commonly associated with childhood at that time. Singing and dancing featured within the curriculum and he employed a small group of musicians to play to the children from a musicians' gallery. Music has always been a strand of child-centred curricula.

> **Activity 3** **The role of music in children's development**
>
> Consider the role of music in your workplace setting. What is its purpose? How does it help children's cognitive, social and emotional development?

Owen's curriculum did not include craft, now more commonly referred to as design technology. We may think this highly unusual, given young children's propensity for creativity, but Owen considered that there would be time enough for such activity in later employment!

Where Owen's approach differs from the current Foundation Stage curriculum (QCA, 2000) is in the pace at which the curriculum is experienced as well as the content.

> *The children were not to be annoyed with books, but were to be taught the uses or nature of common things around them by familiar conversation when the children's curiosity was excited so as to induce them to ask questions.*
>
> Owen, quoted in Silver (1969: 65)

Current emphasis in the English curriculum for the early years is on individuals meeting set targets. This was not present in Owen's nursery school and in this respect his approach bears a closer relationship to European models for the education of the very young than the present English model.

Blenkin (1994:29) indicates a remarkably similar approach to Owen:

> *Rates of development and learning are at their most rapid during this stage of education, and they are highly susceptible to environmental constraints or advantages. The young child, therefore, needs to be stimulated by a wide range of experiences rather than confined to a narrow and restrictive programme.*

The following extract is from a report written by the Duke of Kent's personal physician following a visit to Owen's school at New Lanark:

> *The youngest, or infant class, under the age of five, are of course occupied only in the amusements which are suitable to their age, playing about in the area before the school, when the weather admits it, under the charge of a male and female superintendent, and whose principal office it is to encourage amongst them habits and feelings of good-will and affection towards each other.*
>
> (McNab, 1819)

There are many aspects of Owen's curriculum that will be familiar to those who have worked in 'free flow' play settings: for example, where children have choice over the pace and areas of their learning; where there is an emphasis on outdoor as well as indoor activity; and where there is an emphasis on the development of social skills and support for individual needs.

Social development as an essential element of child-centred models

Social development has been regarded as an essential element of many child-centred curriculum models, as it is now in many of the curricula, most notably that of New Zealand. Owen advocated this and there is some evidence to support the success of his methods, as in the following extract from a report produced by Leeds Poor Law Guardians of 1819.

> *In the education of the children the thing that is most remarkable is the general spirit of kindness and affection which is shown towards them, and the entire absence of everything that is likely to give them bad habits, with the presence of whatever is calculated to inspire them with good ones; the consequence is, that they appear like one well regulated family, united together by the ties of the closest affection. We heard no quarrels from the youngest to the eldest; and so strongly impressed are they with the conviction that their interest and duty are the same, and that to be happy themselves it is necessary to make those happy by whom they are surrounded, that they had no strife but in offices of kindness.*
>
> Podmore (1923:148)

Owen's vision: a lasting contribution

Many of Owen's social experiments were short-lived, but as Silver (1969) indicates, his vision of education inspired generations of activists. Owen was undoubtedly a man ahead of his time, and his principles could not be sustained at a time of rapid industrialisation when many cared little for the welfare of workers. On his death-bed Owen is reported to have indicated that:

> *My life was not useless; I gave important truths to the world. And it was only for want of understanding that they were disregarded. I have been ahead of my time.*
>
> (quoted in Siraj-Blatchford (1997:62)

Owen was undoubtedly a difficult and, at times, pompous man; his responses to issues were sometimes autocratic and paternalistic. Although his approach was soon eclipsed by other more formal and didactic approaches to early childhood education and care, his vision did not vanish. Nursery and infant education was established as a sociological need. The informal approach to early childhood education initiated at New Lanark emphasised early childhood and nursery education as a distinct phase. This obviously has parallels with the thinking of Froebel, Montessori and Steiner. Owen put this into action in Great Britain. The development of the Foundation Stage, drawing the reception year of infant education once more into an early childhood framework with nursery education and care, may be seen as a tribute to Owen's life work.

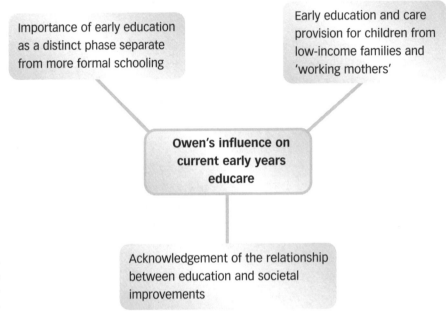

Figure 1.5
Current practice in early years educare: Owen's influence

Importance of early education as a distinct phase separate from more formal schooling

Early education and care provision for children from low-income families and 'working mothers'

Owen's influence on current early years educare

Acknowledgement of the relationship between education and societal improvements

> **Activity 4** **Owen's work in the social context**

Undertake a web-based search to find out more about Owen's work in the social context. Based on the findings of your research and your own practice in the workplace, answer the following questions:

1 Owen recognised the link between children's social welfare and early learning. Is this still important today?

2 Which aspect of Owen's work do you find most attractive or interesting?

The work of Margaret McMillan

Margaret McMillan, like Robert Owen, was distressed by the living conditions of the poor. Although they lived at different times, both saw education and social care as being the answer to a changed order in society. Neither was 'typical' of his or her time and social group; both could be regarded as 'outsiders'.

Margaret McMillan
(1860–1931)

Margaret McMillan, who was influenced by Froebel's teaching, saw nursery education, health and social care as of equal importance. With her sister, Rachel, she founded the first school clinic (1908) and the first 'open-air' nursery school in 1914. The nursery school proposed by McMillan was intended to address the physical, health and educational needs of disadvantaged children. In both the curriculum and the design of the buildings, these 'open-air' nurseries were seen as a means of offsetting the appalling conditions that many children suffered in urban industrial areas.

McMillan was a Christian Socialist at a time when social class was breaking down but society was still rife with social convention. Although McMillan was a member of the Froebel Society, the most active group in her time for those interested in early childhood, her agenda was very different from many other members of the group (Steedman, 1990). Her approach was regarded as radical and socially orientated, which contrasted with the 'safe' and socially conventional approach to change promoted by other members of the group.

The equal importance of nursery education, health and social care

Concern for children's health and well-being as well as their educational development features as a prominent strand, with different levels of emphasis, in the work of both Owen and McMillan. Social and health care for young children is now readily available and is taken for granted and yet the need for vigilance is still present, as recent media coverage indicates.

Margaret McMillan saw nursery education, health and social care as being of equal importance. Recent trends in educational and care provision in England have taken a more unified approach to meeting the needs of young children. Sure Start initiatives have spiralled from small-scale intervention projects to major training and implementation initiatives. This unified approach so central to McMillan's approach is clearly seen in the Sure Start (2003) Framework to Support Children in their Earliest Years, which provides:

> *Support, information, guidance and challenge for all those with responsibility for the care and education of babies and children from birth to three years.*

> Sure Start (2003:4)

As a member of the Independent Labour Party, McMillan was on the School Board in Bradford, which in her time was an industrial city with extensive slums. The School Board, a precursor of the Local Education Authority, provided a platform for McMillan to promote the welfare as well as the education of poor children. Free school meals and health checks were seen as essential prerequisites of education. Children could learn effectively only once they were healthy and adequately nourished.

Open-air nursery schools

There is a tangible link with some of these early educators. Schools visited or founded by McMillan are still in active operation. Margaret and her sister, Rachel, devised, developed and promoted the idea of the 'open-air nursery school'. The purpose of the school was to promote the health and well-being of the child. Those who work in these school buildings today will not have experienced the full force of the elements as those first pupils did, as the verandahs have been largely closed up! Cusden (1938) provides good graphic evidence of the layout of these schools, which were designed to provide space; the schools were 'open' in spatial terms as well as open to the air.

> *Children want space at all ages. But from the age of one to seven, ample space is almost as much wanted as food and air. To move, to run, to find things out by new movement, to feel one's life in every limb, that is the life of early childhood ... In the open-air Nursery Schools nine hours is a reasonable nurture day. Not five out of the twenty-four but nine; and this is the minimum if the work is to be really effective.*
>
> (McMillan, 1930:10–11)

Concern with health was evident in the design of school buildings; for example, as can be seen from Figure 1.6, each room had its own bathroom.

Margaret McMillan drew together ideas she had shared through articles and lectures in *The Nursery School*. This book was first published in 1919 and it is important to place this in the context of its time. After the First World War social conditions were changing. There were huge numbers of young widowed women, and women had taken more responsibility for many aspects of life previously undertaken by men because of their absence during the war.

The relationship between the community and school was crucial. The London County Council Annual Report of the School Medical Officer (1930:44) indicates that the Rachel McMillan Nursery School closed for only six days during the summer period. It was noted that this strategy resulted in much healthier children at the end of the usual summer holiday period than was previously the case.

Margaret McMillan was also unconventional in her view of the size of a school. In rural areas, schools would be small and serve the local community, but in urban areas schools could be very large; McMillan had no objection to schools catering for as many as 300 children. Classes would necessarily be small because of the age of the children, and the need for sufficient and well-trained staff was recognised. Large schools were seen as an opportunity to build links with the community. The schools proposed by McMillan would not only provide support for children's well-being, health and education, but also act as a means of helping to rejuvenate the area surrounding the school. Comments made by McMillan in her talks and in her writing indicate her commitment to social change. As a means of promulgating her approach to community enhancement, McMillan was not averse to overemphasis, what we would regard today as 'hard sell promotion and publicity', as the following quotation demonstrates:

> *No one passes the gate without looking in. All day there are groups near the entrance and eyes watching through the paling. They make me think always of the queues waiting to go into a theatre.*

McMillan (1930:13)

Parents were encouraged to come into school, to watch their children at work and play. She encouraged parents to learn from teachers and teachers to draw on the additional knowledge parents have of their own children. Frequent parents' meetings and the use of the school as a community base were important elements in McMillan's approach to interaction between the school and the community it serves. It could be argued that we would do well to revisit some of these ideas; that rather than using parents either as information providers for assessment records, or as recipients of the records, a more meaningful interaction could be negotiated.

The curriculum

McMillan took Froebel's garden metaphors and related them to real gardening. The absence for many children of gardens from their lives (gardens were a rarity in many inner city areas) was felt to be a particularly serious shortcoming by McMillan. Gardens equated with fresh air and robust health. To this end, McMillan proposed that schools be designed so that a verandah would run along the building and the rooms situated so that each would lead directly onto the garden. The garden would be a

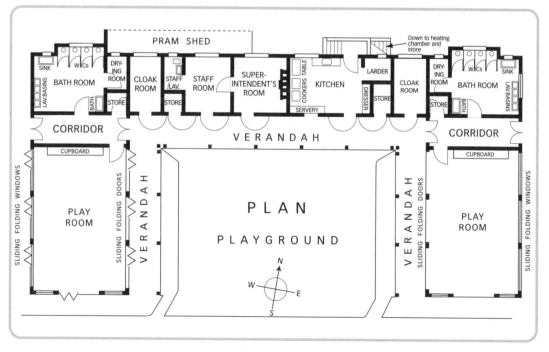

Figure 1.6 *A plan of a McMillan open-air nursery school*

place to grow all manner of flowers and vegetables to stimulate the senses and provide a resource for experiential learning; it would also act as a place where gross motor skills could be developed. The absence of safe and appropriate play equipment in children's home environments would be compensated for by the provision of slides, swings and a playground constructed using many natural materials.

Like Owen, McMillan promoted the inclusion of music in the curriculum and encouraged staff to learn an instrument.

> *If as in one Nursery School some teachers learn the violin it will be a great joy. For very little children appear to have a love of stringed instruments.*
>
> *The flute is also a good instrument, and also the zither and the banjo.*
>
> McMillan (1930:19)

The love of song, rhyme and music is clearly demonstrated by most young children, particularly when gifted practitioners encourage it.

McMillan's influence on present-day practice

McMillan's approach to outdoor play can be seen as a precursor of practice in many mainstream nursery settings today. All-weather surfaces, large tyres, wooden climbing structures would no doubt be approved by McMillan. Finding a working garden is now a rarity, a missed opportunity, as children could experience all of the senses in growing, harvesting and eating produce. With a little imagination, this important aspect of science, health, technology, language, maths and physical development could be revived.

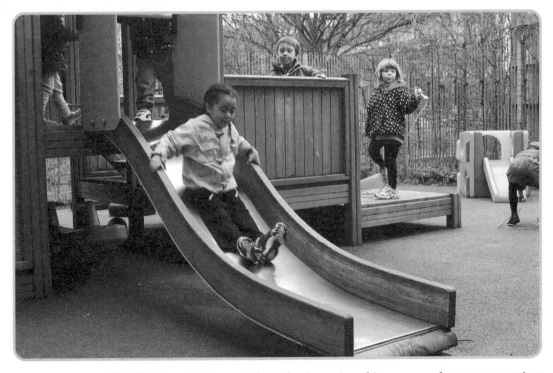

McMillan's emphasis on outdoor play is continued in many modern nursery settings

McMillan had an interesting approach to the use of outdoor areas: outside learning. As well as the resource for areas which would now be linked to Knowledge and Understanding of the World and Physical Development, she also recommended that 'blackboards' (chalkboards) be placed on the outside, as well as the inside, walls of the school in case 'children want to draw or scribble'. In the period before the child's fifth birthday, even in the more formal aspects of the curriculum, a naturalistic approach was taken, and reading and writing was seen as emerging from other activities in a natural and unhurried way. When the child's fifth birthday approached there was no sudden change to more formal methods but more a gradual transition. In some respects, the formation of the Foundation Stage now uses this approach.

> ## Activity 5) Understanding McMillan's curriculum

1 Compare McMillan's curriculum with other early years curricula currently used in New Zealand or Scotland. Carry out your research using the Internet and professional journals such as *Nursery World*.

Consider the following questions:

2 How would you develop gardening as a means of promoting health and social development, and which areas of children's understanding and learning could be fostered?

3 How would you promote 'outside learning'?

McMillan's approach to nursery attendance is interesting in that it foreshadows some aspects of 'wraparound care'. In order that consistent and long-term provision of education and care could be provided, she insisted that the children should attend nursery full time:

> *A short nurture day is in great measure a waste of time and money. The great process which it exists to forward is not possible in short sessions broken by long intervals.*

> McMillan (1930:37)

Training of teachers

McMillan believed a 3-year specialist training for those teachers intending to work with younger children (birth to age 7) was required. The link between theory and practice was promoted by the inclusion of supervised and monitored workplace practice. In McMillan's model can be seen aspects of training that have been used for many years in initial teacher education. The monitoring of practice has always been present in these courses, but the assessment of such practice has been subject to varying degrees of rigour. Teacher competencies, appropriate to different age groups, have been formulated to meet government criteria and curriculum targets. The introduction of **Beacon Schools** and **Early Excellence Centres** may be seen as a means of confirmation of management style and promotion of government-approved practice.

Ideas for further research

McMillan saw nursery education as a means of addressing the terrible social ills of life in the inner city. To what extent is this view reflected in the way in which the Sure Start initiative is addressing the needs of children and families in similar locations today?

McMillan strongly promoted the belief that children should be provided with a suitable learning environment. Although aspects of the healthy lifestyle encouraged in nursery schools in McMillan's day may now have been relegated to peripheral importance, limited space for school rebuilding in inner city areas may encourage more innovative and child-friendly architecture to be considered. What efforts are being made in redesigning, modifying or 'new build' to meet current health needs in childcare and education?

McMillan proposed the view that all children should have access to a nursery with trained staff to look after them. Current trends in England require a minimum qualification for those working in settings with young children. This is currently under review. It would be useful to examine a qualification, for example an NVQ 2, and to consider, in the light of your experience in the workplace, whether the qualification provides adequate training? Justify your opinion.

In McMillan's time it was common for children attending nursery full time to have opportunity for a sleep during the day. Conversations with students on educare courses who are also nursery staff have indicated that many children do need opportunity for sleep and a quiet period during the day. What is your opinion? Is this based on your workplace experience?

Work-related activities: keeping a diary

The diary may be used to provide a commentary about your own personal development alongside your reading and thus support your course of study.

How you set it out will be a personal choice but it does need to be organised! You need to be able to use it for reference – so write clearly and concisely.

Highlight the links between the ideas illustrated in this chapter and aspects of the practice within your workplace as you begin to identify them.

Illustrate your points by specific examples of experience in the form of short stories (vignettes). These may be developed as case studies at a later date (see Chapter 10, Research).

You may wish to focus on one aspect of practice in your setting that reflects the influence of a key figure in the history of early childhood (case study). This will help you to make informed reflections upon recent issues within educare provision.

Remember to reflect and to analyse – and to evaluate your progress.

⟩ Conclusion

> *Habits, in general, may be formed very early in children. An association of ideas is, as it were, the parent of habit. If, then, you can accustom your children to perceive that your will must always prevail over theirs, when they are opposed, the thing is done, and they will submit to it without difficulty or regret. To bring this about, as soon as they begin to show their inclination by desire or aversion, let single instances be chosen now and then (not too frequently) to contradict them. For example, if a child shews a desire to have any thing in his hand that he sees, or has any thing in his hand with which he is delighted, let the parent take it from him, and when he does so, let no consideration whatever make him restore it at that time.*
>
> (Witherspoon, quoted in Swann and Gammage (1993)

We have looked at what we may consider to be the positive influences of key educators and carers on current practice. Practices such as those advocated by Witherspoon, one of the key figures in the development of schools for infants in the 19th century, may be seen as reflecting the values present in Victorian England.

The priority given to values changes within a remarkably short time, as the numerous versions and variations of the National Curriculum illustrate. The fate of National Curriculum Foundation Subjects such as Physical Education, Art and Music demonstrates how a priority in the curriculum, supported by detailed and extensive guidance, may be reduced to a short indicative range of statements with alarming rapidity.

The introduction of the Foundation Stage Profile (DfES 2003) and the tests at the end of Key Stage 1 in England indicate that there is an emphasis on rigorous formal assessment of young children. This may be linked to the ever-changing imperatives of central government in England. Meeting self-imposed government targets may be one reason for such actions. One would hope that at the heart of these actions there is an aim to provide better life chances for children. A very different approach was presented almost ten years ago by the Royal Society of Arts report *Start Right: The Importance of Early Learning*. Christopher Ball, the author, argued for part-time nursery education for 3- and 4-year-olds, which could be part-funded by offering part-time nursery education, rather than full-time schooling, to 5-year-olds and raising the compulsory school age to 6. Nursery education was seen as providing a means of helping to prevent school failure and thereby promoting future success in life.

> *This report ... demonstrates the importance of early learning as a preparation for effective education to promote social welfare and social order, and to develop a world-class workforce.*
>
> (Ball, 1994:6)

Sure Start programmes have blossomed and the concept has now grown beyond its origins in compensatory support for children. However, some questions must still be posed: Is early years education simply

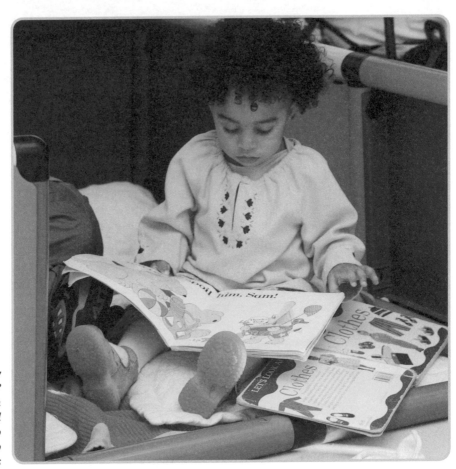

What is early education for? Your own research will help you to find answers to such questions

compensatory? Is this connected with the emphasis placed on increasing the numbers of 3-year-old children entering educational settings in England? Such questions may appear unwarranted. Should not all children have access to 'quality' educational provision?

This chapter may have provided you with grounds for questioning and analysing current approaches to educare in England. Academic criticism should not focus on negativity in its response to an issue. You are encouraged to reflect, to question and to analyse. Current practice in education and care reflects centrally driven policy and legislation and has an influence on many sector settings that were once independent: for example, the pre-schools (formerly play groups), the Pre-School Learning Alliance and Montessori schools. It may be argued that there is little difference between current government initiatives and other intervention strategies proposed by Owen, Steiner and McMillan, or more recent initiatives such as those proposed by the Plowden Committee (DES, 1967).

Based upon your reading you should now be able to provide an argument to support your own views on this subject. What is early education for? What provision should be made? Social contexts have changed dramatically since 1816. Have the needs of children, the type of teaching required and the responsibility of parents in the process of education changed in the intervening time, or are there some trends that are constant? You may now have some answers to these questions.

Developing your skills in research and reading for trends and traditions

You may find a suitable range of books available in your university or college library, but much material is also accessible on the Internet.

Online indexes

Online indexes may be used to find books, journals and newspaper articles about historical aspects of educare. The Internet will also allow you to access media articles about emerging issues.

Keyword search

Use a keyword search. This will help you to locate broad areas of study.

Specific key thinkers can be found by searching, for example: Montessori.org.uk

Use subject headings

The best method of undertaking an initial search is through the use of subject headings. For example:

early childhood education+history

early childhood education+philosophy

early childhood educators+biography

Your research may then be extended by looking at specific thinkers. For example:

pestalozzi+kindergarten

robert owen+education

margaret mcmillan+education

Journal articles

Journals are a good source of relatively current information about your topic. This includes professional journals such as *Nursery World* and the more academic ones, which are now available online.

> **Activity 6** **Self-assessment**

Select from your research one person or trend in the history of early childhood education and care.

1 Consider the era in which the person lived and worked or when the trend began.

2 What major events occurred during the lifetime of the person that may have affected his or her approaches to early childhood education and care?

3 What do you think was the most important personal influence in forming his or her approach to education and care?

4 What do you consider to be the person/trend's major contributions to the development of young children and/or early childhood education?

5 What is the relevance of the trend/work of this person to us today?

6 What lasting aspect of this trend's/person's influence is visible in your workplace setting?

7 Which aspect of studying this chapter have you most enjoyed?

8 How has it affected your personal understanding of early childhood education and care?

9 Will it have an effect on your practice?

References and further reading

Ball, C. (1994), *Start Right: The Importance of Early Learning*. London: Royal Society for the Encouragement of Arts, Manufacture and Commerce

Blenkin, G. and Kelly, A. (eds) (1994), *The National Curriculum and Early Learning: An Evaluation*. London: Paul Chapman Publishing

Bruce, T. (1997), *Early Childhood Education*. London: Hodder and Stoughton

Cusden, P. (1938), *The English Nursery School*. London: Kegan Paul, Trench, Trubner & Co. Ltd

DES (1967), *Children and their Primary Schools*. London: HMSO

DfES (2002), *Early Years Sector-Endorsed Foundation Degree: Statement of Requirement*. Nottingham: DfES

DfES/DfWP (2003), *Birth to Three Matters*. London: Sure Start/DfES

Education Enquiry Committee (1929), *The Case for Nursery Schools*. London: George Phillip and Sons

EYCG (1992) *First Things First: Educating Young Children*. Oldham: Madeleine Lindley

Fisher, J. (1996), *Starting from the Child*. Maidenhead: Open University Press

Hurst, V. and Joseph, J. (1998). *Supporting Early Learning: The Way Forward*. Buckingham: Open University Press

Kramer, R. (1978), *Maria Montessori: A Biography*. Oxford: Blackwell.

London County Council (1930), Report of the School Medical Officer. LCC: London

McAvley, H. and Jackson, P. (1992), *Educating Young Children*. London: David Fulton

McMillan, M. (1930), *The Nursery School.* London: Dent

McNab, H. (1819). *The New Views of Mr Owen, Impartially Examined.* SCCC

Mills, C. and Mills, D. (1998), Dispatches: The Early Years, London: Channel 4 Television

Montessori, M. (1916), *The Montessori Method* (1964 edn). New York: Schocken Books

Montessori, M. (1949), *The Absorbent Mind* (1967 edn). New York: Dell

Podmore, F. (1923), *Robert Owen: A Biography.* London: George Allen and Unwin

QCA (2000), 'Curriculum Guidance for the Foundation Stage'. London: HMSO

QCA (2003), 'Foundation Stage Profile'. London: HMSO

Roberts, R. (1995), *A Nursery Education Curriculum for the Early Years.* Oxford: National Primary Centre

Silver, H. (1969), *Robert Owen on Education.* Cambridge: Cambridge University Press.

Siraj-Blatchford, J. (1997), *Robert Owen: Schooling the Innocents.* Nottingham: Educational Heretics Press

Steedman, C. (1990), *Childhood, Culture and Class in Britain: Margaret McMillan 1860–1931.* London: Virago

Swann, R. and Gammage, P. (1993), 'Early Childhood Education – Where are we now?', in Gammage, P. and Meighan, J. (1993), *Early Childhood Education: Taking Stock.* Nottingham: Education Now Publishing Co-operative

Wells, G. (1987), *The Meaning Makers: Children Learning Language and Using Language to Learn.* London: Hodder Arnold

Useful websites

McMillan

www.spartacus.schoolnet.co.uk/WmcmillanR.htm

Montessori
www.montessori.org
www.montessori.org.uk

Owen and McMillan

http://edheretics.gn.apc.org/EHFHome.htm

Steiner

www.emerson.org.uk
www.steinerwaldorf.org

www.nc.uk.net

The National Curriculum website, run by the QCA. Includes programme of study requirements and teaching resources.

www. high-scope.org.uk

Website run by High/Scope UK, a charitable organisation promoting the High/Scope approach to teaching young children.

The reflective practitioner 2

Elaine Hallet

This chapter discusses the role of the practitioner in an early years setting and how, through being reflective, practitioners and students can develop their knowledge, skills, understanding and practice in order to meet the new opportunities within the developing early years and early childhood studies field.

The chapter explores and discusses:

- ⊃ the role of the practitioner in an early years setting
- ⊃ continuing professional development
- ⊃ studying at undergraduate level
- ⊃ being a reflective practitioner
- ⊃ supporting children's learning
- ⊃ effective communication skills
- ⊃ working in teams and groups
- ⊃ managing change
- ⊃ working with professionals.

After reading this chapter it is hoped that you will be able to:

1 be aware of the different opportunities open to early years practitioners
2 know how to organise your time to get the most from your studies
3 understand the concepts behind reflection
4 understand the importance of developing good communication skills
5 appreciate the significance of becoming a reflective practitioner.

The role of a practitioner in an early years setting

Many practitioners working within early years settings have qualified as nursery nurses. The term 'nursery nurse' emerged from the title of women who worked in children's nurseries during Victorian times. Their role was a nursing and caring one providing for the physical and health care needs of babies and children who attended the nurseries. They were nurses who worked in nurseries, hence the name 'nursery nurses', which is still used today. The role of the nursery nurse has evolved since then as early years settings began to provide a broader raft of services to meet children's educational needs, in addition to their care needs. As a result, a nursery nurse's role has developed into that of a practitioner with a diverse range of responsibilities, working with parents, children, families, and health, educational and social professionals. These roles are often multidisciplinary, crossing health, social and educational areas and include those illustrated in Figure 2.1.

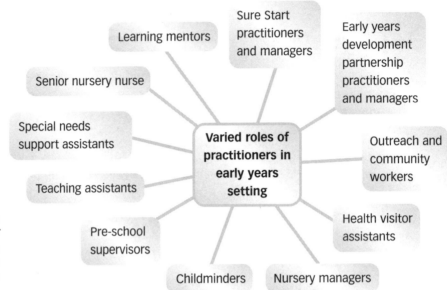

Figure 2.1
Multidisciplinary roles of practitioners working in early years settings

Until the 1990s, a nursery nurse working in a nursery or school would carry out tasks to support the nursery or class teacher's role of teaching the children. These daily tasks may have included setting out activities, displaying children's work, cutting paper, sharpening pencils, tidying up, washing the paint pots and changing children's clothes after an 'accident'. Early years practitioners still undertake these tasks but other roles with differing responsibilities have emerged:

➲ practitioners working in Sure Start projects and as Outreach and community workers work closely with parents, families and their children

➲ nursery nurses working with health visitors assist in clinics and home visits

➲ some practitioners working in Early Years Development Partnerships are involved in developing policy and practice

➲ a variety of roles have developed for early years practitioners working in maintained schools. For example, learning mentors run out-of-school clubs and play schemes, monitor children's attendance, work with parents in developing strategies to improve children's behaviour, and support 'looked after' children in the early years setting. Teaching assistants and nursery nurses support children in literacy and numeracy, and write and implement Individual Education Plans (IEPs) to meet children's individual and special needs.

- ⊃ special needs support assistants work with children who have specific needs, to enable them to access the curriculum
- ⊃ teaching assistants plan and implement activities to help children's literacy and numeracy development
- ⊃ some senior nursery nurses are responsible for the school's nursery class
- ⊃ learning mentors initiate school-based projects to support children's attendance, behaviour and playtime needs.

These roles and responsibilities have emerged in response to the recognition that the early years of a child's life are a significant phase in his or her development. Children's learning and development in these early stages of life underpin much of their future achievements. This has been recognised by those governments that have given a high priority to education.

The DfES has recognised the early years as a significant phase and foundation for children's learning and development. Policy and initiatives have been supported by financial funding and are established to provide standards of provision for children and families. These include the following (Figure 2.2):

Initiative introduced by DfES	Aims and objectives
The National Childcare Strategy	Provides a national approach and framework for childcare provision.
Early Years Development Partnerships	Provide a local base to develop policy and practice within local authorities.
Sure Start	Funds projects in deprived areas for parent and family support.
Beacon Schools and Centres of Early Excellence	Provide professional development opportunities for practitioners.
The National Day Care Standards and Ofsted	Provide high-quality standards in the provision of settings.

Figure 2.2
Initiatives introduced by DfES for children and families

⊃ Continuing professional development

The recognition of the early years as a vital phase of development arose from the Rumbold Report (1990). This report recognised the importance of the early years as a period of 'rapid growth and development, both physical and intellectual. At this stage children's developmental needs are complex and interrelated' (1990:7). The Rumbold Committee researched the quality of educational experience offered to 3- and 4-year-olds. Significant recommendations were made in relation to a pre-fives curriculum, the initial training of practitioners and the continuing professional development of early years practitioners, and these are now evident in the evolving early years field.

The Rumbold Report recognises that the role of the practitioner who works with young children is 'a demanding and complex task. Those engaged upon it need a range of attributes to assure a high quality experience for children' (1990:19). Every child has an entitlement to high standards of care and education. Quality in education and care does not depend solely on government policy, purpose-built schools and nurseries or even funding. The decisive factor in determining it is the quality of the educators. There is a strong link between the quality of training and professional development and the quality of provision for children.

The training and professional development needs of those responsible for the care and education of young children are a key issue. The Rumbold Report proposed multidisciplinary courses in which child health care and education professionals come together. Academic and vocational degree courses in early childhood studies, early years educare and teaching assistance not only provide professional development opportunities, but raise the status of early years workers and signal that high level qualifications are necessary for working with young children.

In 2001 the government identified a national lack of a highly skilled workforce qualified to level 4. Foundation degree studies were introduced to compensate for this, of which work-based learning and assessment form an integral part. As part of their course, Foundation Degree level students use their everyday work with children as a research and evaluation base on which to modify and develop their practice. Work-based mentors play an important role in supporting this learning in the work setting by sharing their expertise and experience with the student. This approach enables students to reflect upon their practice in a relevant and meaningful way, linking theory to practice, so embedding new and developing knowledge and practices within their everyday work. This work-based learning linked to academic study helps the student to become a reflective practitioner or an 'inquiring professional', as Anning and Edwards (2003:34) describe this new practitioner who works in an early years setting.

Both academic and vocational degree-level courses produce a community of learners who:

- ⊃ support each other through their study
- ⊃ exchange ideas
- ⊃ share knowledge, experience and practice
- ⊃ enquire about and challenge concepts, theories, knowledge and understanding in order to reflect upon and develop their provision for children, parents and families.

Degree-level courses provide long-term professional developmental opportunities, but there is also a need for early years practitioners to have an entitlement to short courses in order to update their knowledge, skills and understanding to meet the changing needs of the early years field.

Long- and short-term continuing professional development underpins the various early years roles and responsibilities discussed earlier. It also supports the emerging roles of Senior Practitioners (DfES, 2002) and High Level Teaching Assistants (TTA, 2003). Figure 2.3 illustrates the professional developmental opportunities for early years practitioners working within early years educare and how they support those emerging roles.

Senior Practitioner High Level Teaching Assistant		
Degree level study in early childhood studies, early years educare, teaching assistants	Academic courses leading to:	PhD MA BA BA (Hons)
	Vocational courses leading to:	Foundation Degrees DfES Early Years Sector Endorsed Foundation Degree
Short courses Professional updating	Examples include:	Foundation Stage Child Protection Working with autistic children
Initial training Level 3 qualification	NNEB BTEC National Diploma in Early Years Diploma in Care and Education NVQ 3 Care and Education PLA Diploma	

Figure 2.3
Professional development for early years practitioners

Studying at undergraduate level

Some of those studying early childhood, educare, early years and teaching assistants' courses at undergraduate level are mature students with lots of experience of working with children in a range of settings but who may have had some time out of study; for them returning to study can seem quite daunting. They may ask questions such as 'Can I do it?' and 'Why am I doing it?', particularly during their first semester. Often, when such students get back their first assignment with their grade and tutor feedback, their confidence and self-belief is restored. (Younger students can also feel apprehensive.) It is important to remember your long-term goal and the picture of yourself in cap and gown receiving your degree certificate on a stage in front of your family and friends. A sense of achievement!

An early years degree is a higher education award. The experience of being a university student is different to that of a college or school student. Adult learners returning to study need to develop confidence and strategies in order to become successful independent learners.

What does it take to be a successful student and an independent learner?

One of the important factors that helps a student to achieve success as an independent learner is effective time management. A few tips on how you may manage your time are given in Figure 2.4.

Becoming an independent learner involves:	
Managing your time	Each of us has a busy life. We have a work life, a family life and a social life. Becoming a student means fitting in a study life. How can this be done? The key to this is being able to manage your time, to prioritise and to make effective use of the time available.
Gaining control of your time	Time is precious; it can easily get out of control and disappear. Time can never be regained so you need to control it by planning and organising it.
Creating study time	It is important to identify the time you have available for your studies. This can be done by researching your own weekly timetable and finding out how you will spend your time in a typical working week. Activity 1 below will help you to do this.

Figure 2.4
Independent learning: managing your time

Your time	
Committed time	This is time allocated on a regular basis that cannot be altered: for example, time spent at work, travelling time, childcare arrangements, regular social commitments, meetings and other activities.
Provision time	This is time spent in maintaining the personal needs of your life: for example, shopping, cooking and eating meals, washing, cleaning and sleeping.
Adaptable time	The space left on your time-table is **adaptable time**. This is time that you can use as you wish. In the life of a student some of this becomes study time. How you plan and organise this time determines the effective use of it and your success as a student.

Figure 2.5
Your time: its components

Using your study time in an effective way

It is useful to identify the best time for you to study. Activity 2 has been designed to enable you to do this.

On the timetable below use two different colours of pen to shade and identify the *committed time, provision time* and *adaptable time* that you have. You will need to refer to Figure 2.5, below, for this activity.

My Typical Week

Time (24-hour clock)	Mon	Tues	Wed	Thurs	Fri	Sat	Sun
1.00							
2.00							
3.00							
4.00							
5.00							
6.00							
7.00							
8.00							
9.00							
10.00							
11.00							
12.00							
13.00							
14.00							
15.00							
16.00							
17.00							
18.00							
19.00							
20.00							
21.00							
22.00							
23.00							
24.00							

Activity 2 The best time to study

1 What is the best time for you to study?

Tick the most appropriate statement/s:

☐ I need to work for at least 2 hours to achieve anything.

☐ I can only concentrate for 2 to 3 hours maximum.

☐ I can think and study better in the morning.

☐ I can think and study better in the evening.

☐ I can think and study better at night-time and very early in the morning.

☐ I work better before meals.

☐ I work better after meals.

☐ I find it hard to work in the evenings after work.

☐ I find it better to work for longer periods at the weekends.

☐ I have to be at home to study.

☐ I prefer to study in a library.

☐ I find it easier to study with a friend.

2 Now think about how you are going to organise your study time for successful studying.

Allocate study times

When you have thought about how you study, you can now allocate specific study times on your weekly timetable. This may include negotiating with your partner or family members to carry out tasks, for example, childcare arrangements, so that some of the 'committed' time you have identified is allocated to study time.

Establish long-term goals and short-term tasks

You will read a lot of academic material and write a great deal as an undergraduate student. And it is likely that you will study across several areas. Hand-in dates and deadlines are crucial at university and failure to meet them can result in your failing a module. All this can seem overwhelming so it is important to break your goals down into small and achievable tasks.

In setting a long-term goal, identify what you ultimately want to achieve. It may be to hand in a module on time. Establish some steps or short-term tasks to get there. Your short-term tasks will give you an idea of what you are trying to achieve over the next week and tell you what you need to do when you start a study session. This will stop you wasting time when you sit down because you do not know what to do in the time available. For example, the first goal, 'I will do the assignment by the end of the week', can seem overwhelming and unachievable. The shorter task, 'I will do Question 1 of the assignment in my study time this week', is realistic and achievable.

Make a 'To do' list

Quality use of time is more important than how much is available. It is possible to achieve a great deal in one hour of quality time, particularly if you use a 'To do' list. On this list place everything you have to do before you start. Place the items in order of priority. One of the easiest ways of doing this is to classify the items '1', '2', '3' as follows:

- ⊃ **1** – are the most important and have to be done in that day's study time
- ⊃ **2** – are the next important
- ⊃ **3** – are the least important.

Put a date by each item for when it has to be achieved. Tick or cross out items on the list as they are completed; this gives a great sense of achievement. Compile a 'To do' list at the end of every study time. This revised 'To do' list summarises the work achieved that day and prepares you for the next day's work.

Reminder notes

Write yourself notes to remind yourself of tasks to do. Sticky notes are helpful: they are produced in different colours and can be used to organise different tasks.

Compile a 'Not to do' list

A 'Not to do' list might include jobs or temptations that should not be undertaken as they will use up time allocated for your study time. For example, you may choose not to answer the phone during your studying. This list will help you focus on your studying and use the time effectively.

Avoid substitute activities

These are all things that you might contrive to do before settling down to the main study task in hand. It is easy to be tempted to do the washing up, phone a friend, or watch a television programme, thereby substituting the main study task with other lower-priority activities. Rank the activities in order of importance and do the most important first. The substitute activities can be done after the main task. Discipline is needed for this and maintaining an image of your long-term goal with your degree certificate in hand can help.

Value your time

The purpose behind setting objectives and prioritising activities is to make effective use of your study time. A firm control means extra achievement and satisfaction, leaving you with more time for relaxation in the time left and allocated for it.

Thinking time

It is important to allow 'thinking time' in your study times. This is time when you can reflect upon a university or college session by reading your notes, refer to references and readings you have made or plan for the next part of your assignment.

Challenge interruptions

Challenge any interruptions to your study time so that this is prioritised and is seen to be important to you.

Balance

It is important to balance your work, home, social and study life. You should not be studying to the detriment of the other aspects of your life. The quality of time you give to study is more important than the quantity of time.

Be organised

It is important to have a special place that you can call your own where you can study. You will need a working table, on which you can use your laptop, leave books and notes out and work undisturbed. A notice on the door saying 'I am studying – please do not disturb' may be helpful. In a busy household this can be difficult, but it shows that studying is important to you.

A clear desk

Tidy up after your studying as this helps you keep focused on one task at a time. It also helps you to begin afresh at your next study time.

Keep a diary or journal

By keeping a reflective diary or journal, you will be able to note down your study progress, jot down your thoughts, ideas, feelings, and any relevant work experiences; references to articles you have read or research materials may be put in your journal and annotated with notes. This reflective diary or journal is a personal dialogue and a working notebook, a useful resource to help in writing your assignments. At the end of the course it will be interesting to look back at your journal to see your progress and the development of your ideas.

Cockburn (2001:108) describes how a journal is a useful tool and resource when studying.

> *A journal is a powerful part of an educator's professional development. A journal is a place for reflecting, speculating, wondering, worrying, exclaiming, recording, proposing, reminding, reconstructing, questioning,*

confronting, dreaming, considering and reconsidering. The journal holds experiences as a puzzle frame holds its integral pieces. The writer begins to recognise the pieces that fit together and, like a detective, sees the picture evolve. It is a space for thinking.

Storing your references

When referring to other people's work in your assignments you will need to acknowledge all sources by using the Harvard system of referencing (see the References and Further Reading sections at the end of the chapters in this book). (There are variations within the Harvard system, however, so you will need to clarify the format preferred by the university you are attending.)

As you are writing your assignments it is annoying to find that you have forgotten a reference or cannot find it. It is useful to collect references in one place from the start of your course. This may be in your journal, on disc, in a file or in a box. List the references for books, journals and websites, either under the author or subject headings: for example, Play, The Early Years Curriculum, Special Educational Needs. In your list, include the author's name, date of publication, title of publication, place of publication and publisher's name. This information is then easily accessed for writing your assignment and producing a bibliography.

Filing your notes

Organise your lecture and study notes in separate files so that they are easily accessible. You will find your own way of making notes in lectures and organising them for future reference.

Being an active student

Successful students are active students. It is they who attend lectures, seminars and tutorials. During these sessions they make notes, ask questions and participate in the activities provided in the learning sessions. As an independent learner it is important that you communicate with your tutor and work-based mentor about your learning needs.

Study partners and study groups

Being a higher education student can be quite daunting as you are not always physically present in the university when studying. You may find it useful to establish a study partnership with a supportive friend: someone with whom you can share and discuss your studies, someone you can telephone or email when you are in a panic! You may become part of a study group that meets to discuss their studies, assignment work or research project and to share experiences. You may meet over a cup of coffee in a member of the group's house, while accessing the Internet for information, or you may study together in the library.

Enjoy your studies

This is the main aim of your degree course. Enjoy both your time as a student and your studies, reflect upon your practice, discover new knowledge and develop new understandings and skills within the early years field and gain some new friends.

Being a reflective practitioner

Gervase Phinn, an Ofsted inspector, recounted an incident during one of his inspections (North Yorkshire, 2000). He observed a boy carrying out his daily task of watering the plants in his classroom, which he did before home time each day. The boy came to the last plant in the classroom, which did not have any leaves or flowers on and looked remarkably like a stick in a pot. 'Why are you watering that?', he asked. 'Cos I always do', answered the boy.

The boy's task can be compared to the work of a practitioner in an early years setting. As practitioners we may choose to carry out daily work tasks in a routine way without thinking or considering the impact on the children's learning and development; or we can stop to question and reflect upon our interactions with children, parents and staff and consider how they affect provision for children and, in doing so, be reflective practitioners. The need for reflection, review and evaluation is based upon the changing and evolving job roles derived from internal and external changes. Reflective practice is a process of regularly reviewing our own work and the provision within the work setting, looking for and making improvements. Continuing professional development supports this.

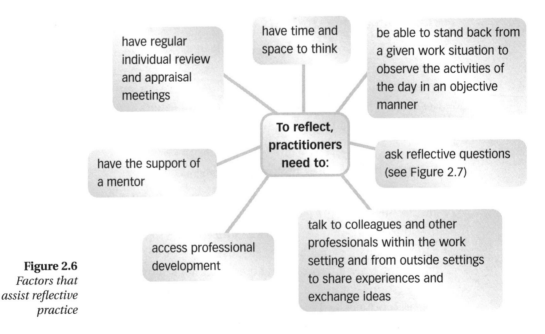

Figure 2.6
Factors that assist reflective practice

Examples of reflective questions are shown in Figure 2.7.

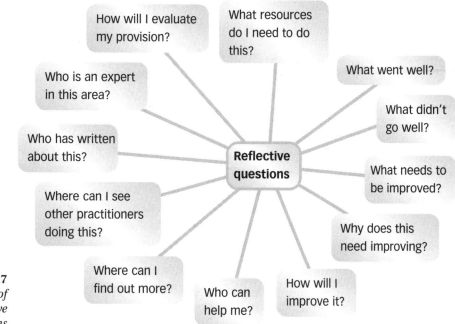

Figure 2.7
Examples of reflective questions

In order to reflect we need to create time from a busy personal and professional life to think about and evaluate our actions.

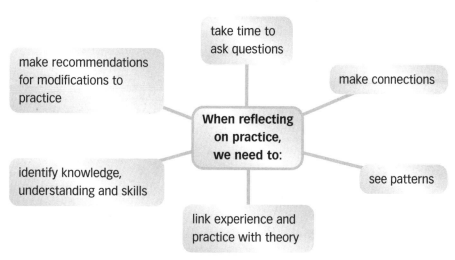

Figure 2.8
Reflecting on practice

Reflection is a learning process; it helps us to make better sense of our practitioner's role and its contribution to the children, parents and families within our work setting and the setting itself. Being a reflective practitioner helps us to increase our skills, understanding and learning. It results in our being more effective practitioners.

Drummond (in Fisher 2002:194) highlights the importance of self-knowledge for the educator and practitioner. She defines effective practitioners as those who understand themselves, their knowledge, their feelings and the framework within which they understand children. Practitioners regularly assess children and it is important that practitioners assess themselves also. Being reflective professionals requires that we continually review and develop our own practice.

Reflective conversations

Reflective conversations are an important part of this evaluation. These can take place at university or college with tutors or within the work setting with colleagues and work-based mentors. Work-based mentors can contribute to the reflective process by sharing their experience and expertise by asking questions and challenging workplace practices in a supportive way. Pollard and Tann (in Fisher 2001:199) suggest that reflective practice, professional learning and personal fulfilment are enhanced through collaboration and dialogue with colleagues.

By reflecting on our thoughts and actions, relating them to those of other theorists and practitioners and taking advice from more experienced practitioners, our workday practice becomes more skilled and 'knowing-in-action', as described by Donald Schon in Cockburn (2001:103). On a daily basis, practitioners make innumerable judgements based upon their understandings, judgements and skilful performances. As practitioners gain experience in their work role they are able to read signs and carry out successful activities based upon their experience. They use their experiences, knowledge, skills and understanding to refine and modify their practice, adapt and make changes as appropriate to meet the needs of children, parents and staff they work with. They will evaluate and reflect upon their work in an ongoing process of review and development.

Case study 1 illustrates a first-year Foundation Degree student's involvement in this reflective process. This is an extract from her assignment 'Reflecting on Personal and Professional Development'.

Case Study 1

Reflecting on personal and professional development

Reflective conversations with other professionals and students, sharing their experiences, listening to their ideas and understanding of education will help me to support or challenge my own perspectives. The way I reflect on my reflections will change as I change and the more I will learn about my professional development. Contact with children and their families, reading relevant publications, examining research reports and engaging in discussions with my tutor, mentor and students will aid my development as a learner, carer and educator. Through self-evaluation, investigating my own practice and developing ways to improve it I will find a way through difficult situations, resolve problems and help to make my work with children and families more successful.

Shirley Collier
Foundation Degree Educare and Early Childhood, University of Derby, 2003

Reflective questioning

Questions are key to the review and evaluation of practice. They enable practitioners to agree, disagree and challenge provision where necessary.

Reflective questions may include considerations about children's learning. Examples of these are shown in Figure 2.9.

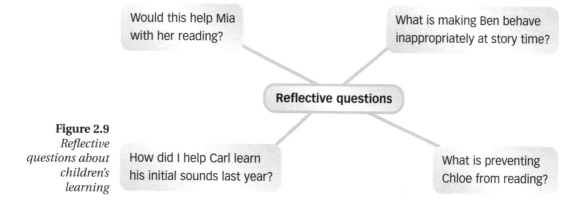

Figure 2.9
Reflective questions about children's learning

Would this help Mia with her reading?

What is making Ben behave inappropriately at story time?

Reflective questions

How did I help Carl learn his initial sounds last year?

What is preventing Chloe from reading?

The words What, Why, How, Can, Where, When and Who are helpful in forming reflective questions in order to review and evaluate practice.

- ⊃ What am I doing?
- ⊃ Why am I doing it?
- ⊃ How am I doing it?
- ⊃ Can I improve it?
- ⊃ Where can I improve?
- ⊃ When can I review my practice?
- ⊃ When can I plan, based upon my review?
- ⊃ Who can help me to reflect?
- ⊃ What resources will help me?

Activity 3 has been designed to help you to evaluate a specific task using these questions as a starting point for reflection and evaluation.

> **Activity 3** **Reflecting upon an everyday task**

1 Choose a task that you carry out each day in your work setting, for example, sharpening pencils, playing a maths game with children, collecting snack money, filling the sand pit, tidying up, making drinks.

2 Reflect upon the impact the task has on the children, parents or members of staff with whom you work by writing notes under the following headings.

- ⊃ What am I doing?

  Is it a general task? Is it an educating task? Is it a caring task? Is it a team task?

- ➲ Why am I doing this task?

  Will it help a child and/or children?

  Will it help a member of staff?

  Will it help the staff team?

  Will it help a parent and/or parents?

  Will it help my work setting?

  Will it help me?

- ➲ How am I carrying out this task?

  Purposefully? Happily? Unwillingly? Routinely? Quickly? Slowly?

- ➲ Can I improve how I carry it out?

  Do I need to alter the way I carry out this task?

  Do I need to alter my interactions with children, staff or parents?

Reflecting upon your role

In reflecting upon your practice you will be reflecting upon your role also, your perception of it and how others perceive it. Figure 2.10 illustrates some of the questions you may ask yourself when considering your role.

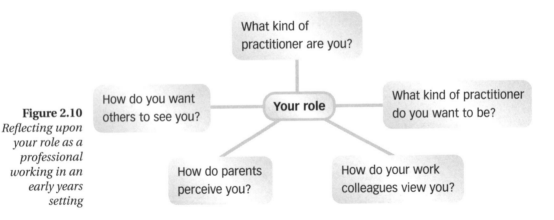

Figure 2.10
Reflecting upon your role as a professional working in an early years setting

To answer these questions you need to know yourself personally and professionally. Some questions that may assist you in this process are given in Figure 2.11.

Your role and responsibilities will vary according to the setting you work within. A practitioner working within a nursery may have responsibility as a key worker for a group of children, be involved in curriculum planning and work closely with parents. However, a practitioner working within an infant school may be involved in implementing curriculum activities and tasks planned by the teacher, rather than initiating them as a practitioner in a nursery may do.

Knowing yourself	
What roles do I have in my life?	I may be a parent, auntie, grandparent, governor, or religious leader. How do these roles influence my role and work with children and parents?
What am I like as a learner?	What was my experience of learning at nursery and school? How has this influenced my approach to learning generally and when providing learning opportunities and experiences for children and parents?
What am I like as an educator and a carer?	Are these roles the same or different? What experiences have shaped me? Who has influenced me? Possibly a significant teacher, nursery nurse, a mentor or parents.
Who am I?	What experiences, influences and people have helped me to achieve as much as I already have? Where do I want to progress to? Some practitioners want to become teachers; some don't, but do want to work with children in a role with more responsibility such as a senior nursery nurse, a learning mentor, a nursery manager, a Sure Start development worker or trainer.

Figure 2.11
Reflective questions about yourself

In developing reflective practice, it is first important to identify the key knowledge and skills needed within a practitioner's role in working with

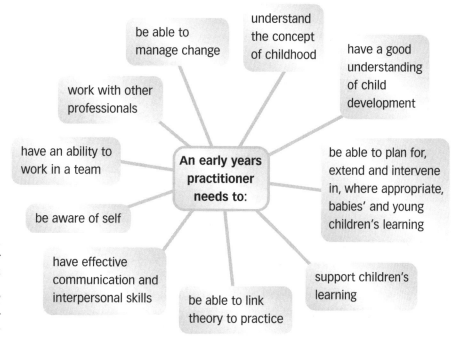

Figure 2.12
Requirements for working as a practitioner with babies and children under the age of 8 years

babies and children under 8 years, their parents and carers, and other professionals.

Supporting children's learning

A practitioner who works in an early years setting on a daily basis with children is a significant adult: a person who plans, supports, intervenes in and extends children's learning. There are many aspects to this role and many ways in which adults support and help children to interact with the environment around them to gain knowledge, skills and understanding from this interaction.

The E Framework shown in Figure 2.13 identifies seven ways in which adults support children's education and learning.

↻ You may like to reflect upon your own role in supporting children's learning using the E Framework

Activity 4) Using the E Framework

Over the time span of one week reflect upon your role in supporting one child's or a group of children's learning using the seven headings in the E Framework.

1 Provide evidence.
2 Identify areas for development.
3 Write an action plan to develop your work.

	Evidence	Area/s for development
EXPERIENCE		
EXTEND		
ENCOURAGE		
ENGAGE		
EDUCATE		
EXPLAIN		
EXAMINE		

The E Framework: a framework for the early years practitioner's role in supporting children's learning

EXPERIENCE	Provide experiences, opportunities, resources inside and outside the learning setting.	For example: **Inside**: planned play areas, cafes, shops, literacy, numeracy, creativity areas **Outside**: chalking boards, walks in the local environment, big toys, playground apparatus
EXTEND	Question, listen, intervene in, and extend children's learning where appropriate.	For example: **Adult during a local walk** Questioning and listening: 'What can you hear?' 'What sound do the leaves make when we walk in them?' **Adult in the home corner** Intervening in and extending a child's play: 'Could you pour me a nice cup of tea, please?'
ENCOURAGE	Praise and value each child's progress in learning. Help children to achieve tasks and activities they may not be able to do on their own.	For example: **Adult writing with a group of children**. 'Josh, I enjoyed reading your story so far. What might the dragon do next? I'll help you with any long words you may need so that you can make your story exciting.'
ENGAGE	Become involved in children's learning experiences. Provide for their individual needs.	For example: **Adult baking with children**. 'You've made some lovely buns. I enjoyed making them with you. Grant wants to ice them, so shall we do that, Grant?'
EDUCATE	Be a role model for children by demonstrating knowledge, skills and understanding.	For example: **Adult at story time**. 'Today I am going to read you one of my favourite stories. I hope you'll like it as much as I do.'
EXPLAIN	Listen to children, answer their questions.	For example: **Adult responding to a child's questions about where the water goes when the bath plug is pulled**. 'The water goes down the plug hole into sewers, which are big tunnels under the street. It then flows along pipes to the sewage works where it is cleaned.'
EXAMINE	Examine children's learning and development through observation and assessment in order to plan for their future development.	For example: Adults meet at the end of the day to review the observations of children they have carried out that day. This review informs planning of the next day's activities to meet children's individual needs.

Figure 2.13
The E Framework

Effective communication skills

A practitioner in an early years setting works in a people-centred service; the service users comprise parents, children and their families. The quality of this service is based upon effective relationships. Practitioners who work in this service are required to have effective communication skills in order to develop relationships with children, staff, parents and professionals. Rodd (1998:40) highlights the importance of practitioners communicating effectively, since 'the way in which early childhood professionals respond to children, parents and staff affects the quality of the interaction'. A people-centred service is built upon effective relationships, and the quality of interactions plays a vital part in this service.

Figure 2.14 indicates the range of people an early years practitioner working in a maintained school or nursery setting communicates with and the context within which they do so.

A practitioner working in an early years setting communicates with:		
Service users	**Immediate context**	**Wider context**
Children	Class or nursery group	Other children in the school or nursery at playtime, assembly time, lunchtime, snack time
Parents	Parents of the children they work with in the class or key worker group	Other parents, for example, parent governors, parent helpers, members of the Parent–Teachers Association
Staff	Class or nursery teacher, nursery nurse, teaching assistant, classroom assistant, support worker	Head teacher, deputy head teacher, other teachers or nursery nurses, the cook, lunchtime supervisors, school crossing patrol, school nurse, school clerk
Other professionals	The school nurse	Speech therapists, psychologists, teaching and support staff in local settings and the LEA

Figure 2.14
The range of people working in a maintained school or nursery with whom a practitioner communicates

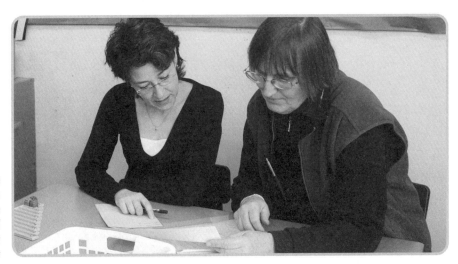

Effective communication skills are essential for all early years practitioners

Defining communication

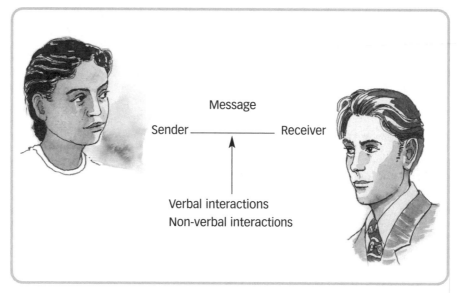

Communication involves giving and receiving messages

Communication is a two-way process, consisting of verbal and non-verbal interactions. Communication is about both giving and receiving messages. The message may give information or communicate feelings. The sender transmits a message through verbal and non-verbal interactions, selecting the form of communication which is most appropriate, with the intention that the receiver will accept it in the way it is intended.

Figure 2.15 lists the forms of communication a practitioner can use.

Forms of communication	
Pre-verbal	Music / Laughter / Sounds / Dance / Dress
Non-verbal	Body language / Sign language
Verbal	Spoken language / Listening / Singing / Recorded speech / Telephone
Written	Letters / Cards / Memos / Poetry / Literature / Fax / Email
Pictorial	Images / Logos and symbols / Sign language

Figure 2.15
Forms of communication

Verbal interactions

Verbal interactions are used throughout a practitioner's day. Carl Rogers (1961) (in Rodd, 1998:40) identified five response styles observed in 80 per cent of verbal communication engaged in by professionals working in human service occupations. These are shown in Figure 2.16.

Rogers' five response styles (1961)	
Advising and evaluating responses	*'What you should do now is ...'*
Interpreting and analysing responses	*'The problem you really have here is ...'*
Supporting and placating responses	*'Don't worry, they all go through that stage.'*
Questioning and probing responses	*'Is everything all right at home?'*
Understanding and reflecting responses	*'You appear to be pleased about how Vikram is progressing.'*

Figure 2.16 *Rogers' five response styles*

> **Activity 5** **Rogers' five response styles**
>
> 1 Do any of the statements given as examples in Figure 2.16 sound familiar? You may like to listen to yourself during a day's work.
>
> 2 What kind of responses do you make in your interactions with parents, staff and children?
>
> 3 How many of Carl Rogers' five responses do you use?
>
> 4 Are there some you use more than others?

Non-verbal communication

Non-verbal communication, or body language, is used in conjunction with verbal communication and helps to convey a message in a positive or negative way.

Body language is just that, a non-verbal language. There are many languages in the world with different concepts and sounds; likewise body language is not the same in every country. It is dependent upon the culture of each country; for example, children in New Zealand greet each other by rubbing noses, whereas this would not be the normally accepted greeting for children living in Liverpool. As practitioners it is important for us to be aware of the different cultural practices of the children we work with in order not to offend service users.

Some examples of non-verbal communication are given in Figure 2.17.

Non-verbal communication includes:	
Facial expressions	Facial expressions may indicate happiness, surprise, fear, sadness, anger, disgust or contempt and interest.
Gestures	Gestures are used to elaborate or to expand upon speech. Some gestures are culture-specific; for example, greetings may involve shaking hands or kissing.
Body movements	While speaking, a person moves his or her hands, body and head continuously. These movements are closely coordinated with speech and form part of the total communication.
Body contact	This includes the use of touch and is used to show affection, support or anger.
Body posture	Attitudes to others are indicated by body posture; for example, a person with folded arms may be putting up a physical barrier to communication.
Physical proximity	The distance a person stands from another indicates intimacy or distance.

Figure 2.17
Non-verbal communication

> **Activity 6** **Body language**
>
> 1 During a session in a working day, write down how you used non-verbal language as part of effective communication in a situation with a parent, child or member of staff.
> 2 Reflect upon how the outcome could have been different if you had used negative body language.

Written communication

Practitioners in early years settings are often required to provide written communication to pass on information to parents, staff and other professionals. This type of communication can be chosen as the most appropriate form for that specific purpose or it can be a requirement of the setting. Practitioners are required to have adequate literacy skills in order to write effectively. Some examples of the different types of written communication produced by a practitioner working in an early years setting are shown in Figure 2.18.

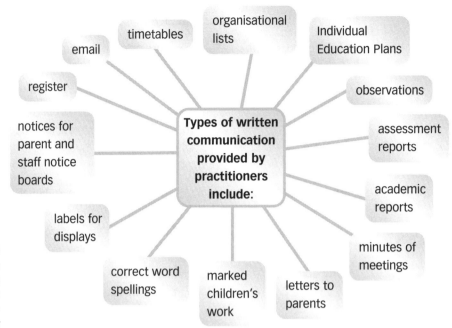

Figure 2.18
Some examples of written communication used in an early years setting

Types of written communication provided by practitioners include:

- email
- timetables
- organisational lists
- Individual Education Plans
- register
- observations
- notices for parent and staff notice boards
- assessment reports
- academic reports
- labels for displays
- minutes of meetings
- correct word spellings
- marked children's work
- letters to parents

The practitioner's readers include:

➲ other staff

➲ parents

➲ professionals; for example, psychologist, LEA, Ofsted

➲ children

Activity 7) Written communication

Consider your own use of written communication.

1 Has there been an occasion on which you chose written communication as a more effective means of conveying your message than verbal communication?

2 Do you use written communication in conjunction with verbal communication? If so, why? Does it make the communication more or less effective?

Active listening

Listening is the most important skill in the communication process. Early years settings are busy places; as practitioners, we do not always have the time to listen attentively to children, staff and parents. Communication will be more successful if the sender gives as much attention to what they hear as to what they say. Being a good listener takes skill and practice. You not only have to hear the words children, staff and parents are saying, but you also have to understand them and then respond in an appropriate way. This means you make listening an active process. Hilton (1994:25) defines this as 'active listening'. Suggestions about how you may become an active listener are given in Figure 2.19.

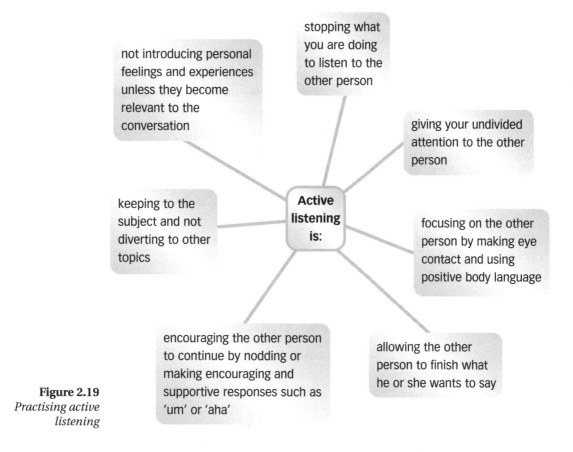

Figure 2.19
*Practising active
listening*

Active listening is:

- stopping what you are doing to listen to the other person
- giving your undivided attention to the other person
- focusing on the other person by making eye contact and using positive body language
- allowing the other person to finish what he or she wants to say
- encouraging the other person to continue by nodding or making encouraging and supportive responses such as 'um' or 'aha'
- keeping to the subject and not diverting to other topics
- not introducing personal feelings and experiences unless they become relevant to the conversation

Activity 8 has been designed to help you to reflect upon your listening skills.

Activity 8   Practise active listening

During the course of a working day select an interaction with a parent, child or member of staff and practise active listening.

1 How did you find this interaction?
2 How did the process of active listening develop positive interactions and relationships?

Barriers to communication

There may be barriers to communication. Linguistic, cultural, physical and emotional issues can prevent effective communication. There may be:

⊃ time constraints

⊃ other stresses within the child's family

⊃ English may be a second language for the child

⊃ sensory difficulties, which may include hearing or sight disabilities.

Practitioners need to recognise possible barriers to communication and provide strategies to overcome them; for example, a bilingual support assistant could help parents to communicate with staff in their child's educational setting. Work settings serve a local community and are usually familiar with community needs. Practitioners working in an early years setting are in the front line of overcoming barriers to communication.

> ## Activity 9 Overcoming barriers to communication
>
> 1 How do you and your work setting overcome any individual barriers to communication?
> 2 What strategies does your work setting use to overcome any community barriers to communication?

Working in teams and groups

Practitioners working within early years settings do not work in isolation but as members of a team and with others in groups or teams. Figure 2.20 illustrates the range of teams that may work together in supporting the learning and development of a child within an educational setting.

Teams and groups within educational settings		
Staff team	Teaching teams	Foundation Stage/Key Stage 1 team / Year teams / Subject specialist teams
	Support teams	Nursery nurses / Teaching assistants / Classroom assistants / Special needs support assistants / Parent helpers
	Ancillary teams	School clerks / Premises/Mid-day supervisors / Catering
	Governors	Sub-committees
Outside agencies		Sure Start/Local Education Authority / Early Years Development Partnership
		Child and family support services, for example, social services and the health service / children's service
Parents and carers		In the nursery or school and in liaison with the home
Children		Indoors and outdoors / in the Foundation Stage 1/Key Stage/Year groups and different classes

Figure 2.20
Teams and groups working together in educational settings

You may recognise some teams that you work in. Practitioners usually work in a number of teams and groups that vary in size. As a member of a team you will have different roles and responsibilities. Team members should have a common aim or aims and it is important for every member to cooperate and share his or her experience to maximise the efficiency of the provision. In order to operate effectively, all teams must have two dimensions:

➲ **The Task** – the job to be done or the problem to be solved

➲ **The Process** – the way in which the task is carried out; it concerns how people bring their knowledge, skills and qualities together.

(in Taylor and Woods (1998:283))

Early years practitioners need to develop strong relationships with individual team members in order to carry out their work effectively and for the team to work successfully within the organisation. This involves effectively communicating to all team members by actively listening, using clear verbal and non verbal communication and supporting all members of the team. According to Woodcock (1986:44), building a team requires:

➲ clear objectives and agreed targets

➲ appropriate leadership

➲ sound policies and procedures

➲ sound inter-group relations

➲ individual development

➲ regular review of team performance

➲ cooperation and constructive conflict

➲ support and trust

➲ openness and confrontation.

Figure 2.21 illustrates some of the differences between effective and ineffective teamwork.

Effective teamwork	Ineffective teamwork
The team should achieve more than the individuals working separately by using the individual talents, skills and specialisms of the team members to the best advantage.	The team may accomplish less than the individuals working separately and may be demotivated. This obviously affects the service the team provides.
Teams can promote creativity, morale and motivation.	Symptoms of bad teamwork may include personality clashes, lack of openness, jobs duplicated or not completed and members failing to support each other.
An effective team may carry out tasks that individuals cannot complete on their own.	

Figure 2.21
Effective and ineffective teamwork

Within the team in which a practitioner works, members take on different roles and responsibilities, based upon their strengths and weaknesses. One team member may develop ideas, another may organise the team and another may actually implement the ideas generated. For successful teamwork, there needs to be a balance of different types of members to take on these roles and responsibilities.

> ## Activity 10   Working in a team

You may like to reflect upon your own experience of working in a team.

1 Was it an effective team, if so why?

2 Was it an ineffective team, if so why?

Leadership

Leadership is a process whereby a person leads a number of other individuals to an agreed set of aims and objectives.

There are now more women in leadership and management within early years settings than in many other professions. This reflects the percentage of female practitioners working within this field. Women leaders can give strong leadership within a collaborative framework. This female approach to power is based upon collaboration, inclusion and consensus building through reciprocal relationships, where the leader seeks to act with, rather than assert power over, others. The woman leader tends to see herself as a member of the team. Leadership becomes an holistic, inclusive and empowering process. Decisions are made in consultation. Issues are thoroughly discussed, with each group member participating fully until a basic agreement that is acceptable to everyone involved is reached. This is considered by many to be the most effective way of making decisions, as it produces 'innovative, creative and high quality decisions' (Rodd 1998:92).

Women lead by empowering, teaching, providing role models and encouraging openness and questioning. Rodd (1998:11) describes four leadership behaviours in Figure 2.22.

Leadership behaviours	
Vision behaviour	Creating a vision and taking appropriate risks to bring about change
People behaviour	Providing caring and respect for individual differences
Influence behaviour	Acting collaboratively
Values behaviour	Building trust and openness

Figure 2.22
Four leadership behaviours, Rodd (1998:11)

Leaders should:

- ⊃ inspire and motivate the staff team
- ⊃ initiate change
- ⊃ take decisions
- ⊃ set objectives
- ⊃ set the pace of the work setting
- ⊃ develop a team culture
- ⊃ facilitate and encourage the development of individuals
- ⊃ inspire loyalty.

Successful leaders reflect, deliberate and plan the organisation of the work setting around values, philosophy, policies and the need to be responsive to change. Effective leadership in early years settings involves creating a community and providing a high quality service. This involves:

- ⊃ influencing the behaviour of others, particularly staff and parents
- ⊃ supporting staff in their personal and professional development
- ⊃ planning for, and implementing, change in order to improve the organisation.

Activity 11 **Reflect upon leadership**

You may like to reflect upon the leaders you have worked with and consider whether there has been one leader, for example, head teacher, nursery manager, playgroup supervisor, who has particularly inspired and motivated you. If so:

1 What qualities did they have?

2 What did they help you achieve?

If there is a leader who has not inspired you:

1 What did he or she do or not do to support you?

2 How could he or she have helped you professionally?

⊃ Managing change

Early years education is undergoing change and is evolving, as are other areas of education. External changes such as the introduction of the Foundation Stage brought internal change to early years settings. Internal changes, too, arise from the needs of individual settings: for example, changing the snack routine or outdoor-play provision. Managing change and surviving it are crucial for every team member. Merchant and Marsh (1998:102) suggest that change should be carefully managed and well planned so that there are not too many demands on colleagues at any one time. Staff should take ownership of change by working in a collaborative way to implement it. Change should also be supported by appropriate staff development and discussion with relevant professionals. Successful change is likely to be lasting when there is a strong element of practicality. An example of this is the number of early years settings that have successfully implemented Story Sacks as a literacy resource to use with children and parents (Griffiths, 1997).

Action Research aims 'to improve and to involve' (Fisher, 2002:199) and is an effective way of managing change. When implementing change, there will be some staff that are resistant to it. The initiating practitioner should lead by example from a sound knowledge base and involve all staff in decisions of 'how' and 'when' the change should be implemented. The following Change Cycle based upon Action Research is a useful way of approaching and managing change.

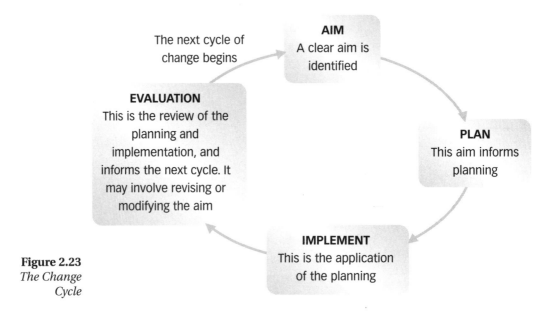

Figure 2.23
The Change Cycle

The next cycle of change begins

AIM
A clear aim is identified

PLAN
This aim informs planning

IMPLEMENT
This is the application of the planning

EVALUATION
This is the review of the planning and implementation, and informs the next cycle. It may involve revising or modifying the aim

> **Activity 12** **A personal role within change**

You may like to reflect upon your role regarding any changes you have experienced.

1 Did you initiate the change?
2 Did you lead the team?
3 Were you a member of the team that implemented the change?
4 Did you resist the change?
5 Has the change been sustained?

Working with other professionals

Practitioners working in early years settings liaise with members of different teams. In the increasing multi-agency work that takes place within early years settings, professionals from health, education and social services work together to meet the needs of children and their families. Practitioners are required to work with other professionals such as health visitors, speech therapists, physiotherapists, educational psychologists, social workers and governors, as well as parents. Supportive and effective relationships need to be developed with all these professionals and with parents too. This is discussed further in Chapter 13. The need for each practitioner to have effective communication and teamwork skills is therefore important.

Practitioners in early years settings work daily with teachers in the classroom or nursery team. This relationship is central to the effectiveness of the work of the early years practitioners and their contribution to the children and parents within their setting. The practitioner should not only be a member of the classroom or nursery planning team and the setting's staff team, but should also be involved in curriculum planning and attend staff meetings. Practitioners should be able to work independently as well as part of a team. Positive feedback about their role and contribution to the setting is important in order to develop a team culture and for practitioners to be viewed as valued members of the school or nursery team. Clear communication and expectations, particularly about behaviour management, are required so that a consistent approach is provided. Open communication within a climate of trust will facilitate the building of an effective relationship between teachers and early years practitioners.

In working with other multi-disciplinary professionals, it is important to define your role and responsibilities, together with those of others within the team and other agencies. Problems may arise in working with other professionals when roles and responsibilities are not clearly defined. Clarification of roles ensures that you know what you are responsible for, what you are required to report and how this needs to be carried out, for example, in a written report or verbally. Practitioners need to be clear about whom to report to in each team. Confidentiality is crucial when working with other professionals. This is particularly important when working with children with special educational needs. Copies of Individual Education Plans, assessments and reports are often required from teaching assistants and nursery nurses at review meetings.

In the following case study, clear roles and responsibilities have been identified in working with professionals to support the child's individual needs.

Supporting a child with special needs

Michael, aged six years, was born with only two fingers and a thumb on his right hand. A need for daily physiotherapy exercises was identified at his paediatric assessment. Michael's support worker helps him with his classroom work and in helping him to undress and dress for PE classes. A physiotherapist met with Michael's class teacher, support worker and parent at the school to show them exercises to carry out daily with Michael at home and at school. His class teacher would take on this role in his support worker's absence. The support worker agreed to keep records of Michael's progress to inform the physiotherapist at their fortnightly meetings. In this case, there was a need for the physiotherapist, the support worker, parent and class teacher to communicate well with each other in order to support Michael's needs.

Activity 13) Supporting a child with special needs

You may like to reflect upon a child you have supported and how you communicated with parents and different teams and agencies.

1 What was successful?
2 What difficulties did you have?

Conclusion

There is a need for flexible services and a range of multi-professional roles to support the changing needs of children and families within the early years field. This chapter has explored and discussed ways that practitioners working within an early years setting may develop their knowledge, skills and understanding in a reflective and evaluative manner, in order to contribute to the new opportunities, roles and responsibilities that are available and emerging within early years settings. Reflecting on their practice enables practitioners to provide relevant and quality services for children, parents and families.

References and further reading

Abbott, L. and Moylett, H. (1997), *Working with the Under Threes: Training and Professional Development*. Maidenhead: Open University Press

Abbott, L. and Pugh, G. (1998), *Training to Work in the Early Years: Developing the Climbing Frame*. Maidenhead: Open University Press

Abbott, L. and Rodger, R. (1994), *Quality Education in the Early Years*. Maidenhead: Open University Press

Anning, A. and Edwards, A. (2003), *Promoting Children's Learning from Birth to Five: Developing The New Early Years Professional*. Maidenhead: Open University Press

Cockburn, A. (2001), *Teaching Children 3–11: A Student's Guide*. London: Paul Chapman

Fisher, J. (2002), *Starting from the Child: Teaching and Learning from 3 to 8*. Maidenhead: Open University Press

Griffiths, N. (1997), *Picture Book Activity and Game Resource Pack*. Swindon: own publication

Hilton, M. (1994), *Interpersonal Interaction*. London: Longman

Kay, J. (2002), *Teaching Assistant's Handbook*. London: Continuum International Publishing Group

Merchant, G. and Marsh, J. (1998), *Co-ordinating Primary Language and Literacy: The Subject Leader's Handbook*. London: Paul Chapman Publishing

Pugh, G. (2001), *Contemporary Issues in the Early Years: Working Collaboratively for Children*. London: Paul Chapman Publishing

Rodd, J. (1998), *Leadership in Early Childhood: The Pathway to Professionalism*. Maidenhead: Open University Press

Rumbold Report, Department of Education and Science (1990), *Starting with Quality: The Rumbold Report of the Committee of Inquiry into the Quality of Educational Experience Offered to 3 and 4 year olds*. London: HMSO

Taylor, J. and Woods M. (1998), *Early Childhood Studies: An Holistic Introduction*. London: Hodder Arnold

Woodcock, M. (1986), *Team Development Manual*. London: Gower Press

Physical development

3

Vicky Cortvriend with a contribution by Maria Robinson

This chapter is designed to provide you with the knowledge and understanding required to enable you to support the physical development of the children in your care. It discusses norms of physical development to assist in your observations of children, which are crucial to the provision of suitable activities that promote children's growth, development and learning.

This chapter addresses the following areas:

- ⊃ human development
- ⊃ theories of motor development
- ⊃ stages of physical development
- ⊃ factors influencing prenatal development
- ⊃ postnatal development.

After reading this chapter you should be able to:

1 review and update your knowledge of the physical growth and development of young children

2 assess the physical development of babies/children in your care

3 understand a range of theories of physical development.

Introduction

An understanding of physical development is essential when studying the **holistic** (all-round or overall) development of children. Children's growth and development enables them to explore their environment, to make sense of their world, to achieve new skills, to change the way others perceive them, and, most importantly, it aids in their development of self. The child who successfully carries out various tasks and develops new skills can achieve a positive self-image. Conversely, children who constantly fail, or who are given the impression that they are failing, have difficulty in developing this positive sense of self. How and why children develop the way they do, and the factors that influence that development is discussed in some detail in this chapter.

Human development

Development is determined by the **genotype** of the child and is also influenced by various external factors, resulting in each child having his or her own personal **phenotype** and developing into a unique person. The genotype refers to the child's genetic makeup, and is entirely hereditary. Phenotype refers to the various environmental factors that influence the child's development.

Human development has, in the past, been studied from a compartmentalised point of view, which tended to lead to an unbalanced idea of the developmental process. Development has been referred to in terms of **areas** or **domains** (cognitive, social, emotional, physical, normative, conative), and periods (prenatal, infancy, childhood, adolescence, adulthood, old age). This unbalanced point of view can result in students concentrating on only one area to the detriment of others, without realising that each area impacts on the rest, and that each stage leads inexorably to the following one.

It is important to view development from an holistic stance, recognising that none of the areas develops in isolation; all areas influence and interact with each other and there is a continuous interaction between the individual's genotype and his or her individual environment. Development is a continuous process, beginning at conception and only ceasing when the person dies.

When studying human development you will come across the terms **growth** and **maturation**; there is a subtle difference between the two (see Figure 3.1).

Growth and maturation defined	
Growth	This is the increase in size, length, and weight.
Maturation	This is the development of the various systems that together form the human body. Examples are the nervous system, circulatory system, and the endocrine system.

Figure 3.1
Development: growth and maturation

Development per se has been defined as 'adaptive change toward competence' by Keogh and Sugden (1985). This suggests that during an individual's lifetime, he or she continually has to make adjustments in order to attain, or maintain, competence, as abilities develop.

> **Activity 1** **Physical development**
>
> 1 Think of a child who can crawl quite competently but who is now learning to walk. The child has to learn how to compensate for the change in the centre of gravity when he or she stands.

In carrying out Activity 1, some examples you may have thought of are:

⊃ walking then being able to hop

⊃ climbing the stairs on hands and knees, then beginning to put both feet on one stair, before finally climbing up as an adult would

⊃ learning how to ride a two-wheeler bicycle after using stabilisers.

In normal circumstances, growth and development are continuous and proceed in a typical, usual, or expected pattern. The term **normal** is used loosely to describe a child who is developing typical characteristics for his age and whose height and weight conform to the average.

There are theories, scales and charts that assist childcare workers in determining whether a child is, in fact, developing according to accepted norms. These include:

⊃ Jean Piaget's developmental milestone theory (see Chapter 5)

⊃ Mary Sheridan's age-related sequences of development (Sheridan, 1975)

⊃ growth charts.

Most developmental scales are based on the work of Arnold Gesell, an American developmental psychologist who researched the development of children in the 1930s (see Theories of motor development on page 72).

Today, when carrying out their routine checks to record the child's progress, health professionals commonly use the Denver screening checklist and development centile, or growth charts, in order to record the child's growth and weight. Copies of the latter are shown in Figure 3.2. Health professionals can then see at a glance whether or not there is any cause for concern. Should there be a problem then the child will be referred to a specialist for further tests.

Practitioners who work in early years settings observe children's physical development and their developing skills as an ongoing integral part of their practice. Should either a parent or an early years practitioner have concerns about a child's development (in any developmental area), then the practitioner needs to be able to provide some evidence that will either refute, or demonstrate, the reasons for these concerns.

Practitioners or parents may express concerns that a child's development is:

⊃ slow

⊃ retarded

⊃ advanced

⊃ precocious.

Carrying out a series of observations on the child, and then evaluating the observations against developmental norms can, in part, provide the

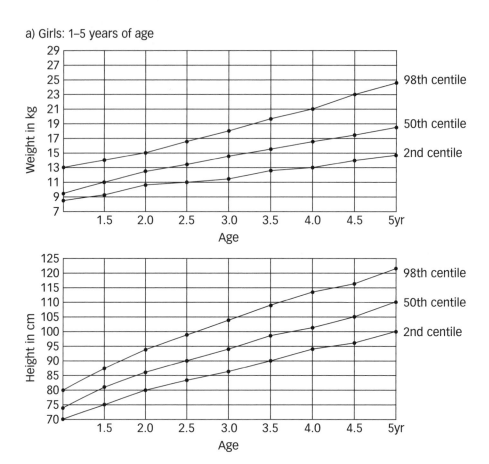

a) Girls: 1–5 years of age

b) Boys: 1–5 years of age

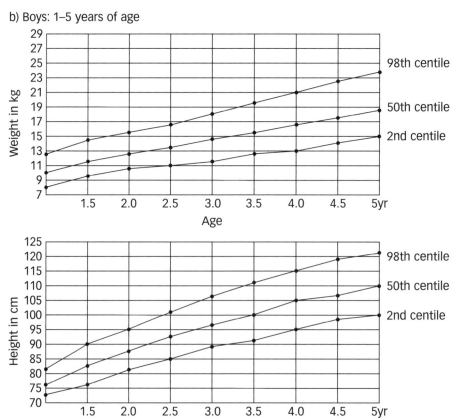

Figure 3.2
Normal weight and height gain falls between the 2nd and the 98th centile lines. The 50th centile line marks the average

evidence for these concerns (see Chapter 9). The practitioner will then be in a position to discuss the issues with the child's parents or carers and have relevant evidence to pass on to other professionals such as child psychologists, paediatricians and health visitors, should the need arise. In addition, this information would be used to plan appropriate activities to support or extend the child's development.

When comparing a child's physical development with the norm, the practitioner observes the child's ability to move and to perform different tasks; this is an important part of the practitioner's role in an early years setting because it enables him or her to know how each individual child is developing, which in turn enables the practitioner to plan and carry out appropriate activities that are designed to allow the child to consolidate skills and extend his or her development (see Chapters 7 and 8). The practitioner in an early years setting is also in a position to provide valuable feedback to the child's parents or carers, and information for other professionals.

Terms commonly referred to when discussing motor skills are **gross motor skills** and **fine motor**, or **manipulative**, **skills** (see Figure 3.3).

Figure 3.3
Terms that describe motor skills

Motor skills	Abilities
Gross motor skills	The ability to move using whole body movements
Fine motor, or manipulative, skills	The ability to perform skills that require hand and eye coordination

Activity 2 Observe children playing

1 Observe a group of children playing for a short period (see Chapter 9 for more information about observations).

2 Describe what they are doing, then evaluate your observation by picking out the fine and gross motor skills used.

3 Explain how the use of these skills enabled the children to socialise with their peers and how they aided the children's developing self-esteem (or not, as the case may be).

4 Plan suitable activities designed to consolidate the children's skills, or, should a child not be progressing as you would expect, plan activities to support him or her in this area of development.

5 Use information from Chapter 4 ('Emotional and social development'), and, if the children are aged 3–5 years, the curriculum guidance for the Foundation Stage (DfEE).

6 If the children are older than 5 years, refer to Key Stages 1 and 2 of the national curriculum. If they are younger than 3 years, refer to developmental milestones.

Theories of motor development

Theories attempt to organise accepted facts in order to give them meaning. They do this by testing known facts, and formulating theories to explore and advance new facts. They try to answer the question why. Theorists are people who conduct research in order to test existing theories or to develop new ones.

There are a range of theories that relate to the physical development of children. These are known as theories of motor development, of which there are three main perspectives.

Maturational theories

These represent the nature side of the nature-nurture debate; they assume that as the brain, nervous system and muscular systems mature and develop, the infant will automatically develop increasingly complex gross and fine motor skills.

Gesell and Ames (1940, quoted in Salter and Lewis, 2002) carried out a longitudinal research programme that followed a group of infants from birth to 9 years of age. They produced findings that concluded that motor development proceeds in an invariant sequence, controlled by a maturational timetable that is present in the central nervous system. These studies still remain an important point of departure for empirical research and formed the basis for the developmental checklists (growth charts) used today.

Their research, however, failed to account for individual differences and also led to the assumption that the entire developmental sequence is predetermined. McGraw (1945) challenged these assumptions, following her own research on newborn babies and longitudinal studies on 82 healthy infants. She also carried out research on sets of twins, where only one twin received enriched motor training. McGraw concluded that walking develops in four major steps (see Figure 3.3).

Phase	Development
First (under 4 months)	During the first phase, sub-cortical reflexes largely control limb movements.
Second (under 4 months)	These reflexes become inhibited by higher cortical mechanisms during the first 4 months and the controlling influence of the sub-cortical reflexes diminishes or disappears.
Third (between 4 and 8 months)	Discrete muscle control is achieved under the direction of the higher cortical mechanisms.
Fourth (between 8 and 14 months)	All sub-cortical and cortical components integrate and the infant achieves the mature walking pattern.
Note: sub-cortical and cortical refer to areas of the brain.	

Figure 3.4
Stages in the development of walking in young children (McGraw, 1945)

Systems theories

Detailed animal experiments conducted by Waddington (1971) provide a strong argument against the maturational theories. His studies, based on the idea that any complex organism is made up of many subsystems, show that each subsystem develops according to its own timetable. Even a minor change in the developmental timing of a subsystem can (under some conditions) result in the emergence of a new species during evolution (quoted in Gould, 1992). This implies that differential growth rates across subsystems, together with other biological variants, may result in the induction of new patterns of motor coordination.

Dynamical systems

These theories concern systems that are influenced by a combination of different factors (similar to the idea of the phenotype) that ensure that the system is inherently unpredictable.

Researchers who are concerned specifically with human locomotion, i.e. the way humans move, have utilised this idea (Thelen, 1989; Thelen and Smith, 1994). Their results showed that there is an important contribution to be made by positive environmental factors in the development of coordinated motor action, such as walking. This development is always the outcome of a complex interplay between all the variables: the central nervous system, musculo-skeletal system, and the environment (Goldfield and Wolff, 2002).

Other theoretical approaches are discussed elsewhere in this book. Important theories include the phase stage theory of which the most well known proponents are Sigmund Freud, Erik Erikson and Jean Piaget; the developmental task theory, developed by Robert Havighurst; and the ecological theories (behaviour setting) of Roger Barker and Urie Bronfenbrenner.

> **Activity 3** **A critical analysis of theories of physical development**

1 Conduct your own research into these different perspectives using the references and websites at the end of this chapter.

2 The only method of confirming research findings, or of making new discoveries, in this field is by carrying out detailed observations on infants. Carry out your own longitudinal observations on one infant, or a group of infants, focusing on an area of motor development that particularly interests you. Conduct your own research (see Chapter 10) into the above theories and using your observations to illustrate your reasoning, write an evaluation that critically analyses the theories of physical development.

Is development continuous or discontinuous?

(See Theories of motor development, page 72.)

This question, together with the nature-nurture debate (nature denoting the effects of genes, and nurture denoting the effects of the environment), has been vigorously discussed and has formed the basis for much research.

Conduct your own research into this area by studying the works of Arnold Gesell (1928) and Myrtle McGraw (1935), who are considered to be pioneers in the study of motor development, and later theorists such as Jean Piaget (1954) and Keogh and Sugden (1985) to help you to decide which point of view you favour.

This could form the basis for an interesting whole-class discussion or debate.

Foetal behaviour

Another area that is now under discussion is that of the function of foetal behaviour. This is the way that foetuses move around in the womb in reaction to certain stimuli, or the way they suck their thumbs, blink their eyes, or move their mouths. You may have seen scans of foetuses demonstrating such behaviour. Why do they do this? This is the question being asked by some researchers. Are there reasons (stress, excitement, pain) for the foetus reacting and behaving as it does, or are the behaviours the result of the maturing of its systems?

Research carried out by Drachman and Sokoloff (1966) suggests that the movements the foetus makes are important for its structural development. It is also thought that the behaviour of the foetus may influence the development of the sensory system and brain. This is an interesting area for further reading and one that has been repeatedly researched by Hepper (see references).

Stages of physical development

In this section, we look at the physical development of a child from conception through to birth.

The developing child

For many years it was thought that the development of the child only really began at birth, and events preceding the birth had little, if any, influence on the child's future development. It is now recognised that the immediate internal environment of the foetus, as well as the development and growth of the foetus, can be influenced by both sociocultural factors, and **teratogens** (a teratogen is an environmental agent that causes disruption in the normal development of the foetus). This results in prominent differences in newborn babies. Even at birth, therefore, babies can differ in their ability to cope with, and adapt to, their new environment.

Cigarette smoke and stress are two factors that are considered to have an influence on the foetus. In the author's experience as a midwife, the babies of the women who had smoked during pregnancy were usually small and the placentas showed signs of calcification on examination after delivery. This is an indication that the baby was under stress while in the womb. Babies born to mothers who lived in poverty were also often small and looked like 'little old men' at birth. A midwife also described the difference between two babies born to the same mother, but ten years apart. The first, born during a time of great stress in the mother's life, when she was 20 years old, was rejected before his birth by the father; he was a very irritable baby, who spent the first year of life crying and did not sleep through the night until 3 years of age. The second baby, however, born 10 years later when the mother was going through a period of calm, and whom both parents wanted, was a quiet and relaxed baby who slept through the night from 6 weeks of age.

Prenatal

The physical development of the child begins at conception. This period between conception and birth, which usually lasts for between 38 and 40 weeks, has been divided into three distinct phases (Moore, 1988). The first is known as the **conceptual or germinal phase**; this starts with the fertilisation of the egg and ends when the pregnancy is established. This is followed by the **embryonic period**, which begins during the second week and ends at the end of the eighth week, when the **foetal period** begins. This continues until the birth of the baby. The period as a whole is referred to as the **prenatal period** ('prenatal' means 'before birth').

Nature-nurture debate

The nature-nurture debate, genotype versus phenotype, is a continuing debate on the relevance and importance of genetic influences on the developing and maturing foetus compared to the influence of environmental and other factors. It is now suggested that development during the prenatal period involves an interaction between genes and the environment, with the environmental influences contributing more to the development of the foetus than was previously thought. It has also been suggested that the actions and reactions of the foetus (that is, its behaviour) will help shape its own development.

Is development continuous or discontinuous?

The question of whether development is continuous or discontinuous asks: When exactly do newborn abilities begin? It was previously thought, for example by the philosopher John Locke (1632–1704), that at the moment of birth the abilities of the baby were suddenly switched on (perhaps in the same way that the lungs begin to work). But it is quite possible that these abilities originate during the prenatal period, thus implying continuous development (Hepper, 1994).

The function of foetal behaviour

Why does the foetus react and behave as it does in the womb and what is the significance of this behaviour? Does its behaviour relate to its development?

- At 7 weeks' gestation, the scan picture of the embryo shows quite clearly the large head, lack of neck, small trunk and tiny buds of growth where the limbs will grow. Movement is just discernible.
- At 8 weeks' gestation, the foetus, as it is now known, is fully formed with all organs present. A startle reflex can be seen and general movement is present.
- At 9 weeks' gestation, the foetus can hiccup and perform isolated arm and leg movements. In a male, the external reproductive organs begin to show.
- Foetal breathing movements begin at around 10 weeks' gestation. Between 8 and 12 weeks' gestation the fingernails, toe nails and hair follicles form. In a female, the development of the reproductive organs begins.

  Bones begin to grow; the foetus can flex arms and legs and can also suck. Sometimes scan pictures show foetuses sucking their hands.
- Between 13 and 16 weeks' gestation the foetus has developed unique hand- and footprints. The spinal cord begins to form and the foetus begins to make eye movements.
- Between 17 and 20 weeks' gestation the foetus becomes covered with the waxy substance known as vernix; its function is probably to protect the skin from the amniotic fluid that constantly surrounds it. The foetal heartbeat can clearly be heard through the woman's abdomen.
- The foetus continues to grow and develop and if born prematurely after 21 weeks' gestation can hear, see and produce crying noises.
- Between 22 and 24 weeks' gestation the foetus responds to sounds by moving.
- Between 26 and 29 weeks' gestation the lungs usually develop sufficiently to allow the foetus to breathe if birth occurs early.
- Between 30 and 38 weeks' gestation the foetus increases its weight by about a half. Fat accumulates, giving the full term 'chubby' appearance. The skin colour turns from red to white to bluish pink for all babies, regardless of their racial origin.

In the space of 38 weeks the baby has developed from a **zygote** (a bundle of cells) to a fully formed baby. This development, however, is not always straightforward as it is influenced by a number of factors. Examples include:

- environmental factors
- genetic factors

- health factors
- age of the mother
- nutritional factors and stress
- pregnancy with more than one foetus in the womb.

Development and maturation of the foetus

There appear to be three main factors that relate to the development and maturation of the foetus. These factors, which are outlined below, have dominated discussion, and continue to raise questions, prompting more research into the development of the embryo and foetus during the prenatal period.

Factors influencing prenatal development

Some of the main factors that affect prenatal development are outlined below.

Teratogens

Teratogens are agents that cause harm to the foetus during its development in the womb (see Figure 3.5).

Teratogens	Effects on the foetus
Rubella	The first agent to be recognised as a teratogen was the rubella virus, commonly known as German measles. In 1941, McAllister Gregg, an ophthalmologist, confirmed that German measles in a pregnant woman often resulted in the baby being born with visual anomalies.
Radiation	The second teratogen to be described was radiation, following reports in the 1940s and 1950s about women who had been exposed to the atomic bomb, and who were reported to have given birth to babies who had birth defects. This, together with reports about research done on animals, implicated radiation as a teratogen (Warkany and Schraffenberger, 1947).
Thalidomide	The drug thalidomide given to pregnant women for nausea in the 1950s and early 1960s resulted in the birth of many infants who had severe arm and leg malformations (McBride, 1961, Lenz and Kapp, 1962).
Other substances	Other substances that are freely taken by mothers today have been identified as having harmful effects on the foetus, alcohol, cigarettes and drugs being the major culprits.

Figure 3.5
Some teratogens and their effects on the foetus

Alcohol

Exposure to alcohol can lead to foetal alcohol syndrome as described by Abel (1989) and first recognised in the early 1970s during observations carried out on babies born to alcoholic mothers (Jones and Smith, 1973). These babies are characterised by growth retardation, abnormal facial features and intellectual retardation. Heavy drinking throughout pregnancy, or binge drinking, is far more hazardous to the developing foetus than moderate drinking, although a safe dose for alcohol consumption during pregnancy has not yet been established. Reports have demonstrated that even moderate amounts of alcohol intake can result in spontaneous abortions, less alert babies and slower learning in newborns.

Foetal alcohol effect is considered to be a milder form of foetal alcohol syndrome, resulting in children who are born with less severe retardation than those with foetal alcohol syndrome, but who may suffer from behavioural difficulties and poor social skills.

Cigarette smoking

Evidence published in the February 2004 report 'Smoking and Reproductive Life', produced by the BMA's board of Science and the Tobacco Control Resource Centre, states that smoking damages the health of both men and women throughout their reproductive life. It can lower fertility rates, and has a detrimental effect on the foetus during pregnancy. The evidence suggests that smoking may increase the risk of cleft lip and palate malformations in the developing foetus. The report confirms the findings from previous studies, suggesting that women who smoke are three times more likely to give birth to low-birth-weight infants. It appears that the number of cigarettes smoked and the length of time the woman smokes during pregnancy are linked to the size of the baby at birth. Spontaneous abortions, stillbirths and neonatal deaths are also more numerous in women who smoke during their pregnancy. Smoking can also compromise breast feeding because women who smoke produce less milk of a poorer quality. There is also substantial evidence to link passive smoking with reduced foetal growth and premature birth.

Prescription and other drugs

Legal and illegal drugs can also have an effect on the foetus. Pregnant women are advised not to take any over-the-counter or illegal drugs during pregnancy. If medication has to be taken, it should only be done so under close medical supervision.

Prescription and other drugs	Effects
Tetracycline	If taken during the second or third trimester of pregnancy, it can cause staining of the baby's teeth.
Streptomycin	This has been associated with hearing loss.
Aspirin	There is a possibility of increased bleeding in mother and infant.
Benzodiazepines	Infants may display withdrawal symptoms at birth.
Vitamin A	Large amounts of vitamin A are known to cause major birth defects.
Retinoids (Roaccutane)	These anti-acne drugs have similar effects on the foetus as vitamin A.
Marijuana	It crosses the placenta and is found in the amniotic fluid surrounding the foetus. It is also probably present in the breast milk of heavy smokers.
Heroin and methadone	Babies suffer withdrawal symptoms at birth. Congenital defects have not been linked directly to either heroin or methadone, but stillbirths, infant deaths and low birthweight in newborns are common among users. Developmental difficulties in infants born to addicts are frequently observed but this may be due to the environment the infant is being raised in, rather than the effects of the drugs when in the womb.

Figure 3.6
Effects of legal and illegal drugs taken during pregnancy

Discussion Point 2

A woman's legal responsibility to her unborn child

Should a woman who is made aware of the possible teratogenic effects that using illegal substances can have on her unborn child, but continues to use them, be prosecuted for child abuse if the child is born with birth defects?

There are various other factors that can have an influence on the effect that a teratogen will have on an unborn baby. You may perhaps cite an example of a woman who smoked 30 cigarettes a day throughout her pregnancy and gave birth to a baby who weighed more than nine pounds! The difficulty lies in predicting who will be affected. This is almost impossible to determine prior to a woman becoming pregnant, but the advent of ultrasound scans and other screening tests means that it is easier to predict the birth of a healthy or possibly damaged baby. As a practitioner in an early years setting, you may be involved in offering advice to expectant parents.

Factors that determine the effect of a teratogen on an unborn baby

The factors outlined below play a part in determining the effect of a teratogen on an unborn baby.

The individual's genetic makeup or genotype

This may affect susceptibility.

The stage of development of the embryo/foetus

The stage of development of the embryo/foetus at the time it is exposed to the teratogen may be significant. There are periods of sensitivity during prenatal development when the embryo/foetus is more sensitive to teratogenic influences than other times. The third to eighth week of pregnancy is a period when many organs and systems are being formed. They are, therefore, very sensitive to toxic agents during this period. The brain, however, continues to grow and develop during the entire pregnancy, which is why exposure to teratogens at any time may have behavioural consequences for the child.

The amount of exposure

Does the type or strength of a teratogen affect the foetus in different ways? It has been documented that the damage tobacco smoke has on the foetus is linked to the amount of cigarettes the mother smoked. But the severity of a disease such as rubella does not always reflect the amount of damage to the foetus. Other factors such as the overall health of the mother play a part in determining the teratogenic effect.

Health conditions and illnesses

A number of health conditions can result in increased risk to the foetus. These include:

- ⊃ Gaucher disease, an inherited condition affecting mainly Ashkenazic Jews
- ⊃ Diabetes
- ⊃ Hypertension
- ⊃ Eclampsia (occurs during some pregnancies)
- ⊃ Rh incompatibility.

All pregnant women should have regular health checks, particularly if they have an underlying condition that may prove to be a risk factor (see Chapter 14, page 457, Screening during the antenatal period). German measles (rubella) is a potential hazard to the developing foetus, and other, severe, viral infections can also be dangerous to the foetus. It is important to refer expectant mothers to their doctor if they are at all at risk.

The websites listed at the end of this chapter provide further information about the above conditions.

Age of mother

Many women, for a variety of reasons, choose to have children later in life. The likelihood of having a child with Down's Syndrome increases markedly with the age of the mother. One in every 1,500 babies born to mothers aged 21 years will have Down's syndrome, whereas in mothers aged 49, the incidence rises to 1 in 10.

Teenagers, however, are also at risk of delivering less healthy babies, according to a study carried out by McAnarney (1987). This is thought to be due to the fact that the ova (eggs) are not fully mature in teenage girls. Teenagers are also still growing themselves and have their own nutritional needs as well as those of the developing foetus.

Nutrition

Nutritional factors can affect the well-being of the foetus, and the need for a woman to eat a well-balanced diet with sufficient protein, vitamins, minerals, and other nutrients during pregnancy is recognised by all health professionals. Women of normal weight for their height are typically advised to gain about 25–35 pounds during pregnancy.

The physical and neural development of the foetus can be severely impaired when a pregnant woman fails to eat a balanced diet. This was clearly demonstrated during the famines that occurred in parts of Holland and in Leningrad during World War Two following invasion by the Nazis. When the malnutrition occurred during the first trimester, death, premature birth and neural defects were recorded. When the malnutrition occurred later in the pregnancy, the babies were likely to be born small.

Stress

Stress has been shown by several researchers to cause harm to the developing foetus (Wadha et al., 1993; Luke et al., 1995, in Bukato and Daehler). Severe stress seems to result in premature births and babies of low birthweight. Anxiety during pregnancy seems to result in difficult births with a higher rate of complications during delivery.

The support given by family and friends has been shown to be a major factor in decreasing the effects of stressors on pregnant women, and so decreasing the harm done to the foetus (Norbeck and Tilden, 1983). Discussing concerns with supportive groups has been found to be an effective method of counteracting the harmful effects of stress.

Educating prospective parents

Consider the following questions.

1 Would education help prospective parents to make the best choices for themselves and their unborn child?

2 Would education help to reduce the incidence of unwanted pregnancies?

3 Would education help to reduce the incidence of premature births and babies born affected by teratogens?

Think about what type of educational experience you would suggest – a series of talks by parents with first-hand experience, perhaps, or lectures by professional experts?

Think about these ideas then carry out the following activities:

1 Plan a series of antenatal sessions for a group of prospective parents. Include all the above information (and further research carried out by yourself) in a format designed to educate rather than frighten the clients.

2 Plan a series of sessions for 14–16-year-olds, again with the idea of educating them about the risks involved in smoking, drinking and drug taking while pregnant.

Postnatal development

A human infant's development in the womb can be influenced by the health, welfare, emotional state and physical wellbeing of the mother. The type, duration and environment of the birth can also influence both mother and baby. The mother's attitude can be influenced by factors including whether how the birth is planned, presence of complications, the level of pain and availability of pain relief, and the proximity of emotional support. A long and difficult birth is stressful for both the mother and her child.

As we saw earlier in the chapter, the baby can be highly active in the womb: in the final three months before birth, the baby moves spontaneously, can respond to sounds and light, and may sucks thumb. At birth, although physically helpless, the baby has a set of reflexes that not only supports its interactions with its carers but also demonstrates that a 'template' for physical activity is in place. In order to understand this, we need to take a brief look at the brain.

The brain has two distinct hemispheres, which, together with the brain stem and spinal cord, are mirror images of each other, although function varies between the left and right hemispheres. There is only one gland – the pineal gland – not duplicated on each side of the brain. The hemispheres are joined by the corpus callosum, which transmits much of the communication between hemispheres. The surface of each hemisphere is covered by the cortex. Its most identifiable features are grooves (sulci) and ridges (gyri) that give the brain its characteristic wrinkled appearance but, more importantly, have characteristics which are unique to each human and which bear the imprint of experience. Each hemisphere is divided into four 'lobes':

- The frontal lobe appears to deal with the most abstract and complex of brain functions, e.g. thinking, planning, conceptualising and in the conscious 'appreciation' of emotion.
- The parietal lobe appears to be mainly involved with movement, orientation, calculation and body image.
- The temporal lobe deals with hearing, language, comprehension, sound and some aspects of memory and emotion.
- The occipital lobe is mostly taken up with visual processing areas.

Our brains ultimately process all information they receive, developing over time. The lobes within the brain develop at different rates, depending on the particular skills they promote. In other words, our abilities and skills depend on the way our brain is 'wiring up'. The concept of physical development is often associated with large or gross motor movements such as walking, running, jumping and dancing, or fine motor movements made with the hands and fingers. However, smooth co-ordinated movements are impossible without support and feedback from our other senses, especially vision and touch. Movement and sensory information are so closely intertwined they should really referred to as a sensorimotor system rather than being divided into the two areas.

One of the most interesting issues about movement is the existence in the brain of 'body maps', which include motor and somatosensory maps. Even though these 'maps' are arranged on a particular part of the cortex, the upward processing of information requires aspects of organisation across the entire cortex and subcortical brain areas (which lie underneath the cortex). A general 'rule of thumb' is that the more precise the movements generated by different parts of the body, the greater the area of the brain devoted to them. Greenfield (2000) describes the hands and the mouth as having an enormous allocation of space on the 'map' compared with the upper arm and the back, which have very little space devoted to them. It is also important to remember that, as Skoyles and Sagan (2002) point out, the brain's 'motor map' is built up by sensory information, including feedback from the position of our muscles and joints. For example, the pre-motor cortex (found in front of the motor cortex) guides movements via information from vision and other sensory feedback systems. The somatosensory maps and the 'motor map' (also known as the somatotopic map) lie close to each other on either side of the central sulcus, the deep ridge which roughly divides the frontal from the parietal lobes. The motor map lies in front of the sulcus and the somatosensory map lies just behind it. Each map displays the same distorted picture of the body, clearly illustrating the overall importance of each body area and the relationships between them.

Key developmental transitions in physical development

The following section concerns the physical changes that occur during the early years; however, children develop at their own pace, achieving each milestone earlier or later than the general 'timeline' of development. In addition, the senses play a part in developing skills in movement: brains are maturing along with bodies.

The section has been divided into groups corresponding to the Birth to Three Matters initiative to provide a broad framework for thinking about the details of physical development. These groups are:

- ➲ Heads up, lookers and communicators (0–8 months)
- ➲ Sitters, standers and explorers (8–18months)
- ➲ Movers, shakers and players (18–24 months)
- ➲ Walkers, talkers and pretenders (24–36 months).

While the focus is on physical development across these age ranges, no aspect of development occurs in isolation and a child's social, emotional and physical environment will also influence the way in which a child develops. For example, a child given no opportunity to explore, or who is deprived of adequate nutrients or who receives little emotional encouragement may not develop optimal motor skills.

Heads up, lookers and communicators

At birth, infants are essentially helpless but by the time they are eight months old, they are able to sit steadily (or with minimal support) and often crawl or make some effort to move independently. While experience does influence development profoundly, a baby is given a 'head start' by the existence at birth of various reflexes. A reflex is an unconscious, spontaneous response to a stimulus. A classic example is if someone taps the knee in a certain place, the leg shoots out. Babies have a number of these reflexes:

- ➲ palmar or grasp reflex
- ➲ rooting reflex
- ➲ sucking reflex
- ➲ moro or startle reflex
- ➲ plantar or foot reflex (stepping reflex)
- ➲ Babinski (curling of the toes).

The first three reflexes support immediate interaction with the mother through touch and feeding. The startle reflex suggests that the baby is 'primed' to respond to surprise or fearful situations, and the plantar and Babinski reflex illustrate a potential 'wiring up' of basic motor movements that have been formed by the baby's actions in the womb. These reflexes all become less obvious over time as the brain matures and the baby becomes more discriminating in his or her responses. As babies get to know their world, they begin to respond more purposefully than the 'global' type of response seen in the new born. For example, the stepping reflex occurs if the baby is held upright with the feet placed on a hard surface. The baby then moves his or her legs as if stepping or walking. Some research has indicated that this reflex does not totally disappear over the next few months but becomes integrated into the patterns of kicking, which in turn bear a similarity to the movements used when walking.

Babies' increasing control of their bodies follow a logical pattern. For example, by about six weeks after birth, babies can usually hold their heads up in line with their bodies when pulled to sit up. By the age of three months, a baby will spend a lot of time moving his or her arms and legs, and hand and finger exploration is notable. By the age of five months, the baby can actively grasp at attractive items such as toys but finds letting go difficult. Even by six months, letting go is usually accidental and the baby loses interest once the toy is out of sight. At the same time, control over the trunk is improving and by the age of four months, babies are able to roll from their backs to their sides. By the age of six months, babies can roll over from their back to their stomach, which incidentally puts the baby in the best position for the 'push ups' required for crawling. Sitting becomes increasingly steady and requires less support. By seven to eight months of age, the baby is usually very active and will change position, push up on his or her arms, move in circles and so on. The grasp is still fairly 'broad' although the baby can pick up objects of different shapes and weights and also start to modify the way in which hand actions are performed: not only banging but patting too.

As stated earlier, it is difficult to separate the child's development of muscular control from the impact of visual input. New-born vision is limited to orientating to single targets, especially faces, but by the age of three months vision appears to be sufficiently integrated for the baby to switch attention from one 'object' to another. This is accompanied by the simultaneous development of such systems as orientation, motion and colour awareness, which all become more sensitive over time. Being able to see the position of a toy, both in relation to the other things around it, and relative to the position of the baby, helps children to learn to reach and grasp. Around the age of five to six months, the baby's visual control of reach and grasp suggests an awareness of 'near visual space', that is, the baby can reach for things close by reasonably accurately. Children of this age can also usually adjust the shape of their hands to accommodate the shape of the desired object. Over the next couple of months, the child's ability to reach with one hand appears to coincide with the child's control of the trunk; the child can usually sit steadily and unsupported by eight months of age.

By the time they reach eight months, therefore, most babies are able to move around freely and with choice and control. Incidentally, getting up is far easier for babies of this age than getting down! In the hands, the emergence of much finer muscle control develops with the emergence of the 'pincer grasp'. Most babies can also sit very steadily by this time and can therefore become involved in careful exploration of play materials. Babies can now also use their forefinger to point. Practitioners may find that babies go through a stage around this time when they do not like being on their backs and will try to sit up as much as possible.

Sitters, standers and explorers

From eight months onwards, both fine and gross motor movements are becoming steadily under the control of the baby. At this age, babies begin to look for an object they have dropped. The skill of letting go emerges at about the same time so babies will often practise this new knowledge by playfully dropping toys and hoping that obliging adults will pick them up so the baby can drop them again! This serves two important purposes. Firstly, the baby gets more practice in the skill of opening the hands in order to 'let go', and, secondly, it reinforces the idea of object permanence. Practitioners may also notice a change in the way the child can balance by no longer having to lean against a chair but standing unsupported and balancing using outstretched hands. Year-old babies have visual control of locomotion, which indicates an integration of physical action, attention, control and awareness of far and near visual space. (Atkinson, 2000). It is only when muscles are sufficiently strong and sufficiently co-ordinated to both support the baby's weight and to follow a specific direction that babies begin to pull themselves up and take a step. The time at which a child walks alone depends on opportunity, the child's own determination, type of encouragement and muscle and balance development, but it is usually between 12 and 15 months (Hall, Hill and Elliman, 1990). It is interesting that it is at about a year old that a child can see clearly to the other side of a room and this coincides with greater mobility – the child can see where they are going. The ability to walk around obstacles requires practice, as does the child's ability to work out his or her body in relation to others. The child will therefore often try to crawl under and around things as well as walk towards desired objects or people. Practitioners may also notice that the child sometimes returns to crawling, as this may still be quicker and easier than the hard work of walking. As the child approaches 18 months, walking becomes steadier and the child wants to climb. Again, this is a practice of motor skills and spatial skills as the child begins to get the idea of up and down. Children also have more control over their bodies by being able to kneel steadily and sit on an appropriately sized seat. All these skills allow for a growing sense of independence and an ability to interact at a number of physical levels.

As with the new skill of walking, fine motor movements require much trial and error. For example, attempts to use a spoon will often require some practice before the trajectory from plate to mouth is fully mastered. (Next time you use a spoon, slow your actions down and notice just how much skill is required to keep the spoon level and upright!). The ability to pick up small items using a pincer grasp also becomes more refined as the child becomes more able to let go of objects and begins to 'post' objects and handle toy bricks. By 18 months of age, children have usually achieved sufficient control over their hands to use them together and to build small towers, to scribble, to use a palmar (whole hand) grasp and to turn the pages of a book. In fact, these are examples of the kind of development test that health visitors often carry out on children aged between 18months and two years.

Movers, shakers and players

Being able to run is the next step in the child's growing set of motor abilities. Running becomes less cautious and more confident as children approach their second birthday, although again there will be individual variations. Children need to feel safe walking before they start running. A new skill such as this engenders activity in various brain areas and as a child practices this skill and becomes more confident at it, the patterns of sensory information, cortical control, instructions to muscles and, ultimately, movements become more refined and so the activity becomes 'automatic'. Children are now confident with stairs but will probably still go downstairs on their bottoms and will need a helping hand or rail when going up. As the months pass, running becomes faster and can change direction. Most children can kick a ball without falling over, and bending down to pick up toys is now quite usual. Fine motor or hand movements are also much more developed, towers can be built higher, and objects can be placed more precisely, assuming, of course, that vision is developing normally too. The use of individual fingers rather than the whole hand is becoming more common. This increases independence as children can begin to try dressing themselves and eating with minimal support.

Walkers, talkers and pretenders

Overall, the next months show a growing refinement of the skills in both large muscle and fine muscle movement. Children aged three have been known to learn to ski or to play a musical instrument, and many children can pedal a tricycle, catch a ball and swim.

Again, individual children will vary considerably both in the type of activity they enjoy and the degree of skill they will reach. It is important that children are given the opportunity to try out their skills but practitioners must remember that children's confidence can be severely shaken if faced with something that they sense is beyond them and they are overly encouraged accomplish it. The abilities to walk, run, climb, throw, catch, build, thread, make marks are all new or 'nearly new' and children will often want to consolidate their skills by repeating some actions over and over. The growing ability to engage in imaginative role play all support children in consolidating physical skills as they imitate domestic and adult activities, or pretend to be imaginary characters who can fly, fight, jump, hop and so on.

To summarise, from infancy onwards children develop motor control over their bodies, becoming increasingly able to move according to their own wishes. Improving physical development supports children in growing into being themselves just as much as any other aspect of development. However, physical development is only one part of development and the child's vision, the proper working of other sensory feedback mechanisms and the realisation that bodies move in space and in relation to other people and objects around them all takes time, practice, opportunity and, most of all, support from attentive adults.

Child's age	Skills
5 months	The baby should have doubled his or her birthweight and can roll over from back to stomach.
12 months	The child can walk unaided, turn the pages of a book and drink from a cup. The child is able to pick up and hold toys.
20 months	The child can kick a ball forwards, and pick it up to throw it overhand to a parent. The child should be able to thread large beads onto a piece of string.
2 to 3 years	The child's fine and gross motor skills develop rapidly. He or she is able to jump using both feet, run and can balance on one foot momentarily. Children of this age can draw or scribble, and when eating can use a spoon confidently.

3 to 4 years 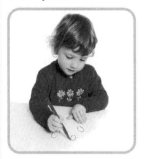	The child can walk upstairs in the manner of an adult, hop and can catch a ball accurately, clasping it to his or her chest. Children of this age are able to dress themselves, putting on a T-shirt, and fastening buttons. They can brush their teeth without help. They can cut items using scissors.
4 to 5 years 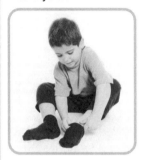	The child can walk downstairs with alternate feet, skip and gallop about, and attempt to catch a ball. Children of this age can eat with a fork and dress themselves without help. They are able to form letters and draw recognisable pictures.
5 to 6 years 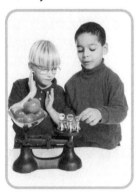	During PE class, the child can balance on a beam, jump about one foot in the air and throw and catch a ball in the same way as an adult. Children can sew simple stitches using a needle and thread.
6 to 7 years	The child develops the ability to tie shoe-laces, and can control a pen sufficiently to write numbers and words. The child can ride a bicycle, has developed ball skills and takes part in running and chasing games.

The development of motor skills has important implications for the holistic development of the child. It is important that practitioners who work in early years settings are aware of the expected norms of development so that they will be aware of any deviation from the norm and can then share their concerns with relevant others (parents, carers, and other professionals).

> **Activity 5** **Skill development**

1 Do early motor skills, i.e. reflexes, pave the way for more complex voluntary activities? Observe a young baby then an infant of perhaps one-year-old. Can you see the link between the early reflexes of the baby and the skills that the one-year-old has developed? Write an account describing your findings.

2 Design a checklist of the above skills for a range of children of different ages. Observe the children to determine whether they are in fact developing according to expected norms. Depending upon your findings, design a series of activities that will either help the children to consolidate their skills, or assist them in developing those skills they are unable to achieve.

Conclusion

Children will grow and develop, usually within expected norms, providing they are nurtured and encouraged to do so. An understanding of human development and theories of motor development is useful to practitioners who work with young children. This knowledge will assist you in your work as you become more aware of the role of significant adults, such as parents and practitioners who work in early years settings, in supporting the physical and overall development of children. A healthy child is the result of a complex interplay of many interrelated factors. An understanding of the consequences of some of those factors that prevent a child from achieving normal development will assist you in defining the steps you can take, as practitioners, should you find, or suspect, that children in your care are not developing in the way you would expect them to.

References and further reading

Abel, E. (1989), *Behavioral Teratogenesis and Behavioral Mutogenesis: A Primer in Abnormal Development*. Hingham: Kluwer Academic Publishers

Atkinson, J. (2000), *The Developing Visual Brain*. Oxford: Oxford University Press

Bee, H. (2000), *The Developing Child* (9th edn). Boston: Allyn and Bacon

Bukatko, D. and Daehler, M. (1998), *Child Development: A Thematic Approach* (3rd edn). New York: Houghton Mifflin Company

Drachman, D. and Sokoloff, L. (1996), 'The role of movement in embryonic joint development'. *Developmental Biology*, 14, pp401–20

Gallahue, D. and Ozmun J. (1998), *Understanding Motor Development*. Boston: McGraw Hill International Edition.

Gesell, A. (1928), *Infancy and Human Growth*. New York: Macmillan

Greenfield, S. (2000), *The Private Life of the Brain*. London: The Penguin Press

Gould, S. (1992), 'Heterochroney', in Keller, E. and Lloyd, E. (eds), *Key Words in Evolutionary Biology*, pp158–65. Cambridge, MA: Harvard University Press

Hall, D.M.B., Hill, P. and Elliman, D. (1990), *The Child Surveillance Handbook*. Oxford: Radcliffe Medical Press Ltd

Hepper, P. (1991), 'An examination of foetal learning before and after birth'. *Irish Journal of Psychology*, 12, pp95–107

Hepper, P. (1992), 'Foetal Psychology: An Embryonic Science', in J. Niehuis, *Foetal Behavior Development and Perinatal Aspects*, pp129–76. Oxford: Oxford University Press

Hepper, P. (1994), 'The beginnings of mind: evidence from the behavior of the foetus'. *Journal of Infant and Reproductive Psychology*, 12, pp143–54

Hepper, P. (2002), 'Prenatal Development' in Slater, A. and Lewis, M. (eds) *Introduction to Infant Development*, Oxford: Oxford University Press

Holt, K. (1991), *Child Development Diagnosis and Assessment*. Oxford: Butterworth Heinemann

Jones, K. and Smith D. (1973), 'Recognition of the foetal alcohol syndrome in early infancy'. *Lancet*, 2, pp999–1001

Keogh, J. and Sugden, D. (1985), *Movement Skill Development*. New York: Macmillan

Lenz, W. and Knapp, K. (1962), 'Foetal malformations due to Thalidomide. *German Medical Monthly*, 7, p253

McAnarney, E. (1987), 'Young maternal age and adverse neonatal outcome'. *American Journal of Diseases of Children*, 141, pp1053–9

McBride, W. (1961), 'Thalidomide and congenital abnormalities'. *Lancet*, 2, p1358

McGraw, M. (1935), *Growth: A study of Johnny and Jimmy*. New York: Appleton Century

McGraw, M. (1945), *Neuromuscular Maturation of the Human Infant*. New York: Haffner

Meggitt, C. and Sunderland, G. (2000), *Child Development: An Illustrated Guide*. Oxford: Heinemann

Moore, K. (1998), *The Developing Human*. Philadelphia: W. D. Saunders

Norbeck, J. and Tilden, V. (1983), 'Life stress, social support and emotional disequilibrium in complications of pregnancy. A prospective multivariate study'. *Journal of Health and Social Behavior*, 24, pp30–36

Piaget, J. (1954), *The Construction of Reality and the Child.* New York: Basic Books

Sheridan, M. (1975), *From Birth to Five Years: Children's Developmental Progress.* Windsor: NFER NELSON

Skoyles, J.R. and Sagan, D. (2002), *Up from Dragons: the evolution of human intelligence.* New York: McGraw-Hill

Slater, A. and Lewis, M. (2002), *Introduction to Infant Development.* Oxford: Oxford University Press

Thelen, E. (1989), 'Self-organization in developmental processes. Can systems approaches work?' In Gunnar, M. and Thelen, E. (eds) *Systems in development: The Minnesota symposia in child psychology, vol. 22,* pp71–117. Hillsdale, NJ: Erlbaum

Thelen, E. and Smith, L. (1994), *A Dynamic Systems Approach to the Development of Cognition and Action.* Cambridge, MA: MIT Press

Waddington, C. (1971), 'Concepts of Development', in Tobach, E., Aronsen, L. and Shaw, E. (eds), The Biopsychology of Development, pp17–23. San Diego, CA: Academic Press

Wadha, P., Sandman, C., Porto, M., Dunkel-Schetter, C. and Garite, T. (1993), 'The association between prenatal stress and infant birth weight and gestational age at birth. A prospective investigation'. *American Journal of Obstetrics and Gynecology,* 169, pp858–65

Warkany, J. and Schraffenberger, E. (1947), 'Congenital malformations induced in rats by roentgen rays'. *American Journal of Roentgenology and Radium Therapy,* 57, pp455–63

Useful websites

www.med.upenn.edu/meded/public/berp
This site from the University of Pennsylvania Health System gives a useful overview of foetal development.

www.pregnancyguideonline.com
An interesting and easy-to-read site providing information and advice about various aspects of pregnancy. Useful for parents and prospective parents.

www.qca.org.uk
This is the official site of the Qualifications and Curriculum Authority. It provides information relating to all aspects of curriculum, including the Foundation Stage.

www.des.gov.uk/foundation
The Department for Education and Skills website provides information on educare. It's also useful for its recent reports on childcare facilities.

www.bbc.co.uk/schools/laac/index.shtml

This interactive website for teachers, parents and children has activities and resources linked to the Foundation Stage.

www.UWO.ca/fhs/pt/PT648.PDF
Theories of early motor development and the therapeutic implications of these.

www.norton.co.uk/gleitman/ch13/basis.htm
This refers to chapter 13 of the book *Psychology* 5th Edition 1999 by Henry Gleitman, Alan Fridland and Daniel Reisburg. This chapter discusses the physical basis of development and includes a definition of genotype and phenotype amongst other relevant definitions and theories.

www.Mostgene.org/gd/gdvol12h.htm
An American site about different aspects of genetics.

www.lifeclinic.com/focus/diabetes/pregnancy_main.asp
A useful site detailing information relating to diabetes and pregnancy.

www.expectantmothersguide.com/library/philadelphia/EPHnutrition.htm
Advice about maintaining good nutrition during pregnancy.

www.vrg.org/nutrition/veganpregnancy.htm
Detailed information about how to ensure that vegan mothers eat a healthy diet during preganancy.

www.cleft.ie/noticeboard/archives/stress090900.htm
The Cleft Lip and Palate Association of Ireland website. This article refers to the link between severe stress in pregnancy and a child born with a cleft lip or palate.

www.psy.pdx.edu/PsiCafe/Areas/Developmental/PhysDev-Child/index.htm
A website provided by the Department of Psychology at Portland State University. The applied developmental psychology section provides a number of links to a range of interesting and useful websites about child development.

Emotional and social development

4

Vivienne Walkup

This chapter aims to explore the emotional and social development of children and the role of the adult in this process. It considers the principles involved in providing an environment in which children may reach their potential and is, therefore, particularly relevant to those practitioners in early years settings who work with and seek to understand children.

The chapter begins by looking at psychodynamic theories of early emotional development and considering how these relate to attachment. Attachment formation is then examined and explored before moving on to a discussion of self-esteem.

The issues involved in children making friends and how these relate to future interpersonal relationships are then discussed.

This chapter addresses the following areas:

- psychodynamic theories of emotional and social development
- attachment between infant and carer
- self-esteem
- children making friends.

After reading this chapter you should be able to:

1 make connections between early aspects of emotional development, attachment formation, self-esteem and making friends

2 understand significant concepts, processes and issues in the development of children's emotional and social development

3 understand the relevance of your knowledge of young children's emotional and social development in your work as a practitioner in an early years setting.

Introduction

The way that children develop emotionally and socially is of prime importance to an understanding of healthy development and learning. It is impossible to separate social and emotional development from other key aspects such as cognitive and physical development, as they are all integrated in the reality of the whole child. It is also difficult to observe these as accurately as other aspects, such as physical development. Therefore, whilst theories help to explain aspects of social and emotional development, it is important to challenge the assumptions they make and acknowledge the part played by interpretation, knowledge of the child and subjectivity.

Psychodynamic theories of emotional and social development

These are based upon an understanding of development as an active process that is influenced by both inborn, biological drives (nature) and social and emotional experiences (nurture; see Chapter 3 for a discussion of the nature-nurture debate).

Both Sigmund Freud (1856–1939) and Erik Erikson (1902–1994) focused upon the development of personality. They considered that the personality developed as a result of psychological conflicts that the developing person must resolve as they occur in a series of stages.

Erikson, however, considered that development covered the lifespan, whereas Freud thought that personality was formed in essence before adulthood.

Freudian theory

This assumes that the individual's personality consists of the **id**, the **ego** and the **superego** (see Figure 4.1).

An individual's personality consists of the:	
Id	This is present at birth and contains the person's inborn biological needs and desires, seeking to maximise pleasure and minimise pain. So the newborn infant consists only of id as he or she seeks to have his or her needs for food, warmth and comfort met by crying.
Ego	This develops as the realistic part of the personality, which finds ways of meeting the needs of the id as well as dealing with external demands, such as those from parents and society. So the young child learns that smiling at mother is an effective way of gaining her attention and meeting his or her needs for food, warmth, comfort, and so on.
Superego	This is the moral and principled part of the personality, which acts as a sort of internalised parent. It consists of the **conscience**, which punishes unacceptable thoughts, feelings and actions with guilt, and the **ego-ideal**, which provides a sense of how we should behave.

Figure 4.1
Freudian theory of personality

Freud suggested that development occurs through a series of **psychosexual stages**, involving conflicts between the id, ego and superego. At each stage, the focus is on a different area of the body (see Figure 4.2).

Stage	Age (approx.)	Description
Oral	Birth to 1 year	The mouth is the focus of pleasure, stimulation and interaction (feeding and weaning involved)
Anal	1–3 years	The anus is the focus of stimulation (toilet training focus)
Phallic	3–6 years	The genitals are the focus of stimulation (gender role and moral development central)
Latency	6–12 years	Period of little sexual activity (shift to physical and intellectual issues)
Genital	12 to adult	Genitals are the focus of stimulation (puberty and mature sexual relationships develop)

Figure 4.2
Freud's psychosexual stages of development

Therefore, according to Freudian theory, development involves resolving these conflicts in a way that is sufficiently balanced for healthy development. If this does not occur, then a person can become **fixated** at a certain stage and **regress** (go back to an earlier stage) when in stressful situations.

Implications of Freud's theory for practitioners

Awareness of the need for balance at each stage suggests that the child should receive enough stimulation (id) but that the needs of the external world should be taken into account (ego), as well as expectations about the values attached. So a child who is allowed to constantly suck upon a dummy or other pacifier may become too dependent upon it and remain 'stuck' at this oral stage of development; but if he or she is completely deprived of the dummy in order to make him or her 'more grown up', the child may still remain fixated because of a constant desire to experience the pleasant stimulation he or she is being deprived of. Therefore, the practitioner might allow the dummy at certain times (such as before a nap) but not at others (such as at lunch or snack time) in order to provide a balanced amount of stimulation.

Erikson's psychosocial theory

This theory places more emphasis upon the social factors that the individual encounters, and proposes that there is a psychosocial crisis at each stage of development. Unlike Freud, Erikson does not stress the role of sexuality but focuses instead upon the emergence of a sense of identity (see Figure 4.3).

Stage	Age range (approx.)	Description
Trust versus mistrust	Birth to 1 year	Focus on oral sensory activity – development of trusting relationships (secure attachment)
Autonomy versus shame and doubt	1–3 years	Development of control over body (toilet training may result in shame if not handled sensitively)
Initiative versus guilt	3–6 years	Testing limits of discovery (becoming more assertive/aggressive)
Industry versus inferiority	6–12 years	Focus on competence and productivity (basic skills including school skills)
Identity versus role-confusion	12–19 years	Identity formation and self-concept (achieving adult identity)
Intimacy versus isolation	19–25 years	Intimate relationships and career (partners, marriage)
Generativity versus stagnation	25–50 years	Creative activity for future generations
Ego integrity versus despair	50 and older	Belief in integrity of life (wisdom) (acceptance of self)

Figure 4.3
Erikson's psychosocial stages

Erikson viewed social forces as an important element of development and considered psychosocial conflicts never to be fully resolved. Therefore, conflicts from earlier stages may continue to affect later development if they have not been dealt with in a generally favourable way. For example, an infant may learn that adults are trustworthy most of the time but that they might sometimes fail to provide adequately for his or her needs.

Implications of Erikson's theory for practitioners

Understanding the importance of the demands that different contexts and cultures place upon a child at particular ages (such as toilet training and school-related skills) is key. So the child is striving for balance between the development of new abilities, leading to greater freedom and autonomy, and the caregiver is concerned with protecting the child from the dangers embedded in this new independence. Again, balance is the solution and the practitioner needs to gradually allow the control to move from him- or herself to the child. For example, a 2-and-a-half-year-old child (autonomy versus shame and doubt) who is keen to try to climb the play frame may need to be supervised and supported initially, but as he or she gains expertise may be allowed to do this independently (with a soft surface beneath to ensure safety). This will ensure that the child moves towards a feeling of confidence in his or her own ability, rather than shame or guilt for falling off or failing to reach the top at the first attempt.

Emotional development

Parents have always claimed that they can read the emotions of their infants, but they have not always been in agreement, either with each other or professionals. One reason for this is that infants cannot use language, so conclusions have to be based upon facial expressions, physiological responses or cries. The ways in which these are interpreted depend upon the subjective response of the observer and what he or she actually knows about the child. For example, a baby's cry may be interpreted by:

➲ an older sibling as the baby wanting the soft toy that has fallen from the pram

➲ the father as a sign of being in need of attention

➲ the health visitor as the baby needing a nappy change

➲ the mother as a signal of hunger.

Innate or inborn emotions

Figure 4.4 lists the range of emotions associated with early childhood and the age at which they are usually experienced.

Category	Age range	Type of emotion
Innate emotions	From birth	Interest, physical distress, pain, disgust and surprise
	Within first month	Sociability (smile)
Primary emotions	7 months to 12 months	Joy, anger, fear and sadness
Secondary emotions	Approximately 2 years	Guilt, envy, shame and pride

Figure 4.4
Early emotional development

Despite difficulties of interpretation, however, there is evidence that infants are born with certain emotions already in place (Izard et al., 1995). These include interest, physical distress, disgust and surprise (in the form of the startle reflex). Soon after this the social smile appears, and by about

7 months old, infants exhibit joy, anger and fear. These latter are known as **primary emotions** because they appear in the first year of life and because there seems to be universal agreement about them. They are said to be innate, resulting from biological programming (Izard, 1994).

Secondary emotions

These appear in the second year (examples include guilt, envy, shame and pride) and require some sophisticated cognitive abilities involving self-awareness. For example, when a child feels ashamed because he or she has wet pants it means that he or she is able to distinguish between him- or herself and others.

Facial expressions

These are an important part of emotional expression and research has shown that infants have an early ability (at 2 or 3 months old) to differentiate between certain facial expressions (Nelson, 1987). After 6 months of age infants seem to understand the meaning behind the emotional expressions of others and by the age of one year they use **social referencing**; that is, they refer to the emotions of other people, communicated through facial expressions, vocal quality and gestures to help them make judgements about events and regulate their behaviour (Hornik and Gunnar, 1988).

Case Study 1

The visual cliff

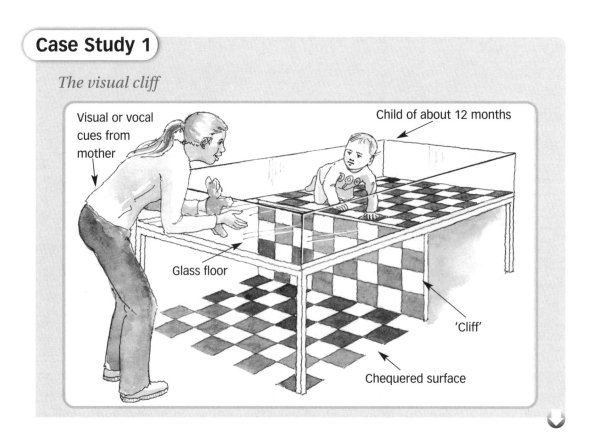

Visual or vocal cues from mother

Child of about 12 months

Glass floor

'Cliff'

Chequered surface

1 A table was designed which looked as though there was a drop (by using chequered material and clear glass) to infants crawling over it.

2 An experiment carried out by Gibson and Walk (1960) to test infant depth perception found that most infants would risk crossing the 'visual cliff' if their mother (waiting on the other side) was smiling or looking happy and interested. However, if she looked frightened or angry very few infants would cross.

3 Interestingly, when the cliff was clearly safe nearly all of the infants would cross without looking at their mothers and, even when the mothers were signalling fear, the babies would ignore her and cross anyway.

It seems from this that infants are most likely to use social referencing when presented with an ambiguous situation. When this is the case they will look for more information before making a decision about action. The visual cliff situation is one that is likely to be quite fear-provoking and so likely to induce this response. Other research into responses to strangers have produced similar findings (Feinman and Lewis, 1983).

This, of course, has much wider implications for personal development in infants and suggests that parents or carers (although mothers were used in this experiment, infants also use fathers and carers as social referents) influence the behaviour of the young more subtly and profoundly than might be assumed.

Adults also use social referencing and, like infants, it is most apparent in ambiguous situations. For example, someone tells a joke that you are not sure about and you look at the reactions of others before deciding whether to laugh.

Smiling

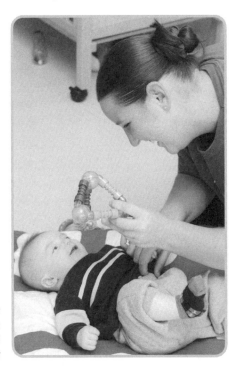

Early interactions can help to build attachment

Smiling is an important social communicator, which appears as a voluntary response at about 3 weeks of age. This suggests that it is not entirely innate because it seems to develop from a non-discriminatory response (where a baby might smile at social and non-social stimuli alike) and towards a response attached to people. The smile is often reinforced by those around and becomes more frequent. So babies may start smiling because they are biologically programmed to do so, but it is the social response (for example, smiling back or talking to the baby) that makes it more likely that babies will repeat the smile.

Discussion Point 1

Effects of smiling upon a carer

Describe the effects that a smiling baby might have upon a carer and how this might affect the way an infant is treated.

For comments on this discussion point, see page 130.

It seems then that these early interactions are mutually reinforcing and may be relevant to the formation of an emotional tie or **attachment** between infant and carer.

Attachment between infant and carer

Attachment, or emotional bonding, is usually formed between an infant and his or her carer during the first year of life and is seen by many as an important base for future relationships. Therefore, it is of major importance in the healthy social and emotional development of the child.

The most famous attachment theorist is **John Bowlby** (1907–1990), who argued that the need for attachment was an instinctive biological need and that mother-love in infancy and childhood was as important for mental health as are vitamins and protein for physical health (1951). Bowlby claimed that babies who were separated from their mothers before becoming securely attached would find it impossible to bond with others and in later life suffer ill effects from this deprivation. Further, based upon his studies of delinquent boys in 1944, he suggested a link between maternal deprivation and juvenile crime.

The work of John Bowlby (1907–1990)

During his lifetime, Bowlby produced the following:

- *Forty-Four Juvenile Thieves, Their Characters and Home Lives* (1944) was based upon case-notes from his work at the London Child Guidance Clinic. The paper linked the affectionless nature of a significant minority of the children to their histories of maternal deprivation.

- He worked with James Robertson in a study of hospitalised children and produced a moving film in 1952 called *A Two Year Old Goes to Hospital*, which played a crucial role in the development of attachment theory and helped to lessen the negative effects of hospitalisation.

- *Maternal Care and Mental Health* (1952) was based on a report he carried out for the World Health Organization looking at the mental health of orphaned children placed in institutions in post-war Europe, which concluded that 'mother love' in infancy was vital for healthy social and emotional development.

➲ *The Nature of the Child's Tie to his Mother* (1957) drew upon ethological theory (that attachment is an essential aspect of human survival which evolved in order to ensure infant survival) and *Separation Anxiety* (1959) discussed the negative effects of separation from the attachment figure.

Considerations of Bowlby's work

Bowlby's work was very influential, not least because of the post-war social-economic climate. Women had been recruited into the workforce during the Second World War, as large numbers of men were serving in the armed forces and when the war ended many women were reluctant to give up the independence that working had given them. Consequently, there were not enough jobs for the returning men.

Bowlby's findings, in *Maternal Care and Mental Health*, that disrupted attachments were damaging to mental health, had the effect of sending many working women back into the home. This was convenient politically and meant that the economic status quo was maintained.

Methodological flaws

There were methodological flaws in Bowlby's work in that:

➲ much of Bowlby's work was based upon research carried out on juvenile offenders. Since this group was not representative of the normal population, the findings cannot be reasonably generalised

➲ the evidence gathered was retrospective, and much of it relied upon memory and accounts of the juveniles' early years. Retrospective data is notoriously unreliable and subjective.

Modifications of Bowlby's views

Bowlby himself modified his views during the course of his long working life and concluded that an attachment could be formed with any **primary caregiver**, not only the child's natural mother, as he had first proposed.

Attachment types

Mary Ainsworth worked with Bowlby at the Tavistock Clinic in London and suggested that attachment could be measured using a laboratory-based 'strange situation' test (Ainsworth and Wittig, 1969). This involved providing an unfamiliar but interesting environment where the child (usually approximately one year old) was motivated to explore but still needed to feel secure (an unfamiliar room with toys). An observer then recorded the child's responses to the departure and return of the mother. This research revealed significant differences between children, which Ainsworth categorised into three major **attachment types**. These are shown in Figure 4.5.

Type of attachment	Child's behaviour
Anxious/avoidant	The child may not be distressed by the mother leaving and may avoid or turn away from her when she returns.
Securely attached	The child may be distressed by the mother's departure and easily comforted when she returns.
Anxious/resistant	The child may be extremely 'clingy' during the first few minutes and become very distressed when the mother leaves. When she returns the child will seek comfort at the same time as distancing him- or herself from the mother, for example, by crying and reaching up to be held but trying to wriggle away when picked up.

Figure 4.5
*Attachment types
(Ainsworth,
1969)*

The importance of forming secure attachment

This has been indicated by many studies that have looked at connections between attachment type and later behaviour and development. These indicate that **securely attached children** are superior on a range of different measures including those identified in Figure 4.6:

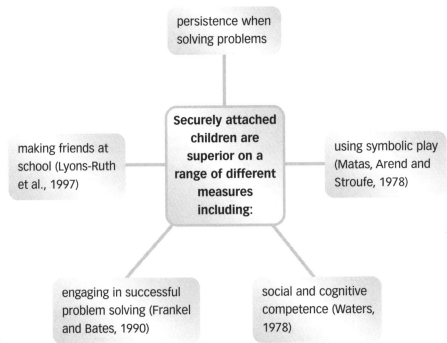

Figure 4.6
*Some of the ways
in which securely
attached
children perform
better*

On the other hand, children classed as **insecurely attached** (anxious/avoidant or anxious/resistant) are:

➲ less effective when mixing with others
➲ succeed less when attempting to master challenging tasks
➲ have more behavioural problems (van den Boom, 1994).

A secure base

Ainsworth suggests that the primary carer needs to provide a **secure base** from which the child can explore the world. If the child develops a sense of trust in the caregiver, he or she is more likely to become independent earlier.

Maternal sensitivity seems to be a key factor here for the child's needs to be met. This includes attentiveness to the child, mutuality of interactions and the mother's ability to stimulate the child.

Mother-infant interaction

Brazleton, Tronick, Adamson et al. (1975) and Brazleton and Cramer (1991) were interested in finding out about the causes of problematic relationships between infants and mothers. They investigated the very earliest interactions in a laboratory setting and found that there was a sort of harmonious 'dance' at times, which involved bursts of attention and then withdrawal. They identified a cycle of interactions, involving joint actions and mutual, continual influence. At times these were synchronised, but at others they were out of time.

Brazleton thought that these bursts of interactions related to the baby's biological need for arousal, which needs to be maintained at an optimal level. Arousal is based upon the need for humans to be stimulated in order to survive and develop. Arousal levels seem to vary between individuals and may be related to temperamental differences. When the baby looks away or fails to respond to the mother's conversation, this is a signal that no stimulation is needed or the infant wants to end the interaction.

Case Study 2

Disrupting interactions

Murray and Trevarthen (1985) tested what would happen if mothers acted in unresponsive or disjointed ways with their babies and used a series of studies to do this:

First study

A mother was asked to remain unresponsive – suddenly still, silent and with a 'frozen face' – in the middle of an exchange of expressions with her baby.

A 2-month-old baby clearly signalled distress but was undisturbed by the mother talking to the experimenter. The infant then seemed to try to regain her attention by noises and gestures.

Second study

A delayed video replay situation was used. In this, the baby saw its mother playing with it on a television screen, acting in a happy, lively manner. However, this was not synchronised (except accidentally) with the actions of the infant.

Again there were signs of distress but the baby was more withdrawn and protested less than in the 'frozen face' experiment.

Third study

A mother and baby interacted through a video link between two rooms. Here, a replay of the infant's part in a previous interaction was substituted (without the mother's knowledge). The mother still thought that she was taking part in a 'live' interaction with the baby, but in fact she was looking at an earlier interaction. This meant that there was activity on the part of the baby, but it was not synchronised with the mother's stimulation.

The mother perceived the baby as being unhappy or perverse, even though it looked quite happy and lively. This is perhaps because she could not engage in a mutual interaction with the infant.

In the first study, the baby is obviously disturbed by the 'frozen face' of the mother but accepts the mother's distraction when talking to the experimenter. This suggests that the baby is used to seeing the mother in conversations with others and uses various means to regain her attention.

The withdrawal of the baby in the second study suggests that the carer needs to be responsive, not just animated, in order for the baby to be happy.

The third study shows the importance of the baby's responsiveness to the mother. If this is not happening, then it suggests that the mother will interpret the baby's actions negatively.

It seems then that these early interactions are relevant for the formation of emotional ties or attachments between infants and caregivers and, therefore, caregivers should be aware of the need for interactions involving sensitive responsiveness when working with infants and young children.

The factors that affect the parent-child relationship are shown in Figure 4.7.

Stranger fear

Babies usually begin to fear strangers at about the age of 6 months and this lasts until the child is about 2 years old. So the baby who happily held hands with strangers and delighted the bus with beaming smiles suddenly starts crying when unfamiliar people appear. **Separation anxiety** peaks

The parent-child relationship is affected by:	
Parent's emotional state	Mental disturbances in the mother or main caregiver may make the child less responsive and the attachment, therefore, less secure. For example, post-natal depression may result in the unresponsive 'frozen face', which Brazleton found related to infant distress. Mothers of anxious children are prone to insecurity, which affects their relationship with the child (Izard, Haynes, Chisholm and Baak, 1991).
Parental attachment status	The way that parents remember their own relationships with their parents seems to provide the basis for expectations about their own role. So, insecurely attached parents may find it more difficult to develop secure attachments with their own infants.
Attitudes and expectations	It seems that the more informed parents are, the more likely they are to do well with their infants. For example, a mother who expects her baby to let her sleep because she is tired is likely to be disappointed and develop negative feelings towards her baby. Help and support from others is also important.
Infant's abilities, temperament and gender	These may also be factors in attachment formation as certain characteristics can help or hinder attachment formation. For example, a responsive baby who smiles happily in response to the mother is likely to evoke more interactions and therefore foster attachment.

Figure 4.7
Factors affecting the parent-child relationship

between the ages of 12 and 16 months. It involves crying and displays of fear such as clinging and distress when the child's parent or caregiver is leaving. Separation anxiety seems to be related to how well the child is prepared for the separation and to his or her past experiences of separation. There is less anxiety if the child is left with familiar people and it is reduced if siblings or favourite toys are present. Whilst it is distressing to all those who witness a child clinging desperately to a parent's leg as he or she tries to leave, it is a clear sign that an attachment has formed and is therefore indicative of the child's ability to form other attachments. Obviously, this is relevant for those working with young children in order that they can anticipate this and minimise the distress involved.

Some of the ways in which you may help reduce separation anxiety in your work as a practitioner in an early years setting are identified in Figure 4.8.

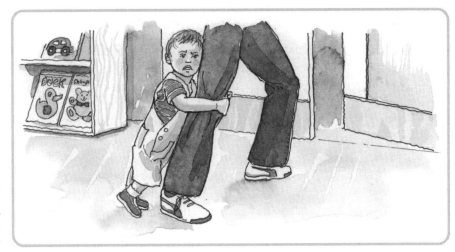

Separation anxiety is distressing for both parent and child

A practitioner working in an early years setting should:	
welcome the child and recognise that parents are also undergoing a change in their contact with the child	Perhaps use a personal place label or poster.
encourage a slow transition from being at home to being in a new environment	If possible, allow the child to get to know you before being left in your care (perhaps by a home visit or having an 'open' policy for parents and children to visit before starting day care). Arrange a gradual schedule, which builds up from perhaps one hour on the first day, then 2 hours on the second day, until the child is staying for a full day.
remind the child that the parent will return	Separation anxiety is often related to fear that the parent may not return, so it is important that the child knows what time the parent is returning. With an older child a clock can be used to indicate this, or some milestone such as 'after juice and biscuits' can be used.
use transitional objects	Items such as a favourite teddy or a blanket can help a child to feel secure because it connects them with the parent. Some children may find photographs or even an article with a familiar smell comforting.
talk with the parents about the child's particular needs	This often helps with anxiety, as does being ready to help to occupy the child when the parent is ready to leave.
warn the child that the main caregiver is about to leave	This helps to prepare the child for the event. Discourage parents from leaving unnoticed, as this adds to the child's anxiety. Sometimes a routine for saying goodbye is helpful so that the child knows that they have three kisses or hugs before the parent leaves.

Figure 4.8
A practitioner's role in helping reduce separation anxiety

Attachment and day care

One of the areas of prime importance here is the question of attachment and day care. Is Bowlby's original assertion that maternal deprivation and disrupted maternal attachment may have serious and long-lasting effects upon the child's later behaviour correct? Or are there other factors that may make this a more benign arrangement?

Perhaps we need to think back to Mary Ainsworth's findings about providing a **secure base**. Surely, if the child has then we can expect him or her to feel confident enough to explore and enjoy a stimulating environment without the fear and distress that might otherwise be the case?

In order to address these and other questions it is useful to examine cross-cultural studies that have looked at attachment. These should provide us with insights about what is 'instinctive' or biologically programmed behaviour and what is learned as the result of being reared in a particular environment (the nature-nurture debate again).

Cross-cultural studies and attachment

It seems that different cultures provide Ainsworth's secure base, but there are variations in the way this is effected. Work by Liedloff (1986) found that all of the women in a community of South American people living in the Amazon rainforest provided security and continuity of care to the infants. Children were certain of comfort and support when it was needed, but there was no primary carer. A study by Troknick, Morelli and Winn (1987) showed that among the Congolese Efe or Pygmy (a people who are hunter-gatherers), infants are raised by multiple women during the first five months of life. Jackson (1993) argued that African-American infants do not exhibit an exclusive attachment, as most of those in the study were reared in two households consisting of approximately 15 people (both relatives and unrelated people).

Continuous care and security

The studies above suggest that attachment is not necessarily **monotropic** (a single attachment between infant and primary caregiver which ties them together, rather like an extension of the umbilical cord) but is much more flexible. It can include a number of people.

The implications for the professional care of children, then, are that these people can become part of the infant's attachment experience. Within a Western culture, many children are reared by mothers, fathers, siblings, grandparents and other family members, as well as receiving care from nursery staff and childminders. The important factors here are **continuous care** and **security**.

Working mothers and day care

Many women still feel guilty about working when their children are small, even though they are often obliged or expected to do so. Perhaps we are still responding to Bowlby's ideas despite the fact that society has now changed significantly. Indeed, Bowlby's ideas have dominated child-care policy and issues for over 50 years (Holmes, 1993). However, there have been considerable changes in the composition of families and their dynamics and these continue. This means that many more children are experiencing exactly that which Bowlby warned against: separation, inconsistency, disruption and loss. There is much greater diversity in terms of family type than at the time when Bowlby first began publishing his work, and currently single-parent and re-formed families are common. Therefore, many children entering day care are not necessarily happy and secure, and this makes it particularly important that emotional security is provided within the context of care.

Generally the findings about **working mothers** or **primary caregivers** can be summed up as follows:

➲ Mothers who work are generally happier, leading to greater life satisfaction, as long as this is through choice rather than necessity (Parke and Buriel, 1998).

➲ Although working mothers have less time at home, they cope by focusing on essentials and becoming more efficient.

➲ Working mothers tend to emphasise independence, which may have positive effects upon children (particularly daughters).

➲ Children with working mothers tend to have better social skills, perhaps because they have been used to mixing with others from an earlier age.

Findings about day care suggest that:

➲ most children are in fact cared for by relatives

➲ some children placed into day care before one year of age exhibit anxious attachment patterns but most are securely attached

➲ poor quality or extensive day care, combined with poor-quality care at home may lead to anxious attachments

➲ there are few differences between the attachment patterns of children entering day care after the age of one year and those of children cared for at home.

Case Study 3

Making childcare arrangements

Jasmine is a single parent with a 3-year-old daughter, Sarah. When Sarah was a baby, Jasmine worked at a number of part-time jobs, while her mother helped out with childcare. However, Jasmine now has a good opportunity to take a job as a paramedic and the additional income will allow them to move to a safer neighbourhood with better schools and facilities. The new job would mean that Jasmine is at work all day and her mother (who is nearly 70) does not feel able to look after Sarah full time. Therefore, Jasmine has to look for childcare but feels guilty at the thought of leaving her daughter for long periods.

How would you advise Jasmine in this situation?

For comments on this case study, see page 129.

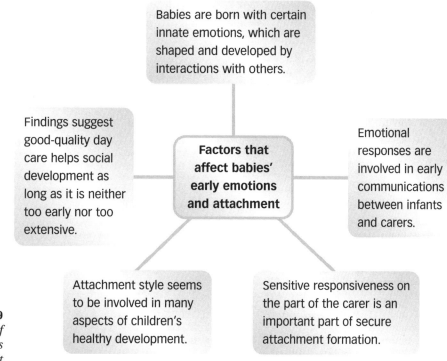

Figure 4.9
Summary of early emotions and attachment

Self-esteem

So far, we have looked at the early emotional development of young children and how this is part of their forming early relationships with others. This seems to form the basis upon which children develop autonomy or the ability to be independent. In other words, it provides them with the security that they are safe and cared for and that those who look after them are trustworthy. Because of this, they do not need to be anxious about the possibility of being abandoned and therefore begin to explore the world more independently, safe in the knowledge that their needs will be met on their return. This is clearly interwoven with another aspect of their social and emotional development: **self-esteem**. This is a central and critical aspect of psychological well-being, which has generated vast amounts of literature and research. In 1998 it was found that there were over 7,000 publications on the subject (Mruk, 1999), which gives an indication of the interest attached to this issue.

Self-esteem usually refers to the way we feel about ourselves. Coopersmith (1967:4) defines self-esteem as 'a personal judgement of worthiness, that is expressed in the attitudes the individual holds towards himself'. Clearly this relates to the development of a sense of self or **personal identity**. Assessing our self-esteem is something all of us continue to do throughout life and involves asking ourselves questions such as what sort of person we are and what we want to be like. When trying to answer these questions, we usually think about how we feel inside as well as the way that others behave towards us, as this tells us how they view us from the outside.

Activity 1) A short description of myself

Imagine you are asked to say what kind of person you are by someone you have never met. Write a short description to convey this to them (approximately 100 to 150 words).

For comments on this activity, see page 132.

Activity 2) Social categories

List the social categories which describe you, in terms of gender, position in family, age, marital status, nationality, religion, occupation, class etc.

Consider how each of these makes you similar to or different from most people that you know.

For comments on this activity see page 132.

Development of self-esteem

There is rapid development of aspects of self during the second and third years of life, and this happens in the context of social interactions and relationships.

Many researchers suggest that without these interactions, this sense of self cannot develop and this is borne out by studies of **feral children** (a term used to describe children who grow up in the wild or are raised in extreme isolation), who seem not to develop a sense of self.

Visual self-recognition

Around 2 years of age, most children display visual self-recognition, which means that they recognise themselves in a mirror or on a photograph. Researchers found that infants up to the age of 15 months did not touch their noses (which had been marked with red rouge without their knowledge) when placed before a mirror, but by the time they had reached 24 months, they did (Lewis and Brooks-Gunn, 1979).

Ability to describe physical self

Increasingly, children become able to describe themselves physically (beginning at about 19 months of age) and by the end of their second year are usually becoming more aware of adult expectations and standards.

Self-evaluation

There are also signs that children begin to **self-evaluate** (or make judgements about themselves or the things they do) towards the end of the second year and they may show satisfaction or pride about building a high tower with blocks or show frustration when they fail.

> **Activity 3** **A young boy's self-description**
>
> Read this example of a young boy's self-description, which has been recorded and transcribed.
>
> My name is Bobby and I am big. I can ride my bike now and be a fire-fighter (makes 'neenah' noise). My Emily is small and can't talk, but she makes a lot of noise. We have to turn the TV up so I can hear it. She goes shouting all the time. My hair is curly, look like this.
>
> ⊃ What would you guess to be Bobby's age and why?

For comments on this activity see page 133.

Competence and self-esteem

Research suggests that more competent children develop a more positive self-esteem as they gain confidence in their own abilities. This then has a snowball effect, allowing them to do more things, more competently, which, therefore, adds to their self-esteem.

This is apparent in the behaviours exhibited by competent children (see Figure 4.10).

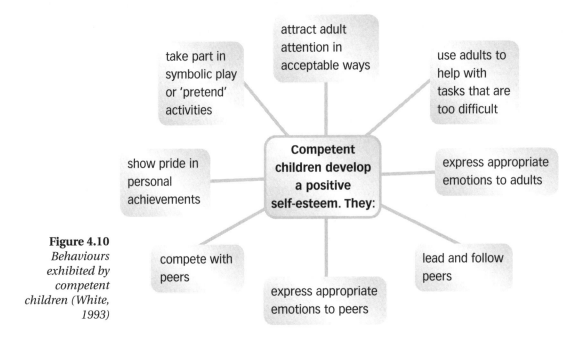

Figure 4.10
Behaviours exhibited by competent children (White, 1993)

take part in symbolic play or 'pretend' activities

attract adult attention in acceptable ways

use adults to help with tasks that are too difficult

show pride in personal achievements

Competent children develop a positive self-esteem. They:

express appropriate emotions to adults

compete with peers

express appropriate emotions to peers

lead and follow peers

Role of caregivers in promoting competence in a child

Again, the influence of the parent/carer/child relationship is seen to be important here. It seems that mothers of children with high levels of competence are more encouraging and supportive when their children wish to investigate and explore, providing a variety of stimulating toys and contexts within which this can take place. They are also more likely to use language and play in a manner that responds to the child's needs, interests and level of development. This sounds very similar to the earlier discussion about **sensitive responsiveness** and attachment formation, and it certainly seems as though this is the most important aspect of a healthy social and emotional development.

Measuring self-esteem

This is quite difficult, particularly in children, because self-esteem is not easy to define. It seems to relate to the picture a child has of him- or herself, which is drawn from two different areas:

⊃ knowing what he or she can do and valuing it

⊃ comparing him- or herself with others.

Harter's (1983) **Self-Perception Profile for Children** identified five different domains. Children were either read a statement, or shown a picture showing a competent or less competent child, and asked to say which is most like them (see Figure 4.11).

Domains of self-esteem	Questions relating to domains
Scholastic competence	How bright do you think you are? How well do you read? How well are you doing at school?
Athletic competence	How good are you at sports? Do you get picked to play? Do you like to try new games?
Social acceptance	How popular are you? Do others like you?
Behavioural conduct	Do you behave in the way that you should? Do adults and other children accept the way you behave?
Physical appearance	How much do you like the way you look? Do you think others like the way you look?

Figure 4.11
Harter's five domains of self-esteem (1983)

Thus, a child can be assessed on these domains and the profile gives a much clearer and more in-depth picture of the child's general self-esteem. However, when trying to understand the way a child feels about himself, it is important to find out which issues matter most to him.

Discussion Point 2

Assessing which factors are important to children

Read the attached self-descriptions and decide which factors seem most important to these children.

1 **Molly** (aged 5 years)
I am Molly. I am the biggest girl in my class. I've got curly black hair and green bobbles. I like some girls, like Jenny and Kali, 'cos they play with me at playtime. I have a reading book, but it's only got pictures – I can't read letters yet. I help my mum at home with the pots and watching Daisy, my baby. My mum says she couldn't do without me. When it's story-time I sit quietly on the mat but Matthew's always getting told off.

2 **Suzy** (aged 7-and-a-half-years)
My real name is Suzannah, but most people call me Suzy. My mum sometimes calls me Nanna 'cos when I was little I used to say 'Sunanna' 'cos I couldn't say Suzannah properly. I am quite small – I want to grow, but even though I eat lots of dinner I am still small. I am on the top table at school, but it is boring. My friend Joanna is always finished first and gets it all right. My brother Patrick is 12 and we are always falling out. It's not fair because he has a bigger bedroom than me and he never gets told off, even though he starts it. I like drawing and painting and my dad likes my pictures.

For comments on this discussion point see page 130.

The role of significant others

The significance of the development of positive self-esteem in children, combined with our understanding of how it develops, means that those working with children have an important part to play in its development.

> **Activity 4**) **Encouraging positive self-esteem**

Read the following account and list ways in which you feel positive self-esteem is being encouraged or discouraged.

The children in Year 1 have recently visited a working farm and are being asked to talk about this during a class discussion.

Teacher: Who can tell me some of the animals we saw? Let's see – Thomas.

Thomas: Pigs and cows and sheeps and dogs.

Teacher: Very good, Thomas, but don't shout. We do see dogs all the time though, don't we, and there is no such word as 'sheeps'. What about you, Katy, you're sitting nice and quietly. What did you see?

Katy: Some chickens and we seed an egg with a chick inside.

Teacher: Yes, we did, didn't we? And chick is the right name for a baby bird. How did you know there was a chick inside, Katy?

Katy: 'Cos the man shined a light and we seed it.

Teacher: Well done. I think you need a sticker for that. Now then, what did you see, Karendeep?

Karendeep: (*mumbles*) Don't know.

Teacher: I can't hear you if you mumble like that. Have you forgotten, perhaps, or don't know the word you want?

(*Karendeep sits with head down and doesn't answer.*)

Look, there are lots of people in this class with their hands up. They all want to tell me. I'll choose Justin.

Justin: Was a goat and it was eating a crisp bag and weeing (*makes hissing noise*)

(*Class giggles.*)

Teacher: Don't be silly and rude, Justin. There were three goats actually, and they usually eat grass. What do goats eat, children?

Class: (*obediently chant*) Grass.

For comments on this activity see page 133.

1 List the qualities that you value in yourself.

2 Are these the ones that you tend to encourage in children?

For comments on this activity see page 134.

How to recognise high self-esteem in children

It is usually fairly clear which children have a positive sense of self-worth, as they tend to be proactive, cheerful and increasingly independent. You might see the following behaviours in these children:

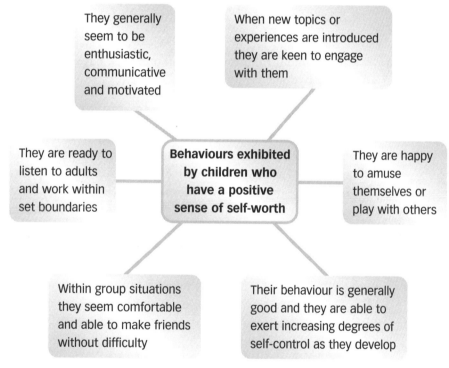

They generally seem to be enthusiastic, communicative and motivated

When new topics or experiences are introduced they are keen to engage with them

They are ready to listen to adults and work within set boundaries

Behaviours exhibited by children who have a positive sense of self-worth

They are happy to amuse themselves or play with others

Within group situations they seem comfortable and able to make friends without difficulty

Their behaviour is generally good and they are able to exert increasing degrees of self-control as they develop

Figure 4.12
Recognising high self-esteem in children

How to recognise low self-esteem in children

These children usually seem to be lacking in self-worth and self-belief. Therefore, they generally seem to be unhappy, withdrawn and reluctant to engage actively with others.

They will sometimes voice their low self-esteem in terms of things they are being asked to do, such as:

⊃ 'I'm rubbish at reading.'

⊃ 'Everybody else can do maths but me.'

Children with low self-esteem view themselves and their future achievements negatively; for example, 'I know I'm gonna come last', or 'I can't do anything right'. This has the effect of actually causing the 'failure' to occur because they do not look at their achievements positively.

Discussion Point 3

Positive and negative self-esteem

Jack and Harry took part in the obstacle race on Sports Day. Jack came third and Harry came fourth. Here is how they reacted to this outcome:

Jack: I told you I was useless – I never win anything.

Harry: I got there before Billy and Jake – yes! Next year I'm gonna get third.

Discuss the role of positive and negative self-esteem here.

For comments on this discussion point see page 131.

How to encourage positive self-esteem

Carl Rogers (1902–1987) was an American psychologist who took a humanistic approach to understanding human personality and behaviour. He suggested that if children are to develop positive self-esteem, they need to have **unconditional positive regard** (UPR) from adults. This means that if the child is to develop his or her full potential, the right conditions are necessary to allow it to grow. This could be compared to planting a number of seeds in the garden, where you need to provide the right conditions for those seeds to develop into flourishing, healthy plants. Some of the seeds might not receive enough sunshine so do not grow as tall or strong as they might have, or they might have to stretch to reach the sun and, therefore, lean over in one direction but not grow in others. Some seeds might lack moisture and fail to thrive, others might be strangled by other stronger plants and not develop in the way they could have.

The important issue here from Rogers' humanistic viewpoint is that all these seeds have the potential to grow into healthy, beautiful plants, but they might not all develop or actualise this potential. Similarly, humans have this same potential, so it is important that the adults around children provide the opportunities for this to happen. UPR does not mean that we never discipline the child, or display anger, but rather that we allow the child to believe that he or she is a *person* who is valued but whose *behaviour* at any one time is not appropriate. For example, the child may be told not to pull the cat's tail because it is cruel to hurt the cat, rather than be told that he or she is a cruel person.

> ## Activity 6 — Acknowledging inappropriate behaviour

Change the following comments so that they do not label the child but rather acknowledge the inappropriate behaviour:

1 *'Ashley, you are a very naughty boy who is unable to sit still and listen on the mat.'*

2 *'There are ways of dealing with bad girls like you, Hayley Atkins – now stop poking your ruler in Chelsie's back.'*

3 *'Be quiet! You are the worst class I have ever had to deal with.'*

For comments on this activity see page 134.

Self-fulfilling prophecy (Merton, 1957)

Labelling the whole child negatively tends to affect the way that the child sees him- or herself and the ways that others perceive him or her. So, if (in the example above) others see Ashley as a naughty boy because he has been labelled as such, then his behaviour is more likely to be viewed in these terms. For example, if Ashley turns round to look at something when he should be listening, it will probably be seen that he is causing trouble by talking to those behind him. If, on the other hand, Chelsie (seen as a 'good girl') does the same, it might be assumed that someone is pulling her hair or causing her to be distracted. Ashley then begins to carry with him this view of himself as naughty and this becomes part of his self-concept, resulting in low self-esteem. This has clear implications not only for children's personal development, but also for their learning experiences. It also relates back to the earlier discussion of the categorical self, where we see children viewed in terms of being like or unlike those they interact with. So Ashley is 'naughty', unlike most of the others in the class, or it might be that he is Asian or Afro-Caribbean. This also makes him different and it is likely that certain stereotypical behaviours may be attributed to him on the basis of this alone. It is important that those working with children are aware of their own preconceptions and attitudes towards gender, social class and race in order that they help, rather than hinder, the development of the children they work with.

Carl Rogers and education

Although Rogers was best known as the founder of 'non-directive' or 'client-centred' therapy, he had much to contribute to education. Rogers stressed the importance of the self and believed that the interpersonal relationship between the teacher/caregiver and child was crucial to the experience of the learner. In his book *Freedom to Learn*, Rogers discusses the following qualities and attitudes necessary to facilitate learning:

Genuineness

The facilitator of learning needs to be self-aware, or 'real', in order to communicate effectively with the learner. Therefore, professionals working with children need to be in touch with their own feelings and attitudes, rather than present artificial or assumed ways of being.

For example, a teacher who is genuinely pleased with a child's behaviour or performance will be much more effective than one who says she is pleased but is in fact irritated because she feels that her view of the child as a troublemaker is being challenged.

Acceptance

Valuing the child as he or she is and accepting his or her thoughts, feelings and opinions is an important aspect of enabling learning to take place. This does not mean that learners are considered to be perfect at all times but that they are prized as individuals with the potential to develop in ways which are right for them.

Empathy

This involves the ability to understand the learner's experience from his or her point of view. Children, like adults, appreciate being listened to and being understood from their own point of view. This involves sensitivity on the part of the facilitator to how the experiences of learning feel to learners. Empathic understanding encourages independence on the part of learners because it allows them to develop confidence in their own reactions and ability to learn.

Discussion Point 4

The practicality of Rogers' suggestions

How practical or possible are Rogers' suggestions? Consider each in turn and discuss with a colleague if possible.

For comments on this discussion point see page 131.

Children making friends

So far we have looked at the early emotional responses of infants and ways in which they develop as part of their early interactional processes. We have thought about how these relate to the formation of attachments with caregivers. We have further discussed the importance of attachment style and the development of positive self-esteem, particularly reflecting upon the role of caregivers and professionals in this. In moving on to another related aspect here, we consider the formation and importance of children's friendships. First, we need to be clear about:

➲ how children make friends

➲ what their friendships are like

➲ how these change as the child develops.

The development of friendships

In general, children become less self-focused, or egocentric (see Chapter 3), as well as less instrumental, or focused upon achieving a particular end for themselves, between birth and 6 years of age as they develop cognitively and acquire experience of social rules. Between the ages of 5 and 10 there is more cooperation involved in their friendships and the beginnings of a more in-depth appreciation of a friend's personal qualities (Bigelow, Tesson and Lewko 1996; see Figure 4.13).

Age range	Friendship patterns
Birth to 2 years	Respond to each other from a very early age, and most parents will find that very young children are fascinated by watching other children, particularly those who are a little older. However, it is not really until the second year of life that they begin to play socially.
2- to 3-year-olds	Generally begin to have playmates, usually children that they meet at nursery or play group, other family members or those who live nearby.
3- to 4-year-olds	Tend to see friends as those they happen to be in contact with or whose toys they like to play with. For example, 'My friend is Christopher at nursery school and we play on the fire engines.' 'Grace is my friend – she has lots of Duplo.'
5- to 6-year-olds	Are still focused upon themselves and their own needs, but they are beginning to understand that others may see things differently and have different needs. Friendship tends to be in short bursts and is based upon contact. For example, 'Ruth isn't my friend any more – she doesn't want to come round and play.' 'Mandeep is my friend 'cos he plays football when I want.'
7- to 9-year-olds	Begin to see friendships as personal and based on personality traits, which may mean that they like or dislike someone because of these. For example, 'A friend is someone who you like and they like you too. They aren't nasty to you and they are kind if you fall over or get upset. I have been Germayne's friend all the time since we've been in Mrs MacMahon's class.'

10-year-olds	Are able to cooperate with their friends and take on their point of view. They might share feelings and be interested in their activities, even though they do not share them. They may exclude others from their friendships. There is an emergent independence as they begin to place more importance upon their friends and less upon their families.
	For example, 'Me and Candice make up dances together. She always comes round when her mum lets her, or I go to hers. We both hate Lauren and Kieran – they're always causing trouble. I tell Candice some of my secrets and she never tells. She's nice.'
12 plus	Have much more complex views of relationships and begin to appreciate them in more depth.
	For example, 'Pravim's a good kid, even though he doesn't like cricket. His family are quite religious, so he has to go to the temple and stuff – we've got different ideas, but we get on great. I tell him about how I'd like to be a rock guitarist and he doesn't make fun of me. We swap wrestling videos and talk about the moves they make and sometimes act them out. We don't hurt each other though, even though my mum says we sound as if we're coming through the ceiling.'

Figure 4.13
Children's changing friendship patterns

Gender differences

Research has established that boys and girls in the pre-adolescent years tend to have different expectations of friendship, with girls reporting higher levels of intimacy, trust and loyalty than do boys in same-sex best-friendships.

Why children's friendships are important

Humans are social beings and, therefore, their social interactions are an integral aspect of their development and well-being. Friendships are an important part of our sense of self-worth as they tell us things about ourselves. They allow us to have a sense of belonging and acceptance. Those children who are unpopular at school are more likely to have problems in later life such as alcoholism, depression, schizophrenia, delinquency, dishonourable discharge from the army and psychosis (Duck, 1991). Some children (one in ten) have a social learning deficiency, which means they do not know how to act in social situations. These children were found to have poor empathy skills and to behave in ways likely to alienate them from others, such as boasting, sulking, cheating and withdrawing from games when losing (Wear, 2000). Clearly then, some children find it difficult to make friends and it is necessary for those working with them to be aware of ways in which friendship making might be facilitated.

Encouraging friendships

As an adult working with and caring for children, you provide a role model of how to behave and react. We looked earlier at the way very young children use social referencing in order to make decisions about ambiguous or novel situations, and this is particularly relevant where other children are concerned. You will be watched for your reactions to a child who is perhaps new to the group, or has failed to become an accepted member of it. Therefore, how you react matters and you need to find ways of working with all children.

Behaviourist approaches

Behaviourist approaches, which focus upon external influences on human behaviour, are useful in terms of understanding ways of helping children to form friendships.

Learning theory (Skinner, 1957)

This theory recognises the importance of rewarding or using **positive reinforcement** when the desired behaviour occurs, in order to increase the chances of it being repeated. So when the child is friendly or helpful towards others, this should be encouraged.

Social learning theory (Bandura, 1977)

This theory suggests that children learn not only from direct reinforcement, but also from observing and imitating the behaviour of significant adults. Therefore, they will learn from your behaviour towards others. So if you are sociable and friendly and you also reward this sort of behaviour in others, children are more likely to behave accordingly.

Discussion Point 5

Encouraging sociable behaviour in children

Think of examples from your own experience where friendly or sociable behaviour in children could be encouraged.

For comments on this discussion point see page 131.

Skills used by children in forming friendships

Making friends is easier for some children than for others and seems to involve the skills identified in Figure 4.14.

Difficulties with friendships

Difficulties with friendships arise for less socially competent children, who may be aggressive, demanding, 'bossy', impatient, whining and inflexible.

Skills	Examples
Ice-breaking	The ability to be the first to make the approach and invite some interaction. For example, 'Hello, my name's Daniel. What are you called? Have you just come into this school?'
Maintaining contact	This can be done in a variety of ways, such as inviting the other child to play, carrying on talking and listening, and generally expressing interest. This is done sensitively by children who have good social skills and this is important, as it does not force contact where not wanted, for example, feeling forced to hold hands or play something the child doesn't want to do.
Managing conflict	Being assertive but not aggressive is an important social skill and allows conflict to be dealt with. For example, 'I was on this bike first – I don't want to get off just yet, so stop pulling it'.
Listening and acknowledging	Recognising that others have feelings and taking this into account. This may involve negotiation. For example, 'If you wait for a bit, I'll let you have a go next. Don't cry'.

Figure 4.14
Skills used by children when making friends

Therefore, there is a cycle of rejection because they have a lack of adaptive strategies at their disposal and they will tend to use less effective ones, such as: 'If you don't let me play I'll tell the dinner lady – so there – and you'll get told off.' It may also be that there are language differences, cultural barriers or special needs that are relevant here, and these may need additional consideration.

Parental involvement

Parents may become involved in helping children to make friends (see comments about reinforcement (learning theory) and modelling the desired behaviour (social learning theory) on page 131, which are relevant in this context too). However, there is also evidence that advice giving and instruction by parents and caregivers can significantly increase the interactive competence of children (Russell and Finnie, 1990). It has also been found that suggestions of positive strategies and non-hostile attitudes resulted in better-liked, less aggressive children (Mize and Pettit, 1997). So parents might encourage children to listen and ask before joining in with other children playing, or offer something which might be used to play with, such as a skipping rope.

Since the evidence above suggests that it is possible to provide advice that can be absorbed on a cognitive level, professionals working with children need to be aware of this when planning tasks, activities and learning experiences.

> **Activity 7** **Friendship building**

1 Plan an activity for 5- to 8-year-olds that includes work on friendship building.

2 How might this fit into other areas of learning?

For comments about this activity see page 134.

Friendships as predictors of social adjustment

It has been suggested that children's friendships are not only relevant to their childhood but are also predictors of social adjustment in adulthood (Nangle and Erdley, 2001). They are seen as a kind of training ground for important adult relationships, including marriage. Parental influence is stressed, not only as role models, reinforcers, and advisors but also as managers of their children's social interactions outside school or nursery. It seems that the children of those parents who provide opportunities for peer contact and participation in activities, as well as monitoring their interactions, are likely to be more socially adept (Hartup, 1979).

However, for those working with children this may not be an area over which it is possible to exert influence. It is thought important for professionals to be aware of those children who are not accepted by their peers and to implement ways of helping them to be so.

The information given in Figure 4.15 may be used to enhance children's social skills and therefore encourage friendship formation.

The role of the practitioner in enhancing social skills	
Provide plenty of opportunities for play with other children	In order that they gain experience of interacting with their peers.
Play with the children yourself in a positive, equal way	Play as though you were another socially competent child, rather than controlling the activity. This might include responding to the child's ideas and responding, listening actively to them, as well as contributing to the action of the play. This enables children to learn from the adult modelling socially competent behaviour, as well as developing confidence in their own ability to contribute to play.

Talk about friendship, social relationships and values with the children	In order to communicate an interest in their well-being in this area, as well as providing them with a place to share information and experiences. This adds to their ability to solve the problems they encounter in this area. (See Circle Time discussion below.)
Tackle difficulties from a problem-solving perspective rather than seeming to know all the answers	Help the child to consider a range of solutions and viewpoints and encourage positive strategies that are relevant to the situation. For example, **Alex**: Well, I could push him over if he gets in my way again. **Adult**: You could. What do you think he would do then? **Alex**: He might thump me back or tell the dinner-lady. **Adult**: What else could you try? **Alex**: I suppose I could ask him to move and say 'please'. **Adult**: That's a good idea. Try that next time.
Encourage resilience to setbacks and a constructive approach to future events	For example, 'I'll try to be careful not to knock their tower over next time.'
Intervene when necessary	But allow older pre-school children to work out their own solutions when possible.
Provide a positive attitude generally for getting along with others	So that the children are encouraged to behave in a friendly way.

Figure 4.15 *Enhancing children's social skills*

Circle Time

Circle Time was popularised by Jenny Mosley, and has its roots in social work and therapeutic approaches. Many schools across the UK now use Circle Time as a means of creating a positive environment and dealing with problems.

Case Study 4

Using Circle Time creatively

Nathan has become increasingly miserable since starting school. He is always alone at playtime and usually tries to force his way into games, which has made him even more unpopular. Most of the other children run away from him now when he approaches and have begun laughing at him and teasing him.

An attempt to solve the problem

Circle Time could be used creatively here in a variety of ways. The teacher could begin after a warm-up exercise by talking about the problem and then ask each child in turn to offer an idea about how to solve the problem. If the issues around 'who did what to whom' arise, then both sides must be heard before, perhaps, a discussion about what should have happened, or other things that could have been done. The teacher might use the discussion to put forward a few suggestions and ask the children to decide which is the best option for them.

Stories, poems and books are often a valuable resource since problems encountered in them can be used to stimulate related discussions.

For example, nursery children might look at a nursery rhyme such as 'Georgie Porgie' and the teacher could ask them questions about why the other children did not want to play with Georgie.

Georgie Porgie Pudding and Pie
Kissed the girls and made them cry.
When the boys came out to play, Georgie Porgie ran away.

With older children the teacher could use books such as Berenstein Bears or Jacqueline Wilson stories, which deal with a wide range of real-world problems including bullying and friendship but within a fictitious framework.

In this way children can be helped with other real problems that they encounter.

An explanation of Circle Time	
Conditions	The children sit in a circle so that everyone can be clearly seen; they often hold something, such as a cuddly toy, to indicate who is speaking.
Role of teacher	The teacher sits with the children as part of the group and ensures that the rules are followed, emotions are protected and appropriate activities are prepared.
Rules	Only one person speaks at a time – the one holding the 'talking object'. If you do not want to speak you can say 'pass'. There are no 'put downs' of people.
Discussion and problem solving	After a 'warm up' consisting perhaps of a pair-game of some kind, the focus can be decided by the teacher. This will depend upon the age, stage and immediate situation of the group. For example, at the start of the year Circle Time might focus upon getting to know each other. It might well be used for dealing with problems such as the child who is being socially excluded or bullied.

Figure 4.16
How to use Circle Time

Conclusion

➲ Emotions are an important part of the infant's initial social and emotional development.

➲ Secure attachments are related to emotional development and seem important for healthy development in a variety of areas.

➲ Self-esteem is key to fulfilling potential.

➲ Friendships help to support children's personal development.

As you read the following, reflect upon the understanding of social and emotional development you have gained by reading this chapter.

Case Study 5

A review

Christopher was separated from his teenage mother, Joanne, at birth, as he was the underweight (just under 5lbs) half of twins. Although it was a full-term pregnancy and he was in good health, he was taken to a hospital 30 miles away, which had a Special Baby Unit. His twin sister, Paula, remained with her mother and was successfully breastfed. He was kept in this hospital for 2 weeks, where he was bottle-fed. During this time, it was possible for his mother to visit him only once.

When he was reunited with his mother and sister, his mother attempted to breastfeed him, but he was used to the bottle by this time and refused to feed from her.

Christopher was a noisy baby, with a loud, persistent cry. He was thin and bald, and wriggled when he was held, comparing unfavourably with his twin, who had black curls and dimples and was plump and contented. Joanne felt that Christopher had rejected her and became increasingly depressed by the way he stiffened his limbs when he was held and his refusal of breast milk. She confessed to a friend, 'Sometimes I feel like throwing him out of the window when he is screaming for food and kicking me away.' Because of the practicalities involved, the father usually fed Christopher, but he was at work for much of the time.

As the twins grew, Paula remained the 'easy' twin and Christopher the 'difficult' one. Joanne found it very difficult to cope with his behaviour, particularly when she became pregnant again when the twins were 8 months old.

When the twins started school, Paula settled in quickly, but Christopher cried most days and had to be dragged to school. This was distressing for all of them and resulted in considerable strain upon Joanne, particularly as Christopher would run to her but then refuse to have a cuddle when he came out of school. The other children at school began to pick on him and call him a baby, which made it even harder to get him there.

1 Were the twins born temperamentally different or was it their experiences that shaped their personal development? (See nature-nurture debate in Chapter 3.)

2 How might your understanding of early emotional development, attachment theory, self-esteem and friendship formation help to shed light upon the case study?

3 How might Christopher and Paula's teacher help him to settle in?

For comments on this case study see below.

⟩ Comments on case studies, activities and discussion ⟩ points

Case Study 3 (page 110): Making childcare arrangements

1 Perhaps you might reassure Jasmine that at Sarah's age, there should be no ill effects in disrupting the attachment, as long as this is currently a secure one. The evidence suggests, in fact, that it will help to improve the child's ability to interact with others.

2 The important things to look for are continuity (so that there is always someone reliable to care for Sarah) and security. It might be possible to arrange a gradual increase in the amount of time spent in day-care, as Jasmine's mother might be happy to share in this. This would allow Sarah to get used to the new situation in a more gentle way and, as long as she feels secure, she might soon enjoy the extra stimulation that it would bring.

Case Study 5 (page 128): A review

1 As these are fraternal or non-identical twins (dizygotic) they will be no more similar genetically than any brother or sister. Therefore, it is possible that there are some temperamental or dispositional differences to begin with. However, the twins experienced different early conditions (one with mother and breastfed, one away from mother and bottle-fed) and these may well have formed the foundation for later developments, which were then reinforced by social interactions.

2 There are a number of issues here and, of course, we can only make an informed guess about some relevant aspects. However, we might start by considering the early interactions between Christopher and Joanne. As she had not been able to have this baby close to her for two weeks, it made it more difficult for early interactions (sensitive responsiveness) to occur. Joanne was able to interact with her daughter, but Christopher had been kept in an incubator and, therefore, had little contact with a 'mother figure'. This, coupled with the rejection of the breast encouraged Joanne to feel that her son did not want her and that she could not supply his needs adequately. Therefore, she saw his crying and stiffened limbs as a rejection of her as an inadequate mother, whereas Paula smiled happily and made her

feel fulfilled as a mother. This could easily have led to the formation of an insecure attachment between Christopher and Joanne, whereas Paula seemed to have formed a secure attachment. Starting school highlighted this and Christopher's insecure attachment might be identified as anxious/ambivalent (running towards her but refusing to cuddle her). It also seems likely that his self-esteem will be low, as he is constantly compared unfavourably with his twin (whether overtly or covertly) and this continues at school, where the other children see Paula's behaviour as acceptable and Christopher's as unacceptable.

3 Circle Time as described on page 126 would be very useful here. The class could be invited to see the world through Christopher's eyes, in order that he and they understand some of the difficulties he faces. Rogers' person-centred approach has much to contribute here. Christopher needs to be accepted for himself and given unconditional positive regard in order to develop his potential. Perhaps it would be a good idea to have the twins in separate classes in order that they develop more as individuals, but this would have to be dealt with very sensitively.

Discussion Point 1 (page 102): The effects of smiling upon a carer

1 If the infant smiles at the carer this is likely to be interpreted as recognition of the carer and his or her care-giving abilities. It signals that all is well and that the baby is fine. This is likely to make the carer feel more confident in his or her own ability to do the job properly. Therefore, the carer will be more relaxed and responsive.

2 This leads to a mutual responsiveness or reciprocal interaction (Bell, 1979) as both parties are reassured by the responses of the other.

Discussion Point 2 (page 115): Assessing which factors are important to children

1 Molly talks about most aspects positively. She seems proud of the fact that she is the biggest and seems pleased with the way she looks (physical appearance). She seems to think that her behavioural conduct is important and feels that she behaves well, particularly compared with others. She also talks about her learning (scholastic competence) and friends (social competence). There is no mention of her athletic competence, however, suggesting that this is not important to her.

2 Suzy seems focused upon her size (physical appearance) and learning competence, again comparing herself with others. She also seems to find behavioural conduct important. There is a more negative feel to her description than Molly's.

3 Both of these descriptions include comparisons with others and it is clear that these comparisons impact upon the security of self-esteem. Suzy's self-esteem is perhaps less secure because she does

not measure up in the ways she sees as important (being physically big and quick academically), perhaps because she compares herself with more competent or older others. However, she does recognise her artistic abilities (valued by her father). Harter stated that significant others have an influence upon the child's self-esteem. So for the school-aged child, not only is the parent or carer involved, but also siblings and peers as well as teachers.

Discussion Point 3 (page 118): Positive and negative self-esteem

1 Clearly Jack has low self-esteem because he sees third place as confirmation that he is a failure, whereas Harry's high self-esteem allows him to enjoy his achievement and view the future with enthusiasm and as a positive challenge.

2 So it is not necessarily the event in itself (because Jack actually achieved more) but the child's perception of it that contributes to self-worth.

Discussion Point 4 (page 120): The practicality of Rogers' suggestions

1 Rogers is often criticised for not taking on board a formal teaching context, where time constraints and class size may make it extremely difficult to adopt a person-centred perspective.

2 Self-knowledge on the part of the teacher may be achievable and is certainly desirable in order to enhance personal and professional effectiveness. However, you may have commented that we do not all undergo therapy and may be unaware of our own attitudes and predispositions. The important thing, perhaps, is to be open to the possibility of our own attitudes influencing the development of children and be ready to address these as they arise.

3 Accepting children as they are is obviously desirable, but it may be that you are constrained by the external demands of the school or educational policies such as SATS. This increases pressure, as there are expectations that children reach a certain standard. Perhaps, you might value each child (UPR) but the system does not seem to.

4 Empathy involves being able to see the world through the eyes of each child. This is difficult when there are 30 children in the class, each with his or her own need for empathic understanding. Rogers worked with clients on a one-to-one basis which allowed for this to happen, but it is obviously much more difficult to achieve when working with groups.

Discussion Point 5 (page 123): Encouraging sociable behaviour in children

1 You may have thought about ways in which you have encouraged children to assist others when they have been struggling with

something. For example, 'Billy, would you hold the door open for Jack, please? He's carrying the lunch boxes for us.'

2 Or you may have thought about occasions when a child has done something helpful without being asked. For example, 'How kind of you to pick up Jake's jacket off the floor. I'm sure he's very grateful.'

Activity 1 (page 112): A short description of myself

1 Your description will probably have included some of your characteristics, such as 'fairly confident' or 'shy'. You might have talked about your interests, such as 'I really enjoy working with children but find it very demanding.' Your account may have included the views of others; for example, 'People always think I am outgoing, but actually I am quite shy, particularly when I don't know people well.' You may also have reflected upon ways in which you would like to be different, such as 'I wish I was more assertive and often feel reluctant to say what I want.'

2 Although your account will obviously be different from this, the process you have gone through to write it will usually be similar. That is, you will have thought about how you feel inside as well as how you feel about the comments that other people have made about you. You may have considered, perhaps, whether you feel differently on the inside from how you appear on the outside. Almost certainly, it will have involved your thinking about how you compare with others. Perhaps you thought of ways in which you might wish to be different, or maybe, ways in which you are happy with yourself.

3 In carrying out this activity, your own description will have been built upon both internal and external information in the same way that children's pictures of themselves are built. It consists of some 'I' statements, known as the **existential self** (or the 'self as I' as William James called it), which is the first part of the self-concept to emerge.

4 Later, the **categorical self** (or self as 'me') emerges and this includes the social categories which describe a person, such as gender, age, ethnicity, size and relation to others.

Activity 2 (page 112): Social categories

1 Let us assume that your list looked something like this:

Woman, nursery worker, single, mother, northerner, Morris dancer, Buddhist.

2 Some of these descriptions might apply to people that you know/work with; for example, many of the people you know may be women, and it is women who predominantly staff nurseries. For a man working in a nursery, this would make him different from his colleagues.

3 Being a mother who is single may mean that you are unlike some of the people you know (who may be married or childless) and many

people that you know may choose to jog or go to the gym rather than Morris dancing. Similarly, your friends and acquaintances may not be of the same (or any) religion. If you are working in London or Cornwall for example, your identity as a northerner (with possibly a different accent and culture) may make you different too.

4 Identifying yourself as different from most of the people you know may have negative effects, particularly if to do so is disadvantageous in some way; for example, if your northern accent is derided or looked down upon by those around you. This has implications for those living in different cultures and from different ethnic origins because it might well influence their sense of belonging (categorical self) and self-worth.

Activity 3 (page 113): A young boy's self-description

You might have reasoned something like this:

1 The child is showing that he has a sense of self – he describes himself physically ('I am big', 'My hair is curly') and is able to compare himself with Emily (who is small) so he must be more than 19 months old. Obviously his use of language would also indicate this.

2 He is able to reflect upon his abilities ('I can ride a bike now and be a fire-fighter') demonstrating that this is something he recognises as an achievement. So this means he is at least 2 years old. He also shows that he is taking on board the expectations about adult standards of behaviour (his sister is shouting all the time which affects TV viewing). This would indicate that he is at least almost three.

Activity 4 (page 116): Encouraging positive self-esteem

1 The teacher here is encouraging those aspects that she sees as important (such as the manner and content of what is said) but discouraging children who have other suggestions and information. This means that those whose perceptions and ways of communicating are different from hers are less likely to develop positive self-esteem within this class. There are important connections here then between the personality of the teacher and the way she responds to the individuals within her class.

2 You may have seen that Katy is being encouraged to develop positive self-esteem here and is being rewarded for her contribution to the discussion.

3 Thomas, on the other hand, receives mixed messages here. He is told that his answer is 'very good' and indeed it contains relevant information, but attention is also drawn to what the teacher perceives as his mistakes. The overall effect may be to reduce his confidence in his ability to contribute (thereby decreasing his self-esteem) because he might get it wrong again.

4 Karendeep seems to have low self-esteem to start with and does not have the confidence to offer an answer, but this is likely to be lowered even more by the teacher's response and comparison with the other children. Her response may be partly due to the cultural differences between her and Karendeep, which she hints at with 'don't know the word'.

5 Justin is not encouraged here although his answer is a graphic one, which could have been built upon by the teacher. Like Thomas, he is treated to critical comments, implying that he has contributed nothing of worth.

Activity 5 (page 117): Qualities that you value in yourself

1 Maybe one of the qualities that you value in yourself is politeness. It may follow that you value polite children more and, therefore, that you encourage their positive self-esteem. The teacher in the extract clearly valued 'sensible' behaviour and therefore discouraged those who were perhaps over-keen to contribute, reluctant to do so, or included 'silly' comments.

2 It is likely that your own experiences and sense of self-worth will influence ways in which you relate to the children you work with, so it is important that you are aware of this.

Activity 6 (page 119): Acknowledging inappropriate behaviour

1 This should involve pointing out that the behaviour is 'naughty' or undesirable because it is distracting to the others, or makes it difficult for the teacher to do her job, but it should not label Ashley as naughty.

2 Hayley is being labelled as 'bad' here, rather than her behaviour – inflicting pain and distracting Chelsie.

3 The entire class is being labelled as the 'worst', rather than their noisy behaviour being dealt with.

Activity 7 (page 125): Friendship building

You could introduce friendship building using discussion or circle time sessions based around a particular question or problem. Keep things unthreatening by putting a number of relevant questions into a bowl and passing them round to be picked out. Role play would often follow naturally from these questions. For example:

'One of your friends is always left out of games in the playground. What do you think you should do?'

'Someone you know is very bad at sharing and always pushes in. What would you do?'

'Your friend is always getting into trouble by arguing. What do you think he or she could do about this?'

References and further reading

Ainsworth, M. and Wittig, B. (1969), 'Attachment and Exploratory Behaviour of One-Year-Olds in a Strange Situation', in Foss, B. (ed.) *Determinants of Infant Behaviour*, Vol. 4, The Data, pp839–78. Hillsdale, NJ: Erlbaum

Bandura, A. (1977), *Social Learning Theory*. Englewood Cliffs, NJ: Prentice-Hall

Bell, R. (1979), 'Parent, Child and Reciprocal Influences'. *American Psychologist*, Vol. 34, pp821–7

Bigelow, B., Tesson, G. and Lewko, J. (1996), *Children's Rules of Friendship*. New York: Guilford

Bowlby, J. (1951), *Maternal Care and Mental Health*. Geneva, World Health Organization: London: Her Majesty's Stationery Office; New York: Columbia University Press

Brazleton, T. and Cramer, B. (1991), *The Earliest Relationship: Parents, infants and the drama of early attachment*. London: Karnac Books

Brazleton, T., Tronick, E., Adamson, L., Als, H. and Wise, S. (1975), *Early Mother-Infant Reciprocity*, Ciba Foundation Symposium 33. Amsterdam: Elsevier

Coopersmith, S. (1967). *The Antecedents of Self-Esteem*. San Francisco: Freeman

Davies, J. and Brember, I. (1995), 'Change in Self-Esteem Between Year 2 and Year 6: A longitudinal study'. *Educational Psychology*, Vol. 15, No. 2, pp171–9

Dowling, M. (2000), *Young Children's Personal, Social and Emotional Development*. London: Paul Chapman

Duck, S. (1991). *Friends for Life*. Hemel Hempstead: Harvester-Wheatsheaf

Feinman, S. and Lewis, M. (1983), 'Social Referencing at Ten Months: A second-order effect in infants' responses to strangers'. *Child Development*, Vol. 54, pp878–88

Frankel, K. and Bates, J. (1990), 'Mother Toddler Problem Solving: Antecedents in attachment, home behaviour and temperament'. *Child Development*, Vol. 61, pp810–20

Harter, S. (1983), 'Developmental Perspectives on the Self-Esteem', in Heatherington, M. (ed.), *Handbook of Child Psychology: Social and Personality Development* (vol. 4). New York: Wiley

Hartup, W. (1979), 'The Social Worlds of Childhood'. *American Psychologist*, Vol. 34, pp944–50

Heard, D. and Lake, B. (1997), *The Challenge of Attachment for Caregiving*. London and New York: Routledge

Holmes, J. (1993), *John Bowlby and Attachment Theory*. Routledge: London

Hornik, R. and Gunnar, M. (1988), 'A Descriptive Analysis of Infant Social Referencing'. *Child Development*, Vol. 59, pp626–35

Izard, C. (1994), 'Innate and Universal Facial Expressions. Evidence from developmental and cross-cultural research'. *Psychological Bulletin*, Vol. 115, pp288–99

Izard, C., Fantauzzo, C., Castle, J., Haynes, O., Rayias, M. and Putnam, P. (1995), 'The Ontogeny and Significance of Infants' Facial Expressions in the First Nine Months of Life'. *Developmental Psychology*, Vol. 31, pp997–1013

Izard, C., Haynes, O., Chisholm, G. and Baak, K. (1991), 'Emotional Determinants of Infant-Mother Attachments'. *Child Development*, Vol. 62, pp906–17

Jackson, J. (1993), 'Multiple Caregiving among African Americans and Infant Attachment: The need for an Emic approach'. *Human Development*, Vol. 36, pp87–102

Lewis, M. and Brooks-Gunn, J. (1979), *Social Cognition and the Acquisition of Self*. New York: Plenum Press

Liedloff, J. (1986), *The Continuum Concept*. Harmondsworth: Penguin

Lyons-Ruth, K., Easterbrooks, M. and Cibelli, C. (1997), 'Infant Attachment Strategies: Infant mental lag and maternal depressive symptoms: Predictors of internalizing and externalizing problems at age 7'. *Developmental Psychology*, Vol. 33, pp681–92

Matas, L., Arend, R. and Stroufe, L. (1978), 'Continuity of Adaptation in the Second Year: The relationship between quality of attachment and later competence'. *Child Development*, Vol. 49, pp547–56

Merton, R. (1957), *Social Theory and Social Structure* (rev. edn). Glencoe: Free Press

Miell, D. and Dallos, R. (eds) (1996), *Social Interaction and Personal Relationships*. London: Sage/Open University

Mills, R. and Duck, S. (eds) (2000), *The Developmental Psychology of Personal Relationships*. Chichester: John Wiley and Sons

Mize, J. and Pettit, G. (1997), 'Mothers' Social Coaching, Mother-Child Relationship Style and Children's Peer Competence: Is the medium the message?' *Child Development*, Vol. 68, pp312–32

Mosley, J. (1996), *Quality Circle Time in the Primary Classroom: Your essential guide to enhancing self-esteem, self-discipline and positive relationships*. Wisbech: LDA

Mruk, C. (1999), *Self-Esteem: Research, theory and practice* (2nd edn). London: Free Association Books

Murray, L. and Trevarthen, C. (1985), 'Emotional Regulation of Interactions between Two-month-olds and their Mothers', in Field, T. and Fox, N. (eds), *Social Perception in Infants*. Norwood, NJ: Ablex

Nangle, D. and Erdley, C. (eds) (2001), *The Role of Friendship in Psychological Adjustment*. San Francisco: Jossey-Bass

Nelson, C. (1987), 'The Recognition of Facial Expressions in the First Two Years of Life: Mechanisms of development'. *Child Development*, Vol. 58, pp889–910

Roberts, R. (2002), *Self-Esteem and Early Learning* (2nd edn). London: Paul Chapman

Rogers, C. (1990), *The Carl Rogers Reader* (edited by Kirschenbaum and Henderson). London: Constable

Rogers, C. (1994), *Freedom to Learn* (3rd edn). Upper Saddle River, NJ: Merrill

Rubin, Z. (1980), *Children's Friendships*. London: Fontana

Russell, A. and Finnie, V. (1990), 'Preschool Children's Social Status and Maternal Instructions to Assist Group Entry'. *Developmental Psychology*, Vol. 26, pp603–11

Skinner, B. (1957), *Verbal Behaviour*. New York: Prentice Hall

Troknick, E., Morelli, G. and Winn, S. (1987), 'Multiple Caregiving of Efe (Pygmy) Infants'. *American Anthropologist*, Vol. 89 (1), pp96–106

Van den Boom, D. (1994), 'The Influence of Temperament and Mothering on Attachment and Exploration: An experimental manipulation of sensitive responsiveness among lower-class mothers and irritable infants'. *Child Development*, Vol. 65, pp1457–78

Waters, E. (1978), 'The Reliability and Stability of Individual Differences in Infant-Mother Interactions'. *Child Development*, Vol. 49, pp483–94

Wear, K. (2000), *Promoting Mental, Emotional and Social Health: A whole school approach*. London: Routledge

White, B. (1993), *The First Three Years of Life*. New York: Simon and Schuster

Useful websites

➲ http://users.stargate.net/~cokids/Circle.html

This website provides a platform for teachers to share ideas about Circle Time as well as links to other sites.

➲ www.antibullying.net

This website contains a bank of information on bullying and easy access to searching within it for particular issues and narrowing the search.

➲ www.kinderstart.com/index.html

Go to this useful and comprehensive website for information and links – again you can search within it for particular areas, for example, social and emotional development.

5

How children learn

Vivienne Walkup

This chapter aims to explore theories of cognitive development and their relevance to early learning contexts. Its purpose is to encourage the development of students' critical thinking skills in considering how best to support children's cognitive development.

This chapter addresses the following areas:

⊃ the work of Jean Piaget

⊃ the relevance of Piaget's ideas for the care and education of young children

⊃ the work of Lev Vygotsky

⊃ the relevance of Vygotsky's ideas for the care and education of young children

⊃ information processing approaches to cognitive development

⊃ applying information processing principles in learning environments.

After reading this chapter it is hoped that you will be able to:

1 critically assess the theories of Piaget, Vygotsky and the information processing approach to cognitive development

2 understand the relevance of the theories of Piaget, Vygotsky and the information processing approach to the care and education of young children

3 evaluate your own experiences of, and insights into, early cognitive development in the light of this learning.

Introduction

The term 'cognition' is generally used to refer to any intellectual process within the human experience and covers a wide range of related areas including attention, perception, memory, thinking and problem solving. It can be thought of as being about the way the 'cogs' within our brains work. There are whole sections of libraries devoted to various aspects of cognitive psychology for those with specialised interests, but the purpose of this chapter is to consider aspects that are important to those working with, and supporting, young children. So what follows is a discussion of the three main theoretical views of cognitive development and a consideration of how these relate to our understanding of children.

The work of Jean Piaget
(1886–1980)

Piaget is the best known and perhaps most influential of the cognitive theorists (Bjorklund, 2000) but he is also the most criticised. Just as with Freud, it is always easy to find lots of things he did that were methodologically flawed, but nevertheless we are left with interesting and valuable insights that add to our understanding of children.

Piaget, a Swiss biologist, first became interested in cognitive development as a result of his observations of molluscs existing in different environments. These caused him to ponder issues of flexibility and adaptation and he suggested that children's brains adapt to their environment through experience. He proposed that humans **construct** their own knowledge through their experiences of the world and that they learn by doing this rather than being told or given information. His work is therefore often referred to as a **cognitive constructivist** approach.

Summary of Piaget's theories of development

Piaget believed that:

- development proceeds through **maturation** and **adaptation**
- adaptation occurs because of **assimilation**, **accommodation**, and **equilibration**
- **schemas** allow knowledge to be shaped and stored
- **cognitive development** occurs in **stages**.

Maturation refers to changes related to biological maturity over which the environment has little control. For example, a child's first teeth begin to develop around six months of age and there is little that can be done to change this. However, the quality of the child's teeth may be affected by environmental factors such as maternal diet or an excess of sugary drinks.

Adaptation describes ways in which the child is shaped by its environment in order to survive within it. For example, the child with poor teeth may learn to suck food thoroughly rather than biting it.

Assimilation is the term Piaget used to explain the way that existing knowledge is used when we are confronted with problems we need to solve. For example, the child with poor teeth who has learned to suck biscuits will also suck an apple when first given one.

Accommodation is the process of changing what we already know to work in order to solve new tasks effectively. For example, the child finds that sucking the apple does not allow it to be eaten effectively and so begins to use his gums to break up the apple.

Equilibration is Piaget's term for the continual attempt at balance between **equilibrium** and **disequilibrium**. If new knowledge can be assimilated into our current knowledge easily, without having to change it, we are in a state of equilibrium. We feel steady and in control. However, if we have to accommodate our knowledge, we exist in a state of disequilibrium or unsteadiness until we have modified our cognitive structures. Thus, we strive for equilibrium but learning involves disequilibrium. For example, the child who finds that her apple does not respond to being sucked in the same way as the biscuit is disconcerted by this and may become distressed. She strives to find a way round this and eventually discovers that using her gums works. Therefore, the process of equilibration may not always be comfortable but results in more efficient means of understanding the environment.

Figure 5.1
Flow diagram summarising Piaget's theory of cognitive development

Schemas or **schemata** are ways in which our knowledge is stored. They, like all cognitive structures, are abstract concepts and would not appear upon a brain scan, but they are extremely useful ways of understanding the learning process. They are rather like mental files or folders stored in a computer. In them we keep everything that we know about particular aspects of the world and when a new experience is encountered we open that particular folder in order to access the information contained within it. They are constantly being adapted and enlarged as we learn more. For example, a child's schema for eating now includes both sucking and using gums in order to eat food successfully.

> **Activity 1** **Schema for turning on the TV**

Think about your schema for turning on the television at home.

1 How do you modify it when using other kinds of TV or electrical equipment?
2 Identify aspects of assimilation and accommodation.
3 How have equilibrium and disequilibrium been involved?

For comments on this Activity see page 167.

Piaget believed that cognitive development occurred in stages that were related to the maturation of the child. Each of these stages involves a qualitative change that makes it different from the preceding one. The order in which these occur is fixed and applies to all children. It is not, therefore, possible to leave out or skip a stage. Each stage must be in place in order that the next can be laid upon it (see Figure 5.2).

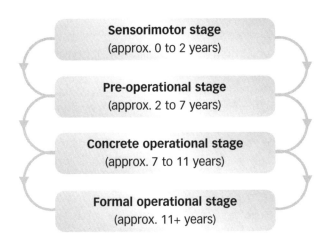

Sensorimotor stage
(approx. 0 to 2 years)

Pre-operational stage
(approx. 2 to 7 years)

Concrete operational stage
(approx. 7 to 11 years)

Formal operational stage
(approx. 11+ years)

Figure 5.2
Piaget's stages of cognitive development

The sensorimotor stage

The sensorimotor stage sees the development of **object permanence**: the realisation that objects still exist even though they are not physically present. It begins to appear between 8 and 12 months. At this age, if an object is hidden under a cloth several times and the child grabs it, and then the object is transferred to another cloth in full view of the child, he or she will still look under the first cloth first because it was seen there most often. This is called the A not B error.

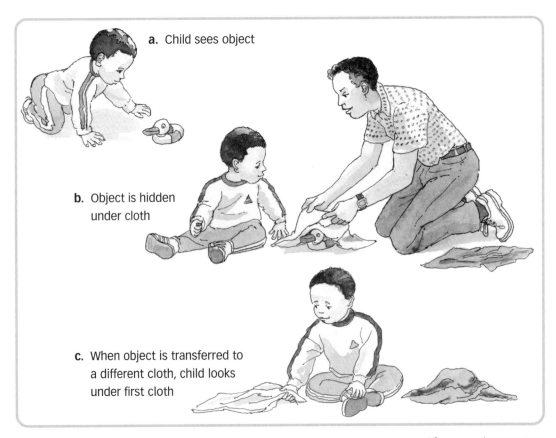

a. Child sees object

b. Object is hidden under cloth

c. When object is transferred to a different cloth, child looks under first cloth

The sensorimotor stage

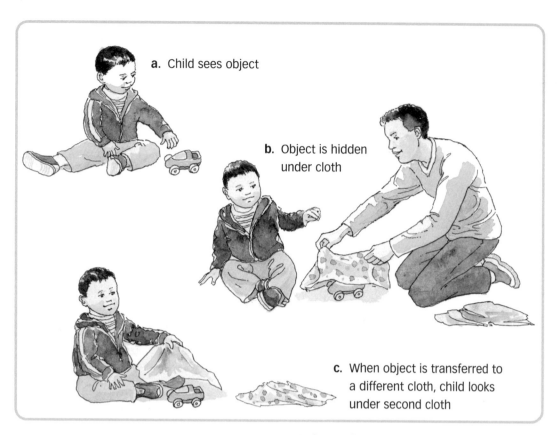

a. Child sees object

b. Object is hidden under cloth

c. When object is transferred to a different cloth, child looks under second cloth

Understanding the concept of object permanence

By the age of 18 months the child is able to **infer invisible displacement** (if an object is seen to be picked up, concealed in the hand, placed in the pocket, taken out and put in the drawer, the child will now look in the drawer even though he or she has not actually seen the object transferred) and develops complete object permanence.

It seems, then, that it is no longer the case that 'out of sight is out of mind' and carers will no longer be able to put things away in full view of the child and be confident that they will not be looked for there. Indeed, once children have grasped this concept, they may become very determined and use resources such as chairs and cushions to allow them to reach the confiscated objects.

The development of language and thought marks the end of this stage and children begin to engage in pretend play.

The pre-operational stage

At the pre-operational stage the child makes considerable headway in the use of symbols to represent aspects of his or her world. Rapid development in language, number, drawing and pretend play occurs as children learn to do this, although there are still some limitations.

There are two parts to this stage: the **pre-conceptual stage** and the **intuitive stage** (see Figure 5.3).

Stages in the pre-operational stage		
Stage	**Age range**	**Characteristics**
Pre-conceptual	2 to 4 years	This is characterised by **syncretic reasoning** (objects are classified according to limited and changing criteria) and **transductive reasoning** (relationships between objects tend to be based upon a single characteristic). For example, a boat may be used in water play one day because it floats on water and then put on the 'blue' table the next day because of its colour. **Animistic thinking** is common. Inanimate objects are believed to be alive particularly if they move, such as the sun and moon. For example, a child may believe that the moon follows him or her to light the way home.
Intuitive	4 to 7 years	This involves the reliance that children have upon what they sense to be true rather than on logic or reason. Children use their senses and imagination freely and may trust these more than the words used. Therefore, they may pay more attention to the apparent sense of what is being said rather than the actual language used. An example of this might be that when shown four toy cars put into three toy garages and asked whether all the garages have a car in them, children at this stage may answer 'no' because they can see that one car still remains. They have failed to 'disembed' the language from the visual sense of the scene and so respond to this rather than the explicit question.

Figure 5.3
Stages in the pre-operational stage

Egocentrism operates in the pre-operational child, who believes that his or her own view of the world is the one seen by others. For example, a child may assume that everyone can see what the teacher has written on the board because this is what the child can see. The child may be quite oblivious to the fact that he or she is blocking the view of others.

The concrete operational stage

At around 7 years of age, children begin to be able to use logical rules to deal with concrete problems. But Piaget would argue that they are still unable to solve abstract problems and that they do not consider all logically possible outcomes. Thinking is limited to real-world scenarios and their own past experiences.

The onset of **conservation** marks entry to this stage. This means understanding that quantities (such as mass, weight and volume) remain stable even though their appearance might change. So a child may no longer assume that pouring a bottle of lemonade into a tall glass makes it more or that a bigger parcel means a more expensive present. At this stage the child is capable of making decisions based upon all aspects of a situation, rather than just on one.

Piaget described this development as moving from **centration** (focusing upon the central aspects of a problem) to **decentration** (attending to the entire problem).

Centration applies to other everyday judgements, too, such as assuming that a friend's mother is older than your own because she is taller.

Class inclusion also appears during this stage and involves the understanding that a class must always be smaller than any more inclusive class that contains it. For example, when asked whether there are more sheep than animals on the farm table (which contains seven sheep, four cows and two pigs), a child becomes capable of answering 'animals'.

The formal operational stage

The formal operational stage (11+ years) is differentiated by the ability to think in abstract terms. This means that children are no longer limited to thinking about concrete objects but can include invention and fantasy unrelated to their previous experiences.

Hypothetico-deductive reasoning is the main factor here and involves being able to deal with possibilities, generate ideas and think in terms of symbols.

Children become capable of thinking scientifically and forming theoretical assumptions about the world, which can be tested and evaluated. For example, they are now able to play chess, begin to understand algebra and plan experiments in science.

> ### Activity 2 — Piaget in action

Complete the table below to identify some behaviours exhibited by children in terms of Piaget's stages. The first one has been filled in as an example.

Behaviour	Age	Stage	Ability
1 Child stirs wooden blocks in plastic saucepan.	18 months	Sensorimotor	Beginning of symbolic play
2 Child brings his favourite toy for Mummy to play with when she is feeling tired.			

Behaviour	Age	Stage	Ability
3 Child believes that the car is covered up at night because it feels cold			
4 Child is happy to have smaller, thicker slice of chocolate cake when sister has larger, thinner one.			
5 Child uses pocket money to buy magazine and chocolate but struggles with addition and subtraction at school.			
6 Child is able to sort and classify football cards according to teams, leagues or players' positions.			
7 Child engages in discussion with family about the pros and cons of war.			

See page 168 for an example of a completed table.

Considerations of Piaget's work

Although Piaget's work has been heavily criticised, it is important to remember that there are also many strengths in his wide-ranging and comprehensive theory. Most significantly, it has succeeded in stimulating decades of research into children's cognitive development, and has provided scientific support for child-centred views of children's learning. Without Piaget's ideas we would lack a framework for understanding and interpreting some of the changes that occur.

Criticisms of Piaget's work

Generally these fall into three categories:

- ⊃ Piaget underestimated the importance of previous knowledge to success in the tasks he set children.
- ⊃ Piaget underestimated children's abilities because his tasks had methodological flaws.
- ⊃ Piaget underestimated the role of culture.

The importance of knowledge

Gagné (1985) found that young children could acquire complex skills once the simpler skills required had been learnt, so children might well have failed some of Piaget's tasks because they just did not possess these prerequisite skills. For instance, young babies might not have demonstrated object permanence because they had not yet mastered the ability to coordinate hand-to-eye movements in order to reach towards the object that had been covered.

It could, therefore, also be argued that development is based upon learning new skills and is continuous not discontinuous as Piaget suggested.

Children's abilities

Piaget underestimated children's abilities because his tasks were methodologically flawed and failed to account for factors such as demands upon memory and physical ability, familiarity with the task and misleading questions.

Demands on memory and physical ability

These are involved in, for example, object permanence tasks, which relied upon infants being able to remember that the teddy was behind the screen and being able to reach out for the teddy at the same time. Young infants may not physically be able to do this. Baillargeon (1987) found that when the task is one that is based upon a visual rather than a reaching response, infants as young as 3 months of age demonstrate object permanence.

Familiarity with tasks

Piaget's tasks may have been too complex, abstract and unfamiliar to allow children to succeed.

Case Study 1

The three mountains task

Children were asked to look at three mountains on a table. They were made of *papier mâché* and each of them was a different size and colour. Something was different on top of each of them: snow, a cross or a house.

A small doll was placed opposite the child, who was then asked which view the doll could see. The experimenter gave the child ten pictures taken from around the table and asked her to pick out the one that showed what the doll could see.

Piaget found that children younger than 7 or 8 years old were unable to do this correctly and usually picked out the view that they could see themselves.

He suggested that they had an egocentric view of the world and were unable to de-centre.

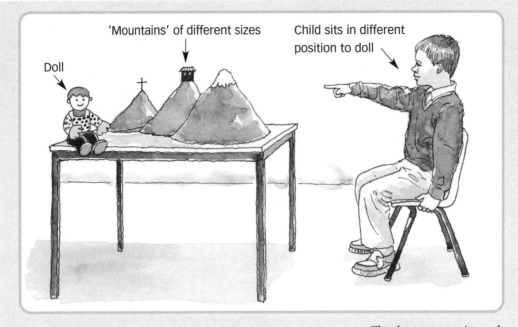

'Mountains' of different sizes

Child sits in different position to doll

Doll

The three mountains task

However, when children were presented with a task involving a boy hiding from a policeman, even three-year-olds were able to say when the boy could be seen by the policeman, even though the viewpoint was different from their own (Hughes, 1975). It seems that tasks that are simpler and more meaningful allow children to show a higher level of competence.

Misleading questions

Donaldson (1978) suggested that children may be misled by, or not understand, the questions being asked.

Case Study 2

Conservation of liquids task

A child was shown two identical beakers, each containing the same amount of water. These were placed in front of the child, who was then asked whether the amount of water in both was the same. When the child was happy that this was the case (after perhaps adjusting small amounts) the experimenter poured the contents from one beaker into a taller, narrower one. The child was then asked whether there was now:

⊃ more water in the new beaker

⊃ more water in the original beaker

⊃ less water in the new beaker, or

⊃ the same amount in both beakers.

Piaget found that up to the age of 6 or 7, children said that there was now more water than before.

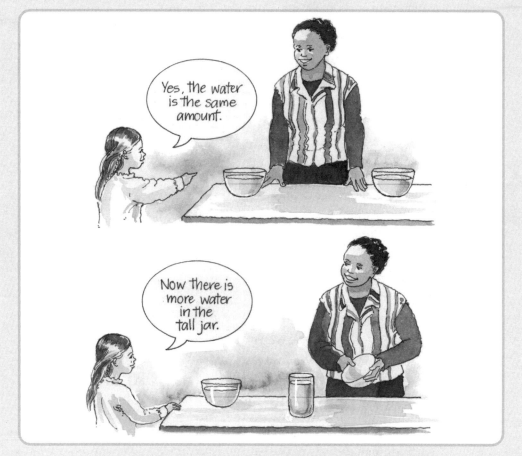

Child performing conservation of liquid task

Perhaps being asked the same question twice led the children to expect the answer to be different. The reason for the changes also seems to be important and when children can make sense of these they are more likely to give the correct answer. When a 'naughty teddy', who was out to make mischief, was used to change things within conservation experiments, many young children were able to conserve. They recognised that changing one aspect of the situation (such as the appearance) did not necessarily mean that other aspects (such as quantity) had also changed (McGarrigle and Donaldson, 1974).

The role of culture

Piaget's tasks were culturally biased because there are differences across cultures in terms of rates of development. Schooling and literacy, in particular, affect rates of cognitive development, and formal operational thinking is not universal.

Studies of illiterate adults in Liberia found that they had difficulty categorising geometric shapes (Irwin and McLaughlin, 1970). This should be an easy task, according to Piaget, as the skill is achieved during the concrete operational stage. However, these adults were able to sort different types of rice successfully. This suggests that their abilities are based on their experiences of learning rather than their maturational level of development. Schooling encourages problem solving that is abstract and decontextualised and for those who do not experience it there is no need for these types of skill to develop.

> ## Activity 3) Adapting tasks

Suppose that you wanted to find out whether two new children in Foundation Stage had the ability to understand the conservation of liquids. How would you adapt Piaget's conservation of liquids task in order to avoid some of the methodological errors?

For comments on this Activity see page 168.

Relevance of Piaget's ideas to the care and education of young children

When Piaget's ideas are applied to the classroom, or early years learning environment, the role of the teacher is to provide an environment that is rich in stimulation for children to explore for themselves, in which they can actively construct their own knowledge (schemas) through their experiences (albeit constrained by social ideologies).

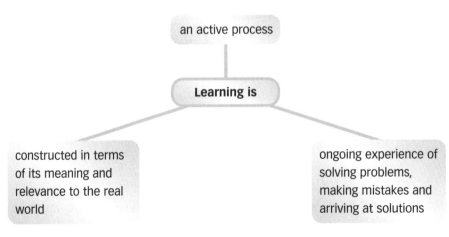

Figure 5.4
Key principles of Piaget's ideas

an active process

Learning is

constructed in terms of its meaning and relevance to the real world

ongoing experience of solving problems, making mistakes and arriving at solutions

Learning environments	
Provide opportunities to construct knowledge through experience	Children need opportunities to construct their own knowledge through their own experiences, rather than being told about things by the teacher. There is less time spent upon teaching particular skills and more emphasis on making learning meaningful. For example, the children might operate a class bank or post office, rather than only doing skill-based numeracy exercises.
Use a particular topic or anchor	Learning and teaching should be centred around a particular topic or 'anchor', which may be a story, a video-clip or situation which is of interest to the children. This will include problems or issues for the children to engage with and resources that can be explored as children decide how to solve a problem. For example, an 'anchor' might be friendship, with the children engaging with problems such as which friends to invite for a sleepover and which not.
Relate something new to what is known	Teaching should involve relating something new to what is already known. Children are expected to learn to read and write in the same gradual way that they learn to talk, without much direct instruction. Learning rather than teaching is stressed and early writing might involve the child describing something familiar to the teacher (perhaps his or her house or neighbourhood) and the teacher writing this on the board or on a large piece of paper.
Use construction kits or toys	Construction kits or toys provide a means for exploration and learning about the properties of objects within a meaningful context. For example, a child may only be able to stick two pieces of Duplo together initially to represent a bus, but the bus has two pieces whereas a car has only one. Therefore, the child is building upon what he already knows (how to connect two pieces of Duplo) in order to solve the problem of representing the relationship of a larger object to a smaller one.

Figure 5.5
Providing different learning environments enhances the learning experience

Lev Vygotsky

(1896–1934)

Vygotsky was an important Russian theoretician who began as a schoolteacher of literature and moved on to become a psychology lecturer in a college of teacher education. Working with colleagues Luria and Leontiev, he created the Vygotskian approach. But Stalin banned his work, as it used some of the assumptions considered to be 'bourgeois pseudo-science'. After his early death from tuberculosis, colleagues and students kept his ideas alive, but it is only since the dissolution of the USSR that Vygotsky's work has become freely available and provoked wide interest.

Vygotsky's approach, like Piaget's, is a **constructivist** one as he sees children as actively constructing their understanding of the world. He drew attention to the external experiences of children, moving away from the Piagetian view of their internal development. His approach is often referred to as **social-cognitive** because it combines elements of cognitive theory (such as Piaget's ideas about children's minds developing through interactions with the world) and social learning theory, which suggests that children learn by watching people model behaviours (Bandura and Walters, 1963). He thought that social interactions with more competent others allow the child to acquire the necessary 'tools' for thinking and learning and that language is one of the most important social tools for shaping the way we think (see Figure 5.6).

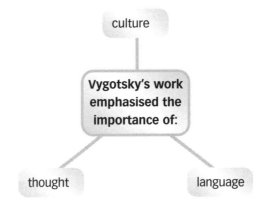

Figure 5.6
Emphasis of Vygotsky's work

Culture

Vygotsky believed that unlearned abilities such as attention, perception and memory are built upon by the culture or context which the child is part of. Culture, he argued, is largely transmitted through language, which is invented by humans. 'Cultural tools' such as language and number systems have to be passed on from generation to generation, as they are complex. Therefore, communication of these tools is an important part of cognitive development.

Vygotsky (1978) provides the example of pointing a finger. Initially, this behaviour begins as a meaningless grasping motion. However, as people react to the gesture, it becomes a movement that has meaning. In particular, the pointing gesture represents an interpersonal connection between individuals, which indicates that one is being singled out.

Language

Vygotsky argued that language begins as external speech in the context of social interactions, with **monologue**, or **overt inner speech**, and then **inner speech**, or **verbal thought** developing later. This gives the child the power to reflect, makes thought possible and eventually controls behaviour. This development proceeds through three stages as shown in Figure 5.7.

Language development		
External speech	0–3 years	The child's use of language is in response to and directed towards the outside world. For example, a child asks for a drink and responds to a question about whether he wants orange or blackcurrant squash.
Egocentric speech (monologue/overt inner speech)	3–7 years	The child thinks aloud. For example, 'I'm putting teddy to bed now and he's going to go straight to sleep.'
Internal speech (inner speech/verbal thought)	7 years onwards	This involves a child thinking silently to him/herself. For example, reflecting upon the day's events at school and the need to take his or her PE kit the following day.

Figure 5.7
Vygotsky's theory of language development

Thought

Thought is therefore shaped by our first communications with others. Once these have been mastered, they become internalised and allow us to think. The language used is part of the culture that invented it and becomes an integral part of that thinking. So if our early carers speak to us in English or French, we learn not only to speak the language but to think in it.

Vygotsky suggested that when children are in a learning environment, they learn best when the material to be learnt is within their grasp but just beyond what they already know. He identified the importance of recognising, therefore, not only what a child knows but also what he or she is capable of understanding at any particular point. Vygotsky called this the **zone of proximal development**.

The zone of proximal development (ZPD)

This is the distance between the child's *actual* developmental level and his or her *potential* developmental level at any one point in time. Full development depends upon adult guidance or collaboration with more competent peers.

At each level or stage, individuals are ready to respond to a particular environment and the people in it, and an interaction occurs between their cognitive structures and the outside world. Therefore, different experiences and cultures shape a child's thinking processes.

Scaffolding

This is the framework which adults or more competent peers provide to enable a child to progress cognitively. (For example, a carer might help a toddler to manipulate shapes in order to post them into a shape-sorting box.)

Scaffolding is most effective when it is within the ZPD but relates to an activity that the child has not yet achieved competence in. The idea is that the adult or peer provides assistance in the form of demonstrations, explanations, questions, corrections and other interactions to allow the child to move from the lower limit of what he or she knows to the upper limits of what he or she is capable of achieving.

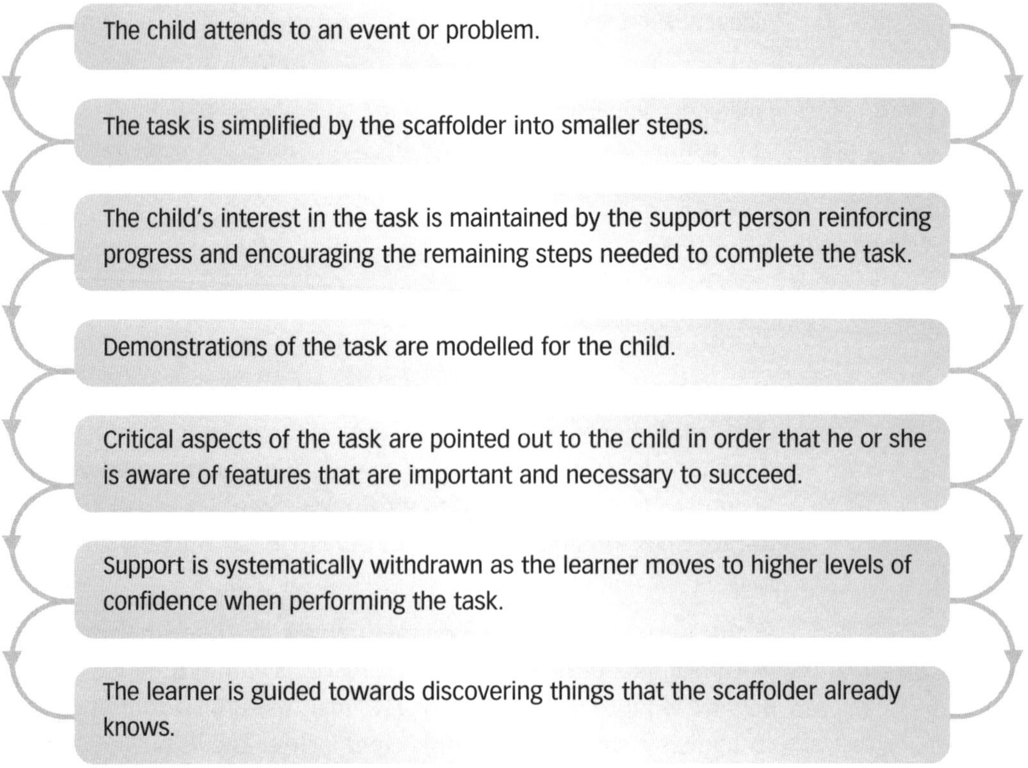

The child attends to an event or problem.

The task is simplified by the scaffolder into smaller steps.

The child's interest in the task is maintained by the support person reinforcing progress and encouraging the remaining steps needed to complete the task.

Demonstrations of the task are modelled for the child.

Critical aspects of the task are pointed out to the child in order that he or she is aware of features that are important and necessary to succeed.

Support is systematically withdrawn as the learner moves to higher levels of confidence when performing the task.

The learner is guided towards discovering things that the scaffolder already knows.

Figure 5.8
Features of scaffolding

Activity 4) Using the concepts of scaffolding

How would you use the concepts of scaffolding to enable a four- year-old child to complete a jigsaw puzzle?

For comments on this Activity see page 169.

Investigations into scaffolding by parents (Pratt, Kerig, Cowan and Cowan, 1988) and older siblings/peers (Azmitia and Hesser, 1993) demonstrated the importance of **sensitive** scaffolding by a more competent other. When scaffolding was responsive to the child's ZPD and sensitive to their needs, the scaffolding was most successful.

There are obvious implications here for teaching and learning relationships including awareness of what the child does know, recognition of effective strategies and finding appropriate ways of allowing him or her to learn more.

Relevance of Vygotsky's ideas to the care and education of young children

Vygotsky's ideas suggest that a child's learning development is affected by the culture, including the family environment, which they are part of. The child's experiences of care and education outside the home usually form part of this culture. Within these experiences:

- ⊃ The curriculum should be designed to maximise interaction between learners and learning tasks. For example, children working together, or in groups, to measure their desk tops.

- ⊃ Children should have opportunities to play, as this allows the developing skills of the child to be practised within safe contexts and providing opportunities to try out new skills and knowledge. For example, when children play at being shopkeeper and customer – developing an understanding of money and their language and social skills – nothing is actually at stake as it would be in a real situation.

- ⊃ Since children can often perform tasks with appropriate help that they cannot do on their own, sensitive scaffolding (where the adult continually adjusts his or her help in response to the child's level of performance) is an effective aspect of teaching, for example, reading.

- ⊃ Assessment methods should take into account the child's current zone of proximal development. What children can do on their own is their actual developmental level and what they can do with help is their potential developmental level. Two children might have the same actual level but given appropriate adult help, one child might be able to solve many more problems than another. Therefore, assessments should take account of both actual and potential levels.

Experiment by Vygotsky (1986)

Two eight-year-olds of average ability were given problems that were a little too difficult for them to solve alone. They were then given help, in the form of hints and leading questions.

With this help, Vygotsky found that one child was able to solve a problem designed for a twelve-year-old and the other reached a nine-year-old's level.

This suggests that some children might not demonstrate their potential unless scaffolded appropriately.

Well-designed instruction should be aimed at a level slightly ahead of what the child can do at the present time in order to draw it towards the next level of learning in the manner of a magnet. Therefore, it is important that the teacher is aware of each child's actual developmental level.

Activity 5) Using scaffolding at different levels

How might a teacher or facilitator provide scaffolding when teaching groups of Year 1 children to play snakes and ladders using a pair of dice?

For comments on this Activity see page 169.

Criticisms of Vygotsky's theory

Whilst there has been considerable research support for aspects of Vygotsky's theory, there have also been a number of criticisms (see Figure 5.9):

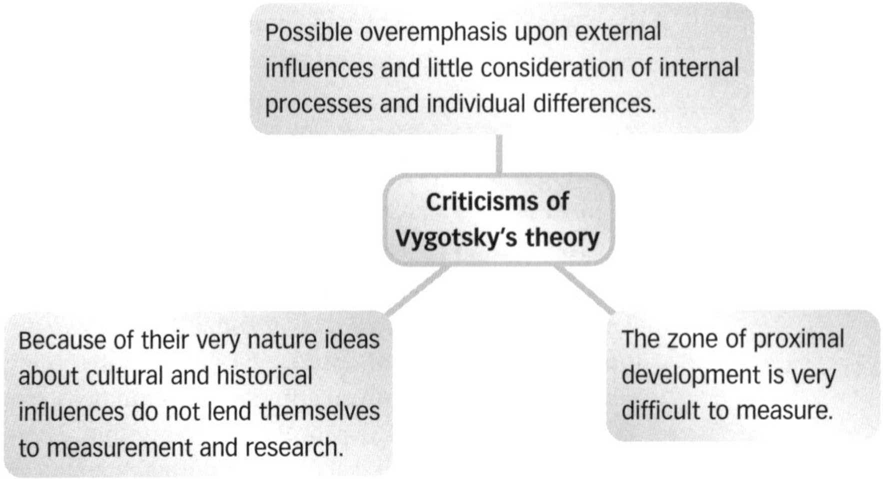

Possible overemphasis upon external influences and little consideration of internal processes and individual differences.

Criticisms of Vygotsky's theory

Because of their very nature ideas about cultural and historical influences do not lend themselves to measurement and research.

The zone of proximal development is very difficult to measure.

Figure 5.9
Criticisms of Vygotsky's theory

Experiences of scaffolding

Think of an example from your own experience of providing scaffolding to enable a child to achieve something he or she could not do without help. Was the scaffolding sensitive? How effective was it?

Piaget and Vygotsky – a summary

A summary of Piaget's and Vygotsky's ideas is shown in Figure 5.10.

Piaget	Vygotsky
Concluded that teaching a child something prevented him or her from learning it on his or her own.	Saw interactions between children and adults within a cultural context as the driving force in cognitive development.
Stressed the readiness idea: a child cannot achieve certain skills until ready to do so. His readiness depends upon his or her stage of development.	Thought that teachers needed to provide demonstrations, explanations and other forms of scaffolding to assist development.
	Emphasised the importance of assessing potential rather than actual abilities.
	Presented a strong argument for the use of challenging instructional materials and methods.

Figure 5.10
A summary of Piaget's and Vygotsky's ideas

Information processing approaches to cognitive development

Information processing approaches do not stem from a single theorist but are based on using the computer as an analogy for the human mind. This is seen as a useful way of understanding cognitive processes, as there are similarities such as encoding information, processing it and storing it for future use. Information processing theorists share the view that the mind, like a digital computer, is a system that uses symbols and works according to certain rules. The assumption is not that humans solve problems or 'think' in exactly the same way as computers but that they both solve complex problems by breaking them down into a series of simpler steps. If this is correct then we can study computers in order to gain insights into the working of the human mind and ways in which cognition develops.

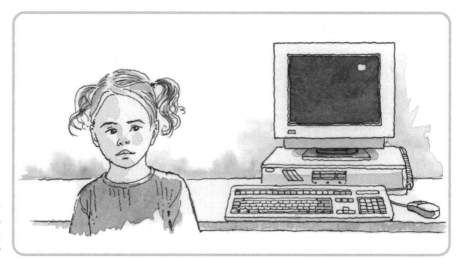

Can a child's mind be compared with a computer?

Cognitive development

We might think of the 'hardware' of the human mind as the physical structure of the brain, including nerves and tissue, and the 'software' as the programmes or strategies we use to deal with the world. Therefore, we need to understand whether there are age-related changes in the basic system and its processing capacity (similar to Piaget's ideas of maturation) and/or to consider the learning needed in order to understand and use the programmes available.

Memory

This is an important part of the computer without which it would be simply a word-processor. Similarly, the human mind depends upon memory in order to learn and develop.

The dominant view of memory is based upon a model proposed by Atkinson and Shiffrin (1968). This is that memory is a theoretical structure and cannot be physically observed within the brain's structure. Three stages are involved in the processing and storage of memory (see Figure 5.11).

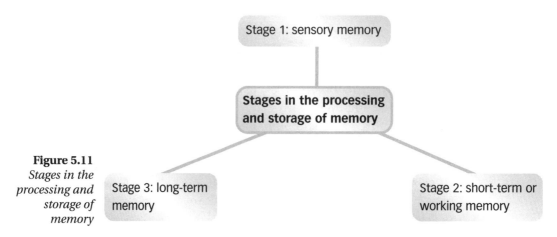

Figure 5.11
Stages in the processing and storage of memory

Stage 1: sensory memory

Stages in the processing and storage of memory

Stage 3: long-term memory

Stage 2: short-term or working memory

Sensory memory represents information in the environment that is experienced through the senses (sight, hearing, smell, taste, touch) and passed to the brain by electrical impulses. The brain then makes sense of these impulses, and in the process of transferring the messages from the senses to the brain a memory is formed. This takes a very short time (approximately half a second for visual information and about three seconds for auditory information).

Children, like adults, are surrounded by sensory stimulation when awake, but the amount of this that is processed is very small.

Activity 7   Awareness

Let your eyes focus upon an object within the room you are in. Now, without moving your eyes become aware of what you can see within your peripheral vision (out of the corners and tops and bottoms of your eyes). You will be aware that there is much more that you could be focusing upon which you are simply not aware of.

Similarly with sounds: if you stop and listen you will become aware of many different sounds in the room. Perhaps you can hear traffic outside, someone moving in another part of the building, your own breathing and so on.

Try this out with what you can feel without moving, or what you can taste or smell.

For comments on this Activity see page 169.

Attention to the information is crucial then if the information is to pass to the next stage. This is most likely if the stimulus is interesting or relates to something familiar.

If attention is not paid then the information will simply be lost.

Stage 2

This is the **short-term**, or **working, memory** (**STM**) and represents what we are thinking about at the present moment. It is a critical part of the memory process because it allows us to process incoming information for storage and to retrieve memories we have already stored. It is, however, very brief (approximately 15 seconds) so if you are attending to the words you are currently reading, they are in your short-term memory but they may be lost (if I ask you to think about your date of birth, for example) and possibly need to be read again.

Short-term memory is also limited in terms of its capacity. Miller (1956) suggested that humans can hold 7 plus or minus 2 chunks of information in the short-term memory at any one time. So if you look up a telephone number (often 6 digits) in the directory you can remember it long enough to dial the number, but will probably have forgotten it by the time you get through. Perhaps this explains also the fact that many of us find it very difficult to remember mobile phone numbers (consisting of 10+ digits). These research findings became known as 'Miller's Magic Seven' as this seemed to be the average number of digits remembered.

Stage 3

This is **long-term memory** (LTM) and represents information stored for longer periods of time, perhaps for a lifetime. This forms the knowledge base of the human mind. It is a complex structure which seems to consist of different types of memories such as those given in Figure 5.12:

Long-term memory comprises:	
Episodic memory	This contains memories of past life events (such as your last birthday or your first day at school).
Procedural memory	This contains stored physical skills or behaviours (such as riding a bike or writing your name).
Semantic memory	This contains non-personal facts (for example, the capital of Australia or the name of the Prime Minister).

Figure 5.12
Constituents of long-term memory

Words that can be easily **visualised** are more likely to be remembered than **abstract** words. So if I read a list of words and ask you to remember as many as possible, you are more likely to remember words that you can 'picture' such as 'balloon', 'river' and 'kitchen' than those which you cannot, such as 'formation', 'reference' and 'summary'.

Retrieval of information from the LTM

This involves **cues**, which allow LTM to be accessed. For example, coming home from work and going upstairs to change may serve as a cue to remind you that you left your missing diary in the bedroom the night before, rather than in the other places you have searched for it.

The best retrieval cues are the same as those present when the information was first encountered or encoded. So being in your bedroom at the same time and in the same situation (or context) as the day before, served as powerful cues to retrieve the memory of putting your diary down there.

Recall and recognition

The difference between **recall** and **recognition** is a significant one, particularly when considering children's learning. Recall involves bringing to mind the information needed, whereas recognition involves being able to select the correct piece of information when presented with others. It might be that when you are spelling a difficult word aloud you need to write it down to see whether it 'looks right'. This allows you to recognise the correct spelling.

Forgetting

According to some theorists, forgetting does not involve actually losing something from our long-term memory. This can only occur if there is damage to the brain. If this is the case, then if we cannot remember something it is either because it was never encoded in the first place (perhaps because we were not attending to it) or because we can no longer retrieve it. So the phone number that we repeated just long enough to enable us to dial is forgotten because it was never transferred to our long-term memory. Probably you still have the first phone number you had when you were a child, stored somewhere in your LTM, but cannot retrieve it. This is probably because of **interference** (all the other phone numbers you have had to learn since then) but you might still recognise it if it was placed with others in a list.

Organisation

The way that material is **organised** affects retrieval. Miller's Magic Seven ignored the fact that we often arrange information to be remembered in different ways, in order to make it easier to remember. So you might remember your mobile number by **chunking** the digits together in twos or threes; for example, 0775860332 then becomes 077, 58, 60, 332. In this way, you are changing the number into four pieces of information rather than ten.

The development of memory

Changes in **processing capacity** may occur as children mature. Perhaps these relate to changes in the physical structure of the brain or increases in speed and efficiency.

Research continues into this area, and work such as that by Kail and Park (1994) supports the theory that there are changes in processing speed and that these are related to some kind of developmental change.

Strategies to aid memory

However, there are other aspects of memory development that occur as a result of children using strategies, or **mnemonics**, such as rhymes (Thirty days hath September, for example), to help them to remember.

> ### Activity 8 Personal strategies that aid memory
>
> Think of a strategy that you use to help you remember something in particular, such as a phone number or the number of days in November. Were you taught this strategy, or did you develop it yourself?

For comments on this Activity see page 170.

The ability to use strategies such as **rehearsal** (repetition; for example look/cover/write/check for spelling), **organisation** (structuring information), **retrieval** (using more explicit cues) and **elaboration** (using association to remember things) increases with age. Young children can be trained to use some of these, but they are less successful than older children, perhaps because of some of the factors outlined below.

Encoding of information and knowledge-base

Age differences in the ability to **encode** information mean that younger children have more limited vocabularies than older children and have a more limited **knowledge-base** about specific events so they may fail to make connections between things in the way that older children do (Brainerd, Kingma and Howe, 1986). So if an adult is given a list of items from a shopping list to remember, he or she would probably sort them into categories such as fruit and vegetables, meat and fish, dairy products, and so on. However, if a six-year-old is given a similar task he or she would probably not do this and would be unable to recall as many items. Even though six-year-olds might be able to classify carrots as vegetables, they do not seem to make connections that identify carrots, potatoes, mushrooms, onions as the vegetables in the list.

Metamemory

Metamemory, or the ability to reflect upon the workings of one's own memory, increases with age. This involves knowing what you do know (such as your own phone number), what you might know (your previous phone number) and what you definitely do not know (the Prime Minister's telephone number).

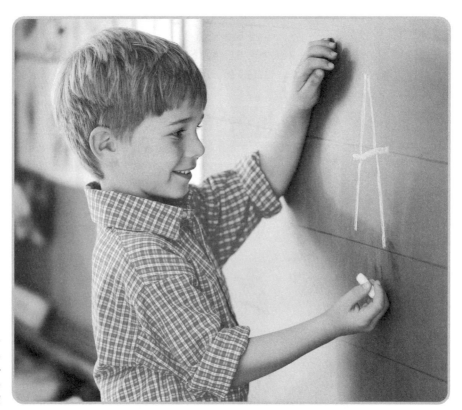

This boy is learning to remember how letters are formed

Developmental theories of information processing

Some theorists such as Robbie Case (1985) suggest that cognitive development is related to increases in the working-memory, or STM, capacity. Case is often described as a neo-Piagetian because he combines aspects of Piaget's theory with information processing concepts. For example, he believes that children become quicker and more efficient at processing information and this allows them to progress to the next stage of development.

Siegler's (1996) model of strategy choice adds an evolutionary perspective to children's cognition, arguing that when faced with a problem, children try a variety of strategies to solve it. They will select these gradually on the basis of speed and accuracy. Which strategies are available at any one point will depend upon the age of the child and the strategies will develop from the simpler ones used by young children to the more sophisticated and complex ones used by older children. This suggests that all children will think differently even when dealing with the same task.

Examples of the means by which practitioners can support young children in learning environments are shown in Figure 5.13.

Applying information processing principles in learning environments	
Gain the learner's attention	This is important. You can do this by perhaps using cues to signal that you are ready to start. Whilst engaged with the learner, keep his or her attention by perhaps moving around the room and varying pitch and speed of voice.
	Do not attempt to maintain children's attention for long periods, as their attention span is not extensive. Although there seem to be no definitive studies measuring attention span in children, it seems that 3 to 4 minutes per year of age is a rough guide. So, a 3-year-old might be expected to concentrate for about 9 minutes and a 5-year-old for about 15 minutes at a time. Obviously, this can vary, not only from child to child but also from activity to activity. Some children who are assumed to be suffering from Attention Deficit Hyperactivity Disorder (ADHD) are still able to pay attention for an extended period of time if the subject is interesting enough, for example, their favourite television programme or video game. Similarly, toddlers may pay attention for longer periods when there are no distractions and the topic is interesting.
	A child's attention span develops in three stages:

	1) Young infants often stare at their mobiles for long periods of time and seem able to ignore other stimuli.
	2) At around 2 years of age toddlers' attention span changes rapidly and spontaneously from one object to another and they rarely play with one toy for an extended period of time.
	3) The school-aged child is able to concentrate for longer periods on a particular task and yet is able to shift this focus when necessary. This is known as selective attention and is required for the child to progress appropriately within educational establishments.
Relate back to things already known	In order to provide something to build upon, you might perhaps talk about the previous lesson on a topic or invite children to recall it as a group.
Pick out important points	By writing important points on the board or on handouts/transparencies, you are encouraging children to attend to these aspects. (This helps to overcome the limitations of sensory memory.)
Organise material	Ensure that material has a logical sequence and progresses from the easiest through to the most difficult.
Encourage categorisation (chunking) of material	Present information in categories. For example, you could present seven groups of seven, rather than 49 separate items. (This helps to overcome the limitations of short-term memory and the fact that only a limited number of chunks of information can be processed at any one time.)
Provide opportunities for both verbal and visual encoding	Although evidence is not conclusive that they are two different systems, it does seem that imaging can help memory.
Include opportunities for children to elaborate upon new information	Connect new information with something already known. This might include a discussion of similarities and differences.
Introduce children to the idea of using encoding when remembering things by devising mnemonics	For material that it is essential to memorise, have fun devising mnemonics with the class in order to encourage deep learning by meaningful association. For example, you could help to support the learning of difficult multiplication tables by associating $7 \times 8 = 56$ with the head teacher's age, or invite the children to find a personal connection such as father's age.

Include repetition	Include repetition within the teaching and learning situation in order to encourage transfer to LTM. Outline, perhaps, the contents of the session beforehand, then engage with children during the session and review at the end. By doing so, there is more chance that the learning will be processed. From time to time it would be useful to review previous learning.
Allow overlearning	This can be achieved through daily repetitions of important numerical facts, for example, or of games and quizzes involving knowledge of basic facts and information.
Arrange for a variety of practice opportunities	This helps the learner to generalise the information so that it can be used outside of the original context within which it was taught.
Help learners become autonomous	Assist children in choosing appropriate learning strategies such as making summaries or asking questions.

Figure 5.13
Supporting young children in learning environments

An evaluation of information processing approaches is given in Figure 5.14.

Evaluation of information processing approaches	
Major strength	A major strength is the way information processing approaches break cognition into separate elements so that each can be thoroughly examined. This can be very useful with conditions such as dyslexia because tests are used to establish the precise problem the child has with reading and then exercises and/or alternative strategies may be suggested to compensate for the deficit. It is also helpful for children and their families to understand precisely where the problem lies and therefore see it as a processing problem rather than a personal failing.
Criticisms	Information processing approaches are often criticised for their biased view of humans in that they take little account of their physical, social and emotional experiences. These are clearly integrated with their mental processes in the real world where, for example, a child's attention may be impossible to gain because he or she is frightened, hungry or angry.
Research findings lack a cohesive framework	As yet, there is no comprehensive information processing theory which links the various approaches together and therefore the research findings lack a cohesive framework.

Figure 5.14
Evaluation of information processing approaches

> **Activity 9** Using principles of information processing

Choose a topic which you want to introduce to the class. Using some of the principles of information processing approaches, make some suggestions about ways in which this could be successfully carried out.

For comments on this Activity see page 170.

Case Study 4

Spontaneous attention

Before speaking to a group of Cert Ed students on a Friday afternoon in November, a guest lecturer began the session by opening a flat, black case and produced pieces of a trumpet, which he proceeded to fit together. He then played a very resounding version of 'Reveille' before putting it all neatly away and launching into a lecture on the history of education. As you can imagine his students were mystified and when they asked him at the end of the session why he had played the trumpet, he replied, 'Spontaneous attention. Remember that when you're in the classroom.' A lesson well learned.

Conclusion

Piaget saw cognitive development as stemming mainly from the child. He stressed the 'readiness' idea, suggesting that a child cannot attain certain abilities until ready to do so. This depends upon the stage of development.

Vygotsky saw interactions between the child and adults/culture as the driving force of cognitive development, so adults need to provide explanations, examples, questions, clues, corrections, and so on, to scaffold/assist this development. Potential must be assessed as well as actual abilities and therefore instructional materials and methods need to be challenging but within reach of the child.

Both Piaget and Vygotsky take a constructivist approach, viewing learning as an active process on the part of the learner.

Information processing approaches use the model of a computer to provide understanding of the way cognition works. Therefore, they stress the importance of processing and storing information.

Discussion Point 1

George

George is six years old and attends a mixed primary school. He struggles to keep up with his peers in both literacy and numeracy and is not popular with his classmates.

1 If we took a Piagetian approach to understanding this boy's cognitive development, how would this help us to provide a suitable learning environment for him?

2 How would Vygotsky's ideas relate to this boy? Outline ways in which his learning might be supported from this perspective.

3 Information processing approaches might provide other insights. Suggest ways in which they would explain George's problems and how they might be applied in the learning situation.

For comments on this discussion point see page 170.

Comments on Activities and Discussion Points

Activity 1 (page 141): Schema for turning on the TV

1 It might be that to turn on your own television, you have to press the red button at the top, but when you decide to use the one at work there is no red button at the top.

2 This unsettles you, as the children are waiting to watch a programme, so you really need to solve this problem (you are in a state of disequilibrium).

3 Perhaps you try pressing the button that is at the top (assimilation) even though it is not red, to see what happens.

4 However, if this does not work, you may try the other buttons or look for a switch elsewhere to turn the television on.

5 Eventually, you discover that there is a switch on the side that has to be pressed in order to use the television (accommodation).

6 Your schema for turning on televisions now includes more information that may be used in future and you return to a more balanced state (equilibrium).

Activity 2 (page 145): Piaget in action

	Behaviour	Age	Stage	Ability
1	Child stirs wooden blocks in plastic saucepan.	18 months	Sensorimotor	Beginning of symbolic play
2	Child brings his favourite toy for Mummy to play with when she is feeling tired.	2–4 years (may be older depending upon experience)	Pre-operational	Egocentrism
3	Child believes that the car is covered up at night because it feels cold.	2–3 years	Pre-operational	Animism
4	Child is happy to have smaller, thicker slice of chocolate cake when sister has larger, thinner one.	7–11 years	Concrete operational	Conservation
5	Child uses pocket money to buy magazine and chocolate but struggles with addition and subtraction at school.	7–11 years	Concrete operational	Ability to solve concrete rather than abstract problems
6	Child is able to sort and classify football cards according to teams, leagues or players' positions.	7–11 years	Concrete operational	Able to understand classification hierarchies
7	Child engages in discussion with family about the pros and cons of war.	11+ years	Formal operational	Able to think in abstract terms

Activity 3 (page 150): Adapting tasks

1 Perhaps small cartons of milk or juice could be used, as children are aware that these are equal and will not need to be asked. You might then pour these into different shaped/sized party beakers and ask the children whether they now both have the same amount.

2 The important thing here is that the children should not be asked twice whether the amounts are equal and that the problem is related to a meaningful situation – one that can be related to the real world which they are part of.

Activity 4 (page 155): Using the concepts of scaffolding

1 First the child must be attending to the jigsaw puzzle, perhaps spontaneously, or the practitioner may have drawn his or her attention to it. Alone, the child may be unable to work out how the pieces fit together, so needs assistance.

2 The carer may suggest that the child looks for corner pieces and show one to the child.

3 Next, the carer may suggest that the child now looks for other edge (straight) pieces, beginning with those that match the colours or pattern of one of the corner pieces.

4 The child may choose some pieces and try to fit them together and on his or her third attempt finds a piece that fits.

5 The carer praises the child and gives encouragement to look for some more.

6 The child does so, but is unable to find any more and becomes frustrated.

7 The carer then selects two pieces and places them close together before asking the child whether these two might fit together. When they do, the child is pleased, smiles and continues to look for more pieces.

8 The carer continues to give words of encouragement and is ready to help if the child gets stuck, but he or she is beginning to understand how this jigsaw works and needs less assistance progressively until he or she is actually working alone.

Activity 5 (page 156): Using scaffolding at different levels

1 The teacher or facilitator will not need to provide much support or guidance to children who are already able to remember number combinations and perform mental arithmetic competently, as they will be able to add the numbers together and move the counter the correct number of places.

2 Children who are unable to do this could be prompted to count the numbers on the dice using simple addition techniques (such as counting all the spots individually and holding up their fingers to show how many spots there are). Modelling might be used to show the children how to do this slowly and methodically.

3 This support would be needed less as the children become more competent and take over the counting themselves. The facilitator has worked within the zone of proximal development to teach them something outside of it.

Activity 7 (page 159): Awareness

The important thing here is that you become aware that there is far more **sensory information** available than you are aware of at any one moment. What you are aware of depends upon what you are focusing upon or attending to at that moment. Without this, there will be no sensory memory or possibility of storage. Obviously it would be impossible to process all of the incoming information, so the brain attends to that which seems the most significant.

Activity 8 (page 161): Personal strategies that aid memory

You may have identified some very personal ways in which you use these strategies (or mnemonics) such as remembering your mobile number in terms of someone's date of birth. You may also have identified some commonly used mnemonics such as Richard Of York Gave Battle In Vain for remembering the colours of the rainbow or the rhyme for the number of days in a month. Those of you who were reared within a different culture from the United Kingdom may have used different ones.

Activity 9 (page 166): Using principles of information processing

1 The attention of the class can be gained by the practitioner clapping, speaking more loudly or standing up, for example.

2 The teacher might then start by talking about where the children live and where the school is in relation to this. He or she might then move on to when their homes were built or who lived in them previously. The aim is to jog the children's memory about things they already know in order to build new information onto it.

3 Important facts could be written on the board or displayed on an OHT, perhaps including pictures, maps or diagrams as well as text. Children could be encouraged to discuss aspects of these facts, such as when their house was built and how this compares with the rest of the class.

4 Basic facts and information should be logically organised and 'chunked' where possible, for example, types of houses, types of building materials, and local facilities, rather than just a flow of information. These facts could be repeated and the children encouraged to learn them, and a quiz held at the end of the topic.

5 Children could be helped to design a simple questionnaire for their parents, about their experiences of the area they live in.

Discussion Point 1 (page 167): George

1 Piaget's approach would suggest that George is in the pre-operational stage of development and, therefore, has not yet learned to de-centre. This might account for his difficulties:

⊃ with numbers (where aspects of problems remain the same whilst others change)

⊃ with language (again where the word might begin with the same letter/s but be different in other respects)

⊃ and with other children (still egocentric).

The fact that most of his peers are already more competent might also suggest that George's basic schemas for carrying out these operations are not yet adequate for dealing with these problems. So his understanding needs to be built up so that he is able to do this. Then assimilation and accommodation will allow him to expand his schemas. Perhaps he is currently dealing with his sense of disequilibrium by ignoring the problem because he does not have enough knowledge to build upon.

Providing situations in which George encounters demonstrations of conservation would help him to acquire this ability, but they should be 'hands on' demonstrations and anchored in a topic that has real-world relevance.

2 Vygotsky's theory suggests that George should be included in group work so that interaction between himself and other learners is encouraged (peer collaboration and scaffolding). Incidentally, although Vygotsky focused on cognitive development, becoming part of a group in the classroom would probably also help with George's social interactions and this might encourage greater integration outside as well. Play might be used to allow him to safely rehearse his developing abilities, and sensitive scaffolding by teachers and other adults should be used to help him perform the tasks he is not currently able to. Perhaps the teaching is not within George's ZPD so he is not able to grasp it at present. Therefore, it is necessary to find out what he can do and what he might be capable of doing with support.

3 Information processing approaches would address George's problem in a systematic way by assessing each of the areas, such as whether he is paying attention in the first place, and how well he is encoding the information. Perhaps it would be useful to present pictorial and visual material alongside verbal information to allow for more opportunities for processing it in STM and transferring it to LTM. George would be encouraged to connect the new information with what he already knows and to repeat the important points regularly. He would also be presented with well-organised teaching materials and allowed plenty of opportunities for practising new knowledge in different contexts. For example, if he learned to add single digits this could be practised in number games, PE scores and post office games.

References and further reading

Atkinson, R. and Shiffrin, R. (1968), 'Human Memory: A proposed system and its control processes', in Spence, K. and Spence, J. (eds) *The Psychology of Learning and Motivation: Advances in research and theory* (Vol. 2). New York: Academic Press

Azmitia, M. and Hesser, J. (1993), 'Why siblings are important agents of cognitive development: A comparison of siblings and peers', *Child Development*, 63(2), pp430–44

Baillargeon, R. (1987), 'Object permanence in very young infants', *Developmental Psychology*, 23, pp655–64

Bandura, A. and Walters, R. (1963), *Social Learning and Personality Development*. New York: Holt, Rinehart and Winston

Brainerd, C., Kingma, J. and Howe, M. (1986), 'Spread of encoding and the development of organisation in memory', *Canadian Journal of Psychology*, 40, pp203–23

Bjorklund, D. (2000), *Children's Thinking: Developmental function and individual differences.* Belmont: Wadsworth

Case, R. (1985), *Intellectual Development: Birth to adulthood.* New York: Academic

Cowan, N. (ed.) (1997), *The Development of Memory in Childhood.* London: London University College Press

Donaldson, M. (1978*), Children's Minds.* London: Fontana

Gagne, R. (1985), *The Conditions of Learning* (4th edn). New York: Holt, Rinehart and Winston

Hughes, M. (1975), 'Hiding from the Policeman', in Donaldson, M. (1978) *Children's Minds.* London: Fontana

Irwin, M. and McLaughlin, K. (1970), 'Ability and preference in category sorting by mano schoolchildren and adults', *Journal of Social Psychology*, 82, pp15–24

Kail, R. and Park, Y. (1994), 'Processing time, articulation time, and memory span', *Journal of Experimental Child Psychology*, 57, pp281–91

McGarrigle, J. and Donaldson, M. (1974), 'Conservation Accidents', *Cognition*, 3, pp341–50

Miller, G. (1956), 'The Magical Number Seven, plus or minus two: Some limits on our capacity for processing information', *Psychological Review*, 63, pp81–97 [available online from *Classics in the History of Psychology*]

Pratt, M., Kerig, P., Cowan, P. and Cowan, C. (1988), 'Mothers and fathers teaching 3-year-olds: Authoritative parenting and adult scaffolding of young children's learning', *Developmental Psychology*, 24, 6, pp832–9

Siegler, R. (1996), *Emerging Minds: The process of children's thinking.* New York, Oxford University Press

Spence, K. and Spence, J. (eds) (1968), *The Psychology of Learning and Motivation: Advances in research and theory* (Vol. 2). New York: Academic Press

Vygotsky, L. (1978), *Mind in Society.* Cambridge, MA: Harvard University Press

Vygotsky, L. (1986; original work published 1934), *Thought and Language* (A. Kozulin, Trans.). Cambridge, MA: MIT Press

Wadsworth, B. (1996), *Piaget's Theory of Cognitive and Affective Development* (5th edn). White Plains, NY: Longman

Useful websites

⊃ http://education.indiana.edu/~cep/courses/p540/piagsc.html

This provides an overview of Piaget's theory.

⊃ http://www.piaget.org/links.html

This website has many links to materials related to Piaget, Vygotsky and constructivism.

⊃ http://129.7.160.115/inst5931/Vygotsky_Analyzes_Piaget.html

This provides an analysis of Piaget's developmental theory by Vygotsky.

Communication and language development

6

Iain MacLeod-Brudenell

The purpose of this chapter is to encourage you to reflect on the development of language and communication in young children. Communication and language have been linked throughout this chapter because we believe that 'language' on its own is too narrow a term to define the means by which children develop skills in communication.

This chapter addresses the following areas:

- ⊃ introduction to the theory of language
- ⊃ language and communication
- ⊃ babies and language
- ⊃ development in language: the early years
- ⊃ the role of parents
- ⊃ accent, dialect and grammar
- ⊃ bilingualism.

After reading this chapter you should be able to:

1 question and reflect upon the development of children's language and communication skills

2 recognise the importance of observation in planning support for children's individual language and communication needs

3 reflect upon current methods and modify practice in the light of your new learning

4 make informed reflections upon recent issues in language and communication within your selected area of educare provision.

The list of issues addressed is by no means exhaustive and provides starting points for reflection on theory and practice rather than detailed specific information, which may be readily accessed elsewhere.

Introduction to the theory of language

Most children use speech to:

- ⊃ express ideas
- ⊃ communicate needs
- ⊃ convey desires
- ⊃ give instructions.

Language is often regarded as being synonymous with the spoken word; this is to deny the use of more visual forms of language such as signing.

How do children learn language?

We do not know exactly how children learn language. The development of language, how it is acquired, how it is used and how children learn language continues to be the focus of much research. Early attempts to explain children's acquisition of speech and of language focused largely on the role of imitation. It has been argued that this is the most natural way to view language development, as babies appear to have an innate ability to imitate sounds. The development from sounds and sound sequences towards language can be seen to be a logical progression as children experience wider opportunities to use language. Reward for correct imitation has figured prominently in the behaviourist approach (Pavlov and Skinner). The behaviourist approach in its most rigorous interpretation held the view that babies are equipped with biological reflexes and all that follows is learned. This extreme approach is now given little credibility but does form a basis for discussion.

In your previous study you will have had opportunities to consider the range of factors that influence children's development and you may be familiar with what is often called the 'nurture / nature debate'. This term is used to indicate two very different perspectives within the study of child development. Theories propose views regarding the effects of genetic inheritance (nature) or contextual factors (nurture) on various aspects of child development. Language development is no exception in this search for answers. You may find that your approach lies between the two views.

Biological, or innate, theory: Chomsky and Slobin

An interesting starting point for reflection would be to consider the biological, or innate, theory, initially proposed by Chomsky (1957) and to relate this to your own experience with children. This theory is based on the principle that the brain has an inbuilt facility for language and that human beings are genetically programmed to develop language. The theory sought to provide an explanation for the means by which a baby develops language skills. Chomsky's theory thus links language skills to the process of maturation. It emphasises the biological control of language development and dismisses contextual factors. However, Chomsky does indicate that in order to trigger this innate capacity for language, children need to hear language spoken. The importance of language as an activity is stressed, rather than the specific language spoken by those in contact with the child. Slobin, who extended Chomsky's approach, noted that babies and very young children respond to language sounds and sound sequences, which he termed operating principles. Research appears to go some way to support this view. Babies do initially respond to sound, tone, intonation and rhythm regardless of the language spoken. This would appear to be a logical answer to the question of how language develops; however, if we were pre-programmed to learn language then all children would learn language in the same way, regardless of the culture in which they were born. It appears that this is not the case.

Cognitive models: Vygotsky and Piaget

Biological models of language development stress the innate ability of children to acquire language; cognitive models focus more on the relationship between the development of children's thinking skills and language development. In Chapter 4, the thoughts of Vygotsky and Piaget on cognitive development are expounded. Their cognitive-related models viewed the acquisition of language in the same way as the acquisition of other areas of knowledge. In terms of language, the approach taken by Piaget differs from Vygotsky in one essential aspect. Piaget considered language development to be primarily an egocentric activity and that the role of the adult was primarily to provide a challenging environment which would stimulate learning.

Heuristic play

There has been a resurgence of interest in Piaget's approach to the role of the adult in early language development, particularly in what has become popularly known as heuristic play.

Heuristic play involves babies and young children exploring a range of objects that will stimulate physical and cognitive development without adult intervention. Goldschmied and Jackson (1994:89) provided babies and children under the age of two with a range of everyday objects to explore, termed a 'treasure basket'. Observers noted that the language that emerged in these contexts was secondary and incidental to the activity; this supports Piaget's approach to language as being a means of children 'thinking out loud', rather than of communicating with others. Heuristic play does appear to encourage egocentric rather than social behaviour, although this does depend upon the context, the other experiences of the children and the nature of the objects that are presented for their

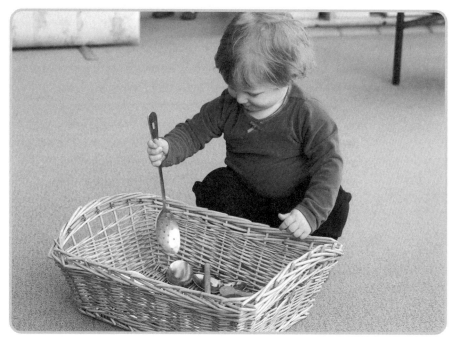

Heuristic play prompts secondary language, e.g. 'this feels hard'

exploration. In many ways, heuristic play presents Piaget's principles quite neatly. The emphasis in heuristic play is upon exploration. In heuristic play, by removing adult influence and interference from an activity, the child is provided with opportunities to become deeply immersed in an activity outside of a social framework. That is not to say that this form of play is not valuable. It most certainly is. Children who are offered this opportunity demonstrate deep and long periods of concentration, and are adept at making choices and decisions.

To Piaget, language was quite separate from actions that led to reasoning. Language is viewed as a system of symbols for representing the world. Piaget's approach would view talking to children in order to explain things before they were at an appropriate stage of understanding as futile. Critics of this approach consider that children's eagerness to communicate is given insufficient acknowledgement and that gauging the precise readiness of children to learn particular skills is thwart with difficulty.

Language takes place within a social framework

Vygotsky's approach takes note of some of the issues raised by Piaget's concentration on the child as a lone individual learner. Vygotsky viewed language as taking place within a social framework and considered that the role of the adult was to actively stimulate in order to support and extend children's learning. Some of the observations made by Vygotsky can be viewed as common sense approaches, which are verified by any practitioner working with young children. To emphasise the part played by the social context of learning language, Vygotsky notes the part played by other and older children in modelling language in a child's development of language and communication skills.

Unlike Piaget, who separates the processes of speech and thought, Vygotsky sees them as being inextricably linked.

For young children, speech is used at first to communicate, to make and share meanings. Later it becomes a tool of thought. By this, he meant that language itself could change the way in which children think and learn. A starting point for reflection on this key issue would be to consider your own view of the relationship between thought and language. Is it possible for young children to talk without thinking? Is it possible for them to think without talking? At first sight, this may appear easily answered, but if one considers children who cannot verbalise or make verbal communication the issue appears more clouded. Does speech have to be audible; can ideas and thoughts be spoken internally?

Inner speech is an essential link between language and thought

Vygotsky believed that in the earliest stages of speech, children talk aloud to themselves and practitioners who work with very young children will verify that this is often the case. Often this talk will involve descriptions of what they are doing. Vygotsky sees this inner speech as an essential link between language and thought in the young child. Inner speech becomes internalised as children become more aware of what they are thinking.

That both of these approaches to learning language are essential in the development of speech is not disputed; it is the degree to which context influences cognition that appears to be the primary focus of debate. It may be argued that heuristic play, 'inner speech' and social aspects of speech provide the basis for language development.

Adult scaffolding, learning and children's language: Bruner

One of the most influential theorists in the area of language development, Bruner focused his early research on the relationship between adult scaffolding, learning and children's language. You will recognise the influence of Bruner in much of the content of this chapter. Key aspects of Bruner's approach are located in the linkage between language and communication and the encouragement of children's understanding of how language works. The holistic approach to language includes visual cues, gestures and body language, turn-taking and the conventions of social use of language.

> ## Activity 1 Language theory

1 Which aspects of this brief discussion of language theory do you find reflect your current perceptions of language development?

2 Which aspects reflect your experience with children?

3 Make notes of your thoughts and revisit these after reading the rest of the chapter to see if there has been any change in your understanding.

Playing with words

Bruner talks about children 'playing with words'. Between 2 and 3 years of age children may use the sound and the meaning of words in a playful way. They may take a familiar rhyme and extend the context of the rhyme whilst using the same format and the same meter.

Another example of playing with words will be familiar to those working with young children in nursery and school: children's jokes. Play with words can extend to early experiments with jokes even with children as young as 2 years of age.

Case Study 1

Children using the sound and meaning of words in a playful way

Henry (aged 2 years) took the following rhyme, which was taught to him by his grandfather, and changed the words to fit a wide range of situations:

'Sausage in the pan, sausage in the pan, sizzle, sizzle, sizzle, sizzle, sausage in the pan.'

When extended to bath time, this became:

'Henry in the bath, splishy splashy ...'

And to his baby sister's sleeping time:

'Poppy in the bed ...'

Following his experiments with changing words to make new rhymes, Henry began to use words with a similar sound but with a different meaning in a humorous way. For example, when Henry's grandmother dropped the gravy powder, she said, 'Oh no, granny dropped the gravy!' Henry responded with 'granny dropped the baby!' This became a joke between them that lasted for several weeks.

1 What does this form of playing with words demonstrate?

2 Note any similar examples of children playing with words – at any age. What conditions support this use of language?

Language and communication

Practitioners in early care and education settings know from their practice that there are increasing numbers of young children who do not have confidence in using language and have delayed development in language skills.

Delayed development in language skills

These children often display difficulty in communicating through language. Conditions such as 'glue ear' or other illnesses that affect hearing are common in young children and this may impact on a child's confidence in speaking. Other physical factors may also impinge on confidence in speaking. There may be links between premature birth and a physical difference that causes delay in maturation and difficulty in communicating through speech. In some cases, young children may have temporary hearing loss. The stage of language development when this temporary setback occurs is crucial and the ability to communicate effectively in language may be hindered. Communication at these points may rely more heavily on gesture to emphasise meaning. Crucially, the ability to communicate through gesture may also be insufficiently developed to compensate for oral language when temporary hearing loss occurs.

In the longer term, some children, for example those with a permanent hearing impairment, may find that communication may not be so readily achievable through the use of spoken language. The absence of auditory response obviously limits their awareness of the sound of spoken language. Where hearing impairment is diagnosed at an early stage and children are encouraged to speak and sign simultaneously, fewer problems are found in communication skills in later childhood.

Non-verbal indicators of confidence

Young children whose speech is difficult to understand may have few problems at home where adult family members and other children are able to 'translate' their words. Problems arise when such children move to out-of-home settings, particularly where there is no support from speech therapists. After initial frustration at not being understood when speaking, children may rely more on gesture when trying to communicate. It is interesting to note that theories of language acquisition tend to focus on spoken language and largely ignore the part played within language development of the role of non-verbal indicators of confidence and, indeed, of body language and gesture. Children communicate their earliest needs through gesture, inflection and emphasis of sounds. As they become more skilled in articulating sounds and using words, gesture may be used less frequently. There appears to be a strong link between the modelling provided by adults and the use of gesture to accompany speech. Tone, volume and emphasis in speech patterns also appear to be acquired in children at an early age. Toddlers will often use the same intonations and phrases that have been modelled by an adult. Children born with a visual impairment will rely on auditory cues, intonation, and the stress placed on words.

Case Study 2

Responding to non-verbal indicators

For many years, a practitioner worked with children who were learning English as an additional language. During that time, he began to notice that there were non-verbal indicators of confidence that would help him to judge a child's readiness to speak on a one-to-one basis or in a small group activity. Children would demonstrate a readiness to use language before attempts were made to communicate verbally. This could be seen through their body language and the eye contact that was made during the often one-way conversations. The practitioner was able to respond to these triggers in order to encourage children to try out using words. This knowledge helped him to plan activities that were most likely to make children feel comfortable enough to talk.

1 Note the ways in which a child demonstrates confidence through body language; for example through eye contact and the way in which the body is positioned in relation to you when the child responds to questions. Do you recognise any difference in the way the child responds when he or she knows the answer?

2 If you work with children with differing needs, in their ability to communicate, note how they reveal confidence.

Awareness of children's understanding

Children's readiness to speak may be indicated by a response to a thought expressed aloud by the adult.

Case Study 3

A child demonstrates understanding ahead of her speech

After a shopping trip, Courtney (13 months) was lifted from her pushchair and went into the kitchen.

'Oh dear, I've left the door open,' said her mother.

Courtney turned around, went back down the corridor and closed the door. This was the first time that her mother recognised that Courtney's understanding was far ahead of her speech.

It has been shown that context is crucial in helping children to understand meaning. Very young children only need to recognise one or two words in context and they can grasp meaning.

Case Study 4

Joining in a conversation without using words

Flora (17 months) screamed when startled by a squirrel dashing past the window. For the rest of the morning, whenever she saw squirrels through the window she screamed and clung to her grandmother. When Flora's aunt came home, the grandmother began to recount what had happened; Flora pointed to the window and shrieked. They were in no doubt that Flora was joining in the conversation.

Adults go through similar stages of language acquisition when on holiday abroad. They will begin by picking out commonly used words in familiar contexts – the bar or restaurant – progressing to experimenting with one or two words and then, depending upon whether the response is positive or negative, attempt more complex sentences in a wider range of situations. Gesture may initially replace and later accompany such requests.

Case Study 5

Recognising different pronunciation

When George was 23 months old, he was able to discriminate between accents. His mother and grandmother both used a 'flat' 'a' in words such as 'bath' and 'grass'. George's father and grandfather both used a 'long' 'a'. Initially, George used a 'flat' 'a' when saying these words. He then switched to a 'long' 'a', as he began to be aware of his gender. He appeared to be using language to identify with males in the family. This continued for some weeks. He then used both forms of pronunciation and has finally settled with a 'flat' 'a'.

The recognition of different ways of saying words is not uncommon. Many children in this country learn more than one language. Some do so from birth, living in homes where more than one language is spoken.

In the case study, George demonstrates another facet of learning a language: the role of gender in the ways in which words are pronounced. There may also be influences on children's attitudes to the use of language that are related to gender.

The ways we use words

We learn words and how to use them at the same time. Children not only learn a word but also any emphasis that may accompany the use of that word to convey subtle differences in meaning. The degree of urgency may be expressed through volume or tone; questioning may be indicated by intonation. Contextual factors are very important in this respect.

Family and cultural patterns of language are naturally acquired at the earliest stages of childhood. Familiarity with out-of-home experiences through contact with other children will not only extend the range of language, but also the use of gestures for communication. The expectations of adults in out-of-home settings for children to conform or adapt to speech conventions will also extend the range of language and communication skills. As adults, we adapt our style and forms of speech (we change the **register**) to match the context in which we use talk. The speech register used in a courtroom will be quite different to that in the pub. The use of register may be further illustrated by comparing the forms of language used during a wedding, where the formal legal or religious language will differ markedly from the family chatter at the end of the ceremony. Children will begin to recognise the changes in register adopted by adults in different settings if they are exposed to a variety of contexts in which they are used – and if adults are skilled in using them. It is not uncommon for children as young as 2 years of age to be able to recognise that adults switch registers in different settings. This may become increasingly obvious in their role play.

Case Study 6

Children match adults in body language, tone and intonation

Practitioners in a nursery were using face painting in a session designed to raise children's self-awareness. Children were asked to paint each other's faces and their language behaviour closely followed that used by staff when applying face paint to the children, including the use of body language, tone and intonation.

1 Have you noticed any similar instances of children copying adult language behaviour in your workplace setting?

2 Write your own account and make an analysis of the things that children are copying.

Body language

It will be seen from this discussion that communication is far wider in scope than spoken language, not just for children with physical differences that prevent spoken language, or conditions that may impede it, such as hearing impairment. Body language to emphasise communication may be formalised as signing, but it is more commonly used in our everyday efforts to communicate meaning to children as well as adults. The importance of body language in everyday communication is often not fully realised. Children are very aware of body language and often use it as a non-verbal cue for action or response. Confusion arises when the spoken language and the body language appear to give conflicting messages. As adults we can recognise this in some of our professional interactions with other adults. The experience may begin in early childhood, for example, when an adult appears through their spoken language to be interested, while their body language gives the opposite impression. Children appear to give messages conveyed by body language precedence over spoken language.

Use of gestures and cues

Language skills and communication skills are interdependent and not mutually exclusive. Sometimes gestures replace rather than emphasise the spoken word.

In their research on language use by toddlers, Acredolo and Goodwyn (1997) noted that gestures were used to replace words even where there was no direct association. Acredolo noted her daughter's use of blowing to represent fish. This gesture was based on Acredolo blowing her daughter's fish mobile (and was in contrast to the use by many toddlers of a popping, blowing bubbles movement of the mouth to represent fish). Gestures relate to experience and contexts and many different signs were uncovered in this research. A key aspect of the use of gestures is that adults recognise and respond to them. Without such recognition, the use of gesture would be abandoned. The use of gesture to replace words diminishes as toddlers become more confident in their use of speech.

Adults usually recognise cues from their children. This appears to help a toddler's language development, particularly when response to gesture is coupled with spoken language.

Young children learn to decipher the nuances of messages conveyed through gesture. Such gestures are often culturally located: they may convey a different meaning from one cultural setting to another. Beckoning with the hand may indicate in one cultural sign language that the child should approach, but in another it may mean that the child should go back. The gap between children who do recognise cues and those who do not appears to widen at the age of 5 or 6. By the age of 6 most children will have knowledge of an extensive range of visual cues which accompany and enhance communication through speech; they may use many cues but also recognise many more. There are exceptions to this; children with autism may have more profound difficulties in learning to communicate and also in reading non-verbal cues, the gesture and body language that add subtlety to a request or instruction. Children who have an autistic spectrum disorder (ASD) also have great difficulty in recognising cues and responses from other children, and their apparent lack of interest can have a negative effect on friendship formation. Eye contact is usually maintained between children and practitioners when engaged in activities and it is usually only as children acquire more awareness of the social conventions of a cultural group that this contact diminishes. An exception to this generalisation will be recognised by those practitioners working with young children who have an ASD and who find making eye contact more problematic.

Producing speech

The act of speaking requires complex physical coordination. An inability to control a group of muscles can result in quite marked differences in pronunciation and clarity of speech. There are over 100 muscles within the mouth that are used during the act of speaking and so it is not surprising that even minor difficulties may emerge. You will become more aware of the difficulties faced by children with this problem if you concentrate on the movements of your own mouth when forming words. Speaking is like riding a bike, but more complex. We make automatic reactions without thinking of the number of distinct and separate tasks that are required. The range of physical tasks involved in speaking is often not fully realised; we take it for granted and expect others to manage in the same way. Children with physical disabilities can have a harder task to learn to speak when their disability directly affects their ability to form sounds through control of their mouth and tongue. It will also often mean that they will take longer to learn to talk. This may be because they find not only the control of tongue and mouth muscles difficult but also the interpretation and decoding of sounds. For some children with learning disabilities, the use of gesture or signing alongside speech will provide more ready access to communication and interaction with others.

Activity 2   Bodily contact

No discussion of gesture and body language in communication would be complete without raising the contentious issue of bodily contact. In recent years contact between practitioners and children has become culturally inappropriate.

1   Note occasions when touching is used to emphasise communication between adults.

2   Note occasions when touching is used to emphasise communication between an adult and child. In a setting where young children come from a range of cultural backgrounds it may be useful to discuss this aspect of communication with colleagues and parents.

Babies and language

Where does it all start? A child's interaction with language begins at birth. It may even be argued that it begins before birth as the baby is exposed in the womb to the sound of the mother's and others' voices.

Babies respond to the human face

Conversation could be said to start as soon as the baby responds to the mother's face. Research appears to indicate that most babies respond to the human face, and it would seem that there might be genetic reasons for this phenomenon. Those of us who have had regular contact with babies will recognise that babies' response to the human face is confirmed by everyday observation.

Close observation of the interactions between a mother and baby who bond well reveals another level of communication that is far subtler and is sensitive to the slightest signal. Language that accompanies such interaction, sound and gesture, forms the basis for social interaction. The interaction between babies and adults has been likened to a form of conversation. This view is justified when one considers that a number of actions adopted by babies are present in conversational interactions of older children and adults. Babies are very aware of the non-verbal cues provided by adults through facial expression. They appear to control the pace of conversation by maintaining eye contact or by dropping their gaze. Either babies or adults may initiate the conversation; however, when babies react to the gaze of an adult and fail to receive a response they lapse into silence. Babies and toddlers need to be able to get adults' attention.

(For further information on this fascinating aspect of communication, see Trevarthen and Murray (1993).)

Adult-led conversation with babies will follow a pattern familiar to parents: initiating interaction through prompts, waiting for a response, allowing time for a response from the baby and then extending the interaction through eye contact or physical stimulation. Between 6 and 14 months of age most babies will produce a wide range of repeated and non-repeated sounds. These sounds and combinations of sounds will be used to represent familiar objects, animals and people. Sounds that are repeated will approximate ever more closely to accurate representation of recognisable words. The range of sounds and 'words' will be culturally located.

Use of songs, rhymes, facial and body gestures

Differences as well as similarities in approaching such conversations will be found in different cultural and social groups. Songs, rhymes, facial and body gestures are used in a variety of ways in different cultural groups, but are commonly used to build and reinforce bonding between the baby and primary caregivers. They may also be seen as a means of inducting babies into the distinct and particular traditions of the culture into which the child is born. Babies who have a rich and concentrated experience of focused speech appear to develop more rapidly in some aspects of their language. This is particularly noticeable in the range and use of communication gestures.

The key to providing an enabling environment is for adults to make opportunities for talk, to make time to talk *with* babies, not just to talk *to* them. Some adults find it difficult to talk with babies; they feel awkward or self-conscious. Playful use of sounds initiated by the baby may be a means of drawing in and involving the adult. The response is crucial. Without response the conversation will fail, as does any conversation. The type of response is equally, if not more, important. As babies explore their range of sounds, they will respond to adult interest. It is important for those working with babies to closely observe how babies develop their language and how body language and gesture are used to reinforce meaning. Observation of the relationship between spoken language and body language is crucial. It forms an essential aspect of communication throughout life. In your observations it would be useful to note if the words used by adults are supported or confirmed by their body language.

Activity 3 · Recognising patterns in language and communication development

1 Do you recognise any patterns emerging in the way children acquire language and communication skills?
2 Are there times when children are particularly receptive to language?
3 Are there contexts or places that you have noted as being helpful in promoting development?

Using oral language to communicate

Speaking requires control of complex groups of muscles in the mouth. Physical differences that are present at birth may indicate the possibility of future problems with learning to talk. These physical differences may be recognised, or identified, at an early stage when feeding. Babies who have difficulty in sucking, for example, may have poor control over muscles in the mouth.

Every aspect of early childhood experience provides the potential for language development, whether this is communicating wants by speaking, signing to others or through internalised speech.

Parents, primary caregivers, family members, friends and other carers use oral language for communication. Children are surrounded by language being used by others and acquire language in a naturalistic way in all the activities they engage in at home. This applies to most children, whatever their backgrounds, cultures or languages. There are, however, exceptions to this. Some families and children with an auditory impairment or a physical or other difference that prevents oral communication will not use verbal language, either from necessity or from choice. Other forms of visual language and communication will be used to supplement or replace speech as a normal part of everyday life.

An indication of the development of children's skills in language is not just demonstrated by what they say, it is also visible in the cues they recognise and in responses that indicate their understanding of what adults say.

> **Activity 4**   **Reflection**

1 Make brief observations of adults talking to children, in the workplace, in the home or outside.
2 Note any evidence of modelling: accent, gesture and body language.
3 Is there a connection between how much the child looks at the adult and the adult response?
4 How can this reflection help you in your planning?

Toddlers' first words

The first recognisable words emerge on average any time between the ages of 12 to 19 months. First words are drawn from their direct experience and there may be a gap between the first recognisable word and any repetition or utterance of other words. Often first words are unexpected.

Case Study 7

First words

Eleanor (15 months) is sitting in the back of the car with her brother Patrick (aged 4) and their grandmother. Patrick says he has been to the pub with his parents.

Granny asks, 'What did mummy drink?'

'Beer,' says Patrick.

'What did daddy drink?' asks Granny.

'Beer,' says Patrick.

'Did you have beer, too?' asks Granny.

'I had lemonade,' says Patrick.

'And what did Eleanor have?' asks Granny.

Before Patrick can respond, Eleanor says, 'Juice'. This is the first clear word she has spoken.

The first words used by children are usually used in a multi-purpose way (holophrases). Often at this early stage, the words will be used with a wide range of intonation to convey a variety of meanings. The same word may also be used to represent a range of things that have a common factor: 'juice' can mean any drink.

Case Study 8

Signing leads to improvement in speech

At 3 years of age, Muhammad was having difficulty with speech. He was monosyllabic and his vocabulary was very small. His words were indistinct and even family members found it difficult to understand him. Eventually, he began to have speech therapy and the therapist suggested using signing to communicate. His confidence in communicating grew through signing and led to improvements in speech.

Development in language: the early years

Parents and carers often use a modified form of language with babies and toddlers. Other older children often follow this modelling when speaking to younger siblings.

Babies seem to respond to language that is simple in structure, is expressive and uses repetitive phrases. Experiments have been conducted using this modified infant-directed speech in languages other than the home language, and babies have continued to respond positively. This would seem to indicate that at this early stage, tone, pitch and pattern in language are more important than the meaning of the words. Modified infant-directed speech is used in many cultures and appears to follow similar rules.

Physical and emotional support is important to language development

Infant-directed speech may improve a baby's language and communication skills as a result of the bonding relationship that is integral to the interactive communication process. Providing the optimum conditions for language development appears to be related to physical and emotional support. Research on mothers who experience depression has shown that although their children do learn to talk, the range and use of language is very restricted. Babies in this situation are often confined and given very little stimulus. Intervention strategies have been successful when mothers have been identified as having this problem and appropriate support has been available.

Showing and giving objects

Children of 18 to 20 months generally demonstrate an ever-increasing interest in showing and giving objects, initially real and then pretend. For example, some children may go through a phase of liking David Pelham's book *Sam's Pizza*; they may pretend to pick out the 'disgusting' things which were added to the pizza – slugs, centipedes and so on – which they might then pretend to spit out. The part that the adult can play in extending the child's understanding and use of language on such occasions is extensive, and is crucial in opening up opportunities, not only for social interaction, but also for subject-located knowledge and understanding, Some of what an adult hears a child say may not be entirely accurate in terms of 'subject' knowledge; however, if the adult has been aware of the context of the child's learning experiences it may be possible to understand where these misconceptions or misunderstandings have come from.

There are some important questions to be asked here. For example, how can *Sam's Pizza* be used for extending scientific knowledge, for encouraging, teaching or finding out a child's understanding of differences between living things, or what can and can't be eaten, if we provide confusing information? Does the 'pretend eating' of objects confuse or reinforce children's understanding of inedible or unsafe things to eat? It is important to consider the types of language that could be encouraged and supported and how they are used.

Books are very useful starting points

Books can be very useful starting points at any age if the adult provides the scaffolding for language extension and modelling of reading behaviour. Pointing out familiar things in books encourages the child to respond, as any parent of a young child will know. Initially, this co-reading will be adult-led. The next stage will be triggered by responses from the child through their intervention: by making sounds, pointing and gesturing. The responsive adult will then extend the input to meet the child's requests and responses.

Young children soon acquire an enthusiasm for a particular book and for its detail. Sometimes this enthusiasm develops to the extent that the parent wishes the child would lose interest and move to another book! Such opportunities provide an ideal setting for language development, linking the everyday and familiar with the unfamiliar and unreal. Extending reading skills in this way may also be used to encourage rich descriptive use of language

Usually, by the time children are approaching their second birthday, they are beginning to demonstrate their developmental stage of short-term memory through fetching and carrying. The stimulus presented to the child by the environment will be readily seen, not only in the range of objects, but also in the language that is used. The modelling provided by adults and older children may motivate extended use of language and gesture.

Memory and communication

Kiran (18 months) occasionally went shopping with his grandmother. By the egg section was a button which, when pressed, produced farmyard noises, including a clucking sound.

Several weeks had passed since Kiran's last visit, but on entering the store Kiran bent his elbows and began to flap his arms up and down. This was his chicken gesture. It was some minutes before his grandmother realised that he was remembering the button that made farmyard noises.

Understanding the purposes and use of speech

For most children the first few months of their second year will be a period of rapid understanding of the purposes and use of speech. Between 18 months and 2 years of age most children will begin to use their first words. This age range is purely indicative of ages that events are likely to occur. Some children may speak at an earlier age, others much later. (Within this book any indication of the ages that events are likely to occur should be taken as a very broad indication of developmental norms.) Again, by this age children will begin to recognise and respond to their name. They also respond to requests related to giving and taking objects.

Toddlers will often structure short phrases from words that elide and combine. Examples of this would be 'heyare', and 'allgone'. The words most commonly used are, of course, those relating to giving and taking. Requests also feature as word combinations, which may be used in a range of situations, and for different purposes. Adults who care for, or work with, children of this age will recognise and respond to these context-related word phrases; to others they may make no sense. Clues to meaning are often provided by gestures as well as changes in tone and intonation in speech, which are modelled on those adults or other children with whom the children are in contact. Over a period of weeks or months, toddlers will respond and adapt to routines and recognise and use gesture and speech to match actions. Describing or commenting upon their own actions can be seen at this stage, especially in their self-directed play. A significant point to note is that toddlers appear to devise, or respond to, rules of language.

You may notice that some children in childcare settings will begin to discriminate between different registers of language. They may use different ways of speaking to adults and to other children or imitate adult speech patterns in some aspects of their role-play.

The range of words used by toddlers may include responses to a modelled social convention, for example, 'Ta', 'bye-bye' and requests for food or drink.

1 Consider the range of the words most commonly used by toddlers in your workplace setting and compare notes with your colleagues.

Many 2- and 3-year-olds respond to words used in more abstract terms, that is, words used outside an immediate context and thus less reliant on non-verbal clues. Memory will feature largely in this stage of development. The events recalled will not only use existing language, but also prompt the acquisition of new words.

2 Reflect upon an incident from your experience that illustrates how 2- or 3-year-old children have used words to remember incidents in the recent past.

Children learn to speak more readily when they are involved in conversations. In this way, new words and phrases become part of the active vocabulary of young children. Where patterns of language experience are adult- directed and -dominated, children's language development will be impeded. A typical example of this approach is when children are sidelined by being talked to rather than encouraged to actively respond.

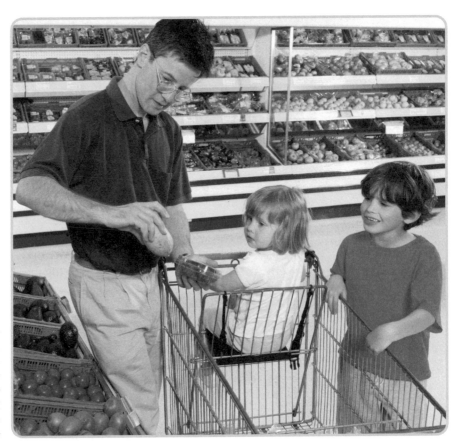

An everyday activity such as a shopping trip can provide opportunities for interaction and language development

Use opportunities while carrying out everyday activities within your workplace setting to speak your thoughts out loud. This helps to involve children more effectively within the thought processes of planning and evaluating their activities. It will build on familiar patterns of learning experience within the home; for example, when an adult helps a child to make a sandwich and describes the actions involved, giving the child a choice of reactions and encouraging response and comment.

By the age of 3 and a half, many children will play with words, exploring differences in meaning, and ask questions in a more focused way. By this age, some children will be able to differentiate between alternative meanings for the same word, and jokes based on word play may emerge.

The interest shown in what young children do and the ways in which they express themselves are key aspects of the provision of scaffolding for language learning. Very young children are focused in the way that they perceive the world around them; they often have strong views, which need to be recognised, acknowledged and understood.

Physical interaction is supported by language

Much of the physical interaction that takes place between parents and primary caregivers and children is supported by language. The interchange of responses in interactions often becomes a complex turn-taking activity with the parent and child responding to each other. Language not only supports, but also extends, bonding and reinforcement of the social and emotional interactions. Bath time, bedtime, shopping and, even watching television with an adult who is attuned to their child's interests provide opportunities for extended and complex conversation. Language may be extended and supported in these familiar situations.

> **Case Study 10**

Extending and supporting language through social and emotional interaction

Shareen enjoys bathing her daughter Aurely (age 4) while her mother looks after the other children. It is a time when Shareen and Aurely are able to spend some quiet, intimate, 'quality' time together. They talk about things that happen during the day.

At nursery, the practitioner notices that Aurely particularly enjoys opportunities to bath the dolls, shampoo their hair and talk to them. She becomes so engrossed in this activity that she is unaware of those around her. Observation of her behaviour led to the practitioner questioning her mother and the links between these activities were recognised.

The earliest experiences of language provide models for the use of language in communication. In these, and many other social contexts, this social function of turn taking will not be entirely possible for some children. Those children with an autistic spectrum disorder may already at 4 or 5 years of age have begun to display an inability to communicate in a conventional way. Their responses to cues from others either in speech or body language may be inappropriate to the context or be open to misinterpretation. This inability to communicate in a conventional way may increase as the child gets older.

Children still learn to talk regardless of their support at home. There are, of course, exceptions, but these are either due to physical differences that impede language development, or are extreme cases of language deprivation. Children who are completely deprived of human conversation, such as feral children, mimic and imitate the sounds they hear around them.

Lack of confidence in using language in pre-school settings

An increasing concern for many practitioners who work in pre-school settings is the number of children who on entry display very limited confidence in their use of language. Concerns for children who have had little stimulus may be addressed through language intervention strategies provided within settings, or by programmes provided by outside agencies. The provision of a home environment that is rich in opportunities for talk should not be confused with social class (see studies by Tizard and Hughes (1984) and Wells (1987)). Parents, whatever their socioeconomic background, can enable their children to acquire language skills which equip them well for pre-school and school through questioning, problem solving and conversation. The conditions that applied to this research in the 1980s have changed with the pattern of language use in homes, which have very different life styles than those that pertained nearly 20 years ago. Anecdotal evidence indicates that language use within the home and relationships between family members have more influence on children's capacity for language than socioeconomic background.

By 3 years of age most children are using language effectively, to communicate their needs, and in ways that demonstrate much wider language skills.

Case Study 11

Language use within the home

Samantha is the youngest child in the family, with an age gap of 10 years between her and her 14-year-old brother. One day, while at nursery, Samantha in a very matter of fact manner stated that her mum was very upset with her brother because the police had been round to their house and that he was in trouble again and it was drugs. Although the subject matter was not what one might expect at nursery it did demonstrate the degree of expertise Samantha had with language.

Too few opportunities for one-to-one experience

McAuley and Jackson (1992) indicate that research shows there is a paucity of sustained conversation between any one individual child and an adult in nursery settings. Experience indicates that opportunities for this one-to-one experience are still difficult to achieve. Much of the language used in early years settings is instructional or organisational. The degree to which this occurs increases as the child gets older when it is even less likely that time will be made available for one-to-one naturalistic conversations within school classrooms. Time constraints imposed by the demands of the curriculum are often presented as the prime reason for the lack of opportunity for quality conversation.

Careful planning can overcome this problem; focused conversation can be used within the delivery of the curriculum to enhance and consolidate learning. Children often find difficulty in responding to tasks when there are few opportunities for checking on, and confirming, the demands made on them by the practitioner. One-to-one conversations allow for matching tasks to a child's ability more readily and more accurately than relying solely upon group conversation, but both types need to be built into the planning cycle in order to test children's understanding and to counter any misunderstanding of concepts. No matter how carefully tasks are presented, some children will struggle with understanding new work within their existing conceptual framework. Children's misunderstandings often have a 'logical' basis, in that they use their existing knowledge to make sense of a situation to arrive at an answer, and children know only too well that an answer is always required when an adult asks a question. Conversation is an effective and possibly non-threatening means of eliciting answers to questions and gauging children's understanding of how they think about the world.

Talking to children about fire engines, trucks and ambulances, lifts, escalators and revolving doors, vacuum cleaners and DVD players can provide them with an amazing number of facts, with many of them being accurately – or partially accurately – understood!

> ### Activity 7   Language specific to an area of knowledge
>
> Collect some examples to demonstrate how children's questions indicate their growing awareness of language specific to an area of knowledge. You may, for example, look at children's understanding of science or technology in the home, in school or in the local environment.

Young children need to be encouraged to explore

There are many ways of encouraging children's exploration of science through language. Adults provide crucial role models and in order that we may effectively help children we need to be explorers with them (Siraj-Blatchford and MacLeod-Brudenell, 1999:14). If we, as practitioners, share children's pleasure in seeking answers to scientific or technological questions, wondering how and why things happen, we will provide models for further reflection.

Case Study 12

Answering children's questions

Holly (4 years, 6 months) loves eating mashed potatoes, but today she is eating crisps. 'What are crisps made from, Daddy?' she asks.

'They're made from potatoes,' he replies.

'Then how do they make them hard?' she asks.

Children see things in different ways to adults, not only from an intellectual viewpoint, but also by reason of their physical stature, from a different height. They notice things that may pass us by. Encouraging talk about everyday things – chairs, car door handles and soft drinks dispensers, for example – can be quite revealing. The detail that is noticed, which may be elicited with carefully supported questioning, often reveals knowledge of the intricacies of mechanisms and materials. Only adults who are sensitive to children's interests will draw out this detail in conversation.

The role of parents

You are probably familiar with the term 'parents are a child's first educators'. Parental influence can provide rich experience in social and emotional development. Indeed, the role parents or primary caregivers play in development of language is crucial. Negative parenting, or poor parenting skills, have a very negative effect on language development. Children who have not received encouragement to speak at home often lack spontaneity in using speech in their play both at home and in out-of-home settings. This can be rectified by providing opportunities for collaborative play, in which children and adults can demonstrate the use of words within an appropriate context.

Young children develop their innate capacity to learn to speak through their experience of language used by adults and other children. Exposure to language used readily and confidently by adults helps young children to understand words and link them to particular and specific contexts. Hearing words used in context also encourages imitation. A key aspect of play for some children is playing with words, revisiting contexts in which they have heard words used. The majority of children who suffer hearing impairment are born to hearing parents. The use of both spoken language and signing is very important for these children's competence and confidence in communication. Using and playing with words in play within everyday contexts is encouraged at as early a stage as possible.

Most parents know what their children are interested in and respond to these interests. It is not uncommon for a 4-year-old child to have a wide vocabulary related to an area of particular interest.

Case Study 13

Children's vocabularies and special interests

Emily's dinosaurs

From the age of two, Emily has been interested in dinosaurs. This interest has developed over time to the present day (4 years, 9 months). Emily uses dinosaur names; recognises physical attributes; knows what they ate; knows they lived a very long time ago; knows about skin and links them with reptiles now; and knows about their skeletons. Emily says that she wants be an archaeologist when she grows up.

Connor's cars

Connor, like many little boys, has an in-depth knowledge of vehicles. This began before he was 2 years old, with an interest in mini-cars. Now aged 3 years and 5 months, his knowledge is wide, and he recognises and names a huge number of cars. Recently, while a passenger in a car that was parked alongside a big green vehicle, he corrected an adult who said that he thought the vehicle was a bit like a Range Rover.

'No, it's not,' said Connor. 'It hasn't got a wheel on the back,' he added.

As he drove away, the adult checked and conceded that Connor was right.

1 Is Connor exceptional in his understanding or is it that he is able to express his thought well because he is highly competent in using spoken language to demonstrate his knowledge?

In essence, the language users around children provide them with scaffolding for early learning (Bruner, 1983). This is addressed in further detail in Chapter 5.

Interactive speech cannot be replaced by simply hearing speech. Watching television is often denigrated as a negative activity for children, but there can be positive aspects to this experience if an adult sits with the child and talks through the experience, much as if they were reading a book together. This social activity could be extended to the use of a computer.

Case Study 14

Using a graphics package to aid language development

When Danny (aged 4) used to visit his grandparents for holidays, he regularly saw flooding en route to their home. Danny had problems with making his words understood and communicating his thoughts. He loved to use his grandfather's computer to draw. He became very adept at using the graphics package and would use the paint spray to make 'dark clouds'. Danny was able to use his painting as a means of prompting talking about his experiences as well as using his imagination. He was able to make up stories from his paintings, even though he had a very limited vocabulary.

1 How could this activity be replicated with children in out-of-home settings?

2 Tizard (1994) notes that extended conversations at home were often at relaxed times – over tea or during a one-to-one story time. Danny's experience illustrates this point. Similar conversations may only happen at Danny's nursery when an adult stays with him to talk through his explorations. Would Danny be able to work on a computer like this without adult help?

Case Study 15

Recognising language awareness

At nursery a practitioner chose *The Very Hungry Caterpillar* by Eric Carle to read to a group of children. A little boy became very excited and exclaimed that he had the video at home. He knew the words by heart and spoke them out loud, imitating the tone used by the narrator in the video, as the practitioner read the book. The next day, when he came to the nursery, he asked for the book and sat with the practitioner while they read it together. This event recurred on several days, until one day the practitioner suggested that he read the book to her. Not only did he do that, but he also gathered a little group of children and read to them, holding up the book to enable them to see the picture. The practitioner gave him a copy of the book to take home.

1 What aspects of language awareness are being demonstrated here?

Case Study 16

Scaffolding

Laura was interested – almost to the point of obsession – in cats. She was very shy and self-conscious and hid behind the persona of her cat. Her reception class teacher found the only way to involve her in classroom activities was through all things feline: drama and movement developed around cats, books and poems about cats and individual maths lessons – which cat is the odd one out?, draw three cats, and so on. As her confidence grew, she developed an interest in birds, but by this time she had begun to use the library to study her interest.

Young children often have very strong interests. How could you harness a child's interests through careful matching of their interest in your planning?

> **Activity 8** **Scaffolding learning**

1 How do you help to scaffold learning?

2 Do you recognise aspects of language support in this chapter's case studies that are reflected in your practice?

3 Which aspects of scaffolding do you find the most effective in your practice?

Accent, dialect and grammar

There are clear and definitive distinctions between accent, dialect and grammar and, at first sight, this appears to be quite a straightforward matter. There are, however, some issues pertaining to this area of study of which we should be aware and which are not generally discussed. For example, the accent we hear and use as children may determine the one we use for the rest of our life.

Earlier in the chapter, note was made of the relationship between manipulation of muscle groups, the tongue and making speech. Although this was in the context of children with physical differences or disability, the issue also has bearing on the development of speech for everyone.

Note how uncomfortable it feels when your mouth muscles are forced to make unfamiliar sounds. Try to concentrate on how your mouth and tongue move when pronouncing words in an unfamiliar way. You will become aware of the difficulties some children may have when trying to change their accent in order to 'fit in' when they move to another area.

The case study demonstrating George's awareness of different pronunciations illustrates a conscious effort to play with words (see page 182).

Standard English

There is an emphasis on the use of Standard English in school. Standard English is a dialect of English which has been selected for general public use throughout the country. It comprises conventions of grammar and spelling that are promoted as being the only acceptable form of language for public communication. Regional dialects are not supported as a means of public communication in this country.

> **Activity 9** **Dialect**

Dialect words may be in general use within a geographical location or be used by a particular age group. The following dialect words are used in parts of Nottingham:

➲ pawpaw: a sore or minor injury

➲ tab: ear

Grammatical conventions

Young children quickly develop an awareness of the grammar, conventions of language and rules of speech used within their community. The forms of grammar used within a family as well as in the community may differ from those found in Standard English. Non-standard grammar and dialect may be acquired by children from their family and from people in the community. Tension frequently occurs when young children move to situations in which Standard English is required and they are expected to conform. It is not uncommon to find variations from Standard English grammar used widely within a community; for example, 'was' rather than 'were' as illustrated by 'we was going'.

Case Study 17

Local accents in the supermarket

Jo, a practitioner who works in an early years setting, is standing in the queue at the checkout in the supermarket, observing a couple and their son, who looked about 4 years of age. Jo's attention moved from the boy to the parents when she heard the father saying to the boy:

'We don't want any of those, we've got some at *om* (at home).'

The mother quickly corrected him by saying, '*at owm*'.

This move on the part of the mother to modify the local accent must prove even more confusing for the child when he goes to nursery and encounters yet another pronunciation of the word.

As children become more confident in using grammatical conventions, they will adapt their own creative and non-standard variations to conform to their understanding of the rules! For example, 'I used to was.'

Children are generally adept at imitation and learn to switch between the types of language that are acceptable for use in different contexts. Usually, by the age of 5, children are beginning to be able to move between different registers of language use with confidence.

Bilingualism

Bilingual speakers have been present in England for many centuries, in fact, for longer than England has been a nation. This fact is often neglected in current discussions on bilingualism, where the issue is often regarded as a fairly recent phenomenon. The use of a language other than English for everyday communication still appears to be regarded with varying degrees of indifference, antagonism or hostility. Bilingualism is more often regarded as an issue relating to recent migrants to England. The recent history of bilingual education in England, therefore, is inextricably linked with attitudes to race and cultural difference.

Recent moves by the United Kingdom government to introduce tests for those seeking British citizenship have raised many issues relating to the role and place of languages other than English in British society. An acknowledgement that tests could be made in Welsh and Gaelic, as well as English, has indicated that these languages have equal status with English. This may be seen as a positive acknowledgement to speakers of these languages. Languages other than English have been used in religious contexts for many years as a means of maintaining religious or cultural identity.

Using a range of languages in the home

Babies will learn the language of their primary caregiver and the acquisition of an additional language may occur in a number of ways. Children who are in daily, or regular, contact with a family member who speaks another language will acquire an understanding of, and varying degrees of competence in, communicating in that language. For children in bilingual families, there may be a range of scenarios of language use within the family as well as in their out-of-home experiences.

The following case study demonstrates the complexity of switching between languages that one child copes with on a regular basis. The example focuses on western European languages but reflects the experiences of many, if not most, children who live in families that communicate through the means of different languages.

Case Study 18

Switching between languages

Gavin's mum was born of Italian parents in Wales. His father was born to Welsh-speaking parents. Gavin's mum and dad speak English to each other and their children. Gavin speaks English to his parents and siblings. He understands Italian and has learned Welsh at school and heard it spoken at his paternal grandparents'. This apparently complex linguistic context is found in very many homes in Britain.

Using a range of languages may be a necessity for some families, but in others it may be a matter of choice. Awareness of the benefits of the ability to communicate in more than one language may not emerge until families feel secure and confident within the wider community, or feel able to demonstrate pride in their ethnicity. If children are encouraged to learn two languages within a bilingual family, each language is often directed to different family members.

Case Study 19

Choosing to use a range of languages in the home

Alison is married to Juan, a Spanish speaker. Of their three children, the eldest, Jaime, speaks only English. Paul speaks English and understands some Spanish, and the youngest, Annabel, is bilingual.

Annabel experienced simultaneous learning of both languages as a young child. Evidence indicates that bilingual children who learn two languages simultaneously may sometimes confuse languages. If there is a clear distinction as to which language is spoken to which individuals within the family, there are fewer opportunities for confusion.

The role of parents is crucial for the development of language. This may be seen even more keenly in those families that have the additional ability to use more than one language in everyday communication. Parents' perception of the importance of the home language is crucial. Without a positive understanding of the benefits that the use of this language provides for their children, opportunities for their children's language enhancement may be lost. The merits of bilingualism must also be recognised by those with whom children come into contact within their out-of-home experiences at school, pre-school or nursery (Karram, 2003).

Research appears to demonstrate that there are positive benefits for children who are bilingual: greater cognitive flexibility, problem solving capacities and linguistic awareness (Hakuta and Pease-Alvarez, 1992).

Learning a second language in an out-of-home setting

Many children learn their second language when they move to an out-of-home setting: nursery, pre-school or reception class settings or on entry to school. The existing language skills of the child should be acknowledged.

Often children will already be confident users of their home language and be able to access a wide range of learning opportunities. Sometimes a child's lack of competence in spoken English is erroneously seen as an indication of a wider lack of understanding; children may choose not to speak!

Conclusion

Communication is more than spoken language, in any of its forms. Interaction between people involves language, gesture and body language. It is hoped that you will continue your reflection on the development of children's language and communication skills within your workplace setting and in conversations with the significant adults in the life of children with whom you work. It is also hoped that you will use the suggestions made in this chapter for further reading and as a basis for ongoing evaluation of your practice. Children's acquisition of communication skills is one of the most exciting developments of early childhood. Encouraging and influencing this development is potentially one of the most rewarding aspects of your professional role.

References and further reading

Acredolo, L. and Goodwyn, S. (1997), *Baby Signs*. London: Hodder and Stoughton

Athey, C. (1990), *Extending Thought in Young Children: A parent-teacher partnership*. London: Paul Chapman

Browne, A. (2001), *Developing Language and Literacy* (2nd edn). London: Paul Chapman

Bruner, J. (1983), *In Search of Mind: Essays in autobiography*. New York: HarperCollins

Carle, E. (1970), *The Very Hungry Caterpillar*. London: Puffin Books

Chomsky, N. (1957), *Syntactic Structures*. The Hague: Mouton

Cousins, J. (1999), *Listening to Four Year Olds*. London: National Early Years Network

Donaldson, M. (1978), *Children's Minds*. London: Fontana

Goldschmied, E. and Jackson, S. (1994), *People under Three*. London: Routledge

Grieve, R. and Hughes, M. (eds) (1990), *Understanding Children*. Oxford: Blackwell Publishers

Hakuta, K. and Pease-Alvarez, L. (1992), 'Enriching our views of bilingualism and bilingual education', *Educational Researcher*, 21, pp4–6

Karram, S. (2002), ' "Auntie-ji, please come and join us for an hour": The role of the bilingual education assistant in working with parents with little confidence', in Devereux, J. and Miller, L. (eds) (2002), *Working with Children in the Early Years.* London: David Fulton

Meadows, S. and Cashdan, A. (1988), *Helping Children Learn: Contributions to a Cognitive Curriculum.* London: David Fulton

Mukherji, P. and O'Dea, T. (2000), *Understanding Children's Language and Literacy.* Cheltenham: Stanley Thornes

Nutbrown, C. (1994), *Threads of Thinking: Young children learning and the role of early education.* London: Paul Chapman

Pelham, D. (1996), *Sam's Pizza.* New York: Dutton Juvenile

Siraj-Blatchford, J. and MacLeod-Brudenell, I. (1999), *Supporting Identity, Diversity and Language in the Early Years.* Maidenhead: Open University Press

Siraj-Blatchford, J. and MacLeod-Brudenell, I. (1999), *Supporting Science, Design and Technology in the Early Years.* Maidenhead: Open University Press

Sutherland, P. (1992), *Cognitive Development Today: Piaget and his critics.* London: Paul Chapman

Tizard, B. and Hughes, M. (1984), *Young Children Learning.* London: Fontana

Trevarthen, C. (1993), 'The function of emotions in early infant communication and development', in Nadel, J. and Camaioni, L. (eds) (1993), *New Perspectives in Early Communicative Development.* London: Routledge

Whitehead, M. (1996), *The Development of Language and Literacy.* London: Hodder and Stoughton

Whitehead, M. (1999), *Supporting Language and Literacy Development in the Early Years.* Maidenhead: Open University Press

Vygotsky, L. (1978), *Mind and Society.* Cambridge, MA: Harvard University Press

Play and parenting – developmental experiences in children aged 0 to 3 years

7

Janet Kay and Elaine Hallet

In this chapter, the key theme is the differential developmental experiences of young children aged 0 to 3 years, and the impact these have on the individual child's ability to learn and develop within early years settings from age 3 onwards. The role of parents in promoting their young children's holistic development will be explored, with reference to the role of play in development and the ways in which parents can support this. Parenting and play is a focus of the discussion in the age range of 0 to 3, in order to critically examine the influence of parenting on pre-school children. Differences in the ways in which children are reared are discussed, and the implications of these for children entering pre-school, early years settings (nursery, pre-schools, childminders) is appraised. The chapter also focuses on the transitions that children make between home and early years settings, with reference to the wide range of cultural experiences and developmental stages at this age.

The chapter concludes by examining how early years settings can respond to the wide range of children's needs and stages of development they encounter, and the ways in which transitions from home to early years setting can be effectively supported. The main issues affecting transitions will be identified and discussed, including children's language development, their different early experiences and home cultures, their experiences of play and how these impact on the child and the early years setting.

This chapter addresses the following areas:

- ⊃ the family and context of parenting
- ⊃ parenting styles and child-rearing
- ⊃ play in the age range 0–3 and the role of adults
- ⊃ play with parents
- ⊃ transitions to educare early years settings
- ⊃ making the transition work.

After reading this chapter you should be able to:

1 recognise how parents influence children's early development

2 understand the role of play in early development in the home

3 identify the impact of different early experiences and their role in children's access to early years settings

4 evaluate the ways in which settings can best respond to a wide range of needs and stages of development.

Introduction

It is critical to understand the role of parenting in children's development in the first 3 years is if we are to understand the skills, abilities, knowledge and understanding of the environment that individual young children bring with them into pre-school early years settings. Acknowledging that parents are children's first educators is a starting point, but parents also influence many other aspects of their children's development, and all of these developmental aspects contribute to the child's ability to access more formal learning situations. Play is an extremely important medium through which parents support their children's learning and development; and the encouragement of play in the home is one of the child's most significant early experiences.

Child-rearing styles and approaches to parenting vary considerably and children will, through both genetic factors and their early experiences, vary significantly in their stages of development when they enter their first educare setting. Children will have reached different stages in their aptitudes and skills; their speech and language; physical development and ability; social skills and emotional maturity; and comprehension of their environment. Some children may have more extreme developmental delays, while others may need to acquire a second language in order to access the early years curriculum. These variations pose a significant challenge to practitioners in the Foundation Stage and beyond.

The ways in which early experiences are incorporated into the child's activities and learning in early years settings are crucial to ensuring that children have positive experiences of care and education on which to build in their school years. This first transition from home to an early years setting is vital in determining how children perceive their learning environment. The role of play is central to ensuring that there is continuity between home and the early years setting, and that the early years setting encourages the child to use home experiences as a basis for learning. The variety and range of these early experiences will differ according to the child's parenting, the culture, language and situation of the family, family type and any significant events affecting a family. As such, each child's experience is unique, and this presents every early years setting with the challenge of both acknowledging the validity and equal importance of each child's unique experiences, and ensuring that play and activities are relevant to them all.

The family and context of parenting

This section discusses the notion of a 'family' and its changing composition, in addition to considering families as systems.

Defining the family?

In British culture, children are usually raised within families, but in the early-21st century asking the question 'What is a family?' poses some difficulties. For a start, we may have difficulty defining 'family' , as diversification over the last 50 years has led to a much broader range of family types than were previously common. The family may be more fruitfully thought of as a social construct, in that defining a family realistically may be dependent on self-definition; for example, 'we are a family because we think of ourselves as a family'. This type of definition gets us away from the idea of listing characteristics of families in order to define them, and acknowledges that families are very diverse in both structure and functions.

Changing family types

Family types are now less stable, with increases in divorce and remarriage leading to a shifting pattern of lone parent and 'blended' families (Thurtle, 1998). Over the last 20 years there has been a decrease in the number of couple-headed families, corresponding to the increase in lone-parent headed families. However, although lone-parent families are a fast-growing category of family type, the majority of lone parents re-enter marriage or cohabitation, often with partners who have children of their own. So 78% of children still live in traditional households headed by a couple. Some of these households are stepfamilies, which constituted 8% of all families in 2000–1. These statistics cannot really reflect the changing patterns of family type that many individuals experience. However, falling marriage rates and increased numbers of children conceived outside marriage (over 50% in 2000) confirm the possibility that many children do not spend their whole childhood with two married biological parents. This is supported by the fact that two-fifths of all marriages are remarriages (Summerfield and Babb, 2003). It can be concluded that many children are raised in a range of family types within their childhood; for example, when families separate, operate as lone-parent families, and then become part of 'blended' or 'reconstituted' families.

A small percentage of children are raised within the care of local authority social services. Many of these children will experience more than one change of family, with some experiencing three or more foster care placements, as well as parenting within their family of origin. Some children who enter the care system will be placed in adoptive families and lose their legal ties with their birth families, although, increasingly, adopted children are maintaining contact with birth family members throughout their childhood. Greater numbers of children are being raised in lesbian and gay households by parents who may or may not be related to them biologically. The advent of scientific and technological developments in the fields of fertility and conception have also influenced the ways in which parenting can be achieved.

Thus, there are many more complex ways in which the link between parent and child is created, other than biological parenting.

Families as systems

Families can be analysed as a series of separate relationships or as systems. The application of systems theory to the study of family behaviour and relationships underpins our understanding of the complex interplay of relationships within families and the reactions and adjustments family members make in their dealings with each other. In studying the role of parenting in the development of children in the early years, it is important to recognise this complex interplay within families. Children are no longer viewed as 'lumps of clay' to be moulded and socialised by others, but as active participants in determining the parenting styles within their families (Bee, 2000; Messer and Millar,1999).

Practical experience tells us that events affecting one member of a family will affect the family as a whole. Examining patterns of influence within families can give us an insight into how different child-rearing styles develop and the impact that various approaches to parenting can have on young children's development. For example, the serious illness of a parent can produce anxiety and distress in both the parent's partner and the children. The illness of one parent combined with the anxiety of the other parent could make the children feel insecure and anxious. At a time like this, the children may receive less attention and less parental focus. This may add to the children's feelings of insecurity and anxiety. The children may seek to redress the balance and gain parental attention through demanding behaviour, 'clinginess' and openly expressed distress. In dealing with this, the parents might not have the time and energy to focus on child-centred approaches in their response and may be more authoritiarian than usual, adding to the children's feelings of anxiety and insecurity.

> ### Activity 1 Feedback loops
>
> Think of a family you know that has recently been subject to change, for example, in employment patterns, addition of new members or bereavement. Consider how the change has affected all parts of the family and how 'feedback loops' may have developed as outlined in the example above.

Influence of other systems on the family

As well as viewing the family as a system in itself, it is also important to recognise that families are influenced in their behaviour by other systems outside the family, which may affect family functioning directly or indirectly. These influences could include the social and work situation of the parents, the support systems that adults and children have access to, and the stresses on the family, which may include economic status, housing situation and health status. Bronfenbrenner's ecological approach (1979, 1989) cited in Bee (2000) is a useful model with which to explore family systems. This model reflects the 'complex, interactive and interdependent nature of environmental influences on a child' (Woods, 1998). Bronfenbrenner described the influences on families as:

- **microsystems**: the child's direct contacts; mainly family, daycare, school
- **exosystems**: factors that influence the child indirectly; for example, parent's work, social contacts, income, local environment
- **macrosystems**: include the wider culture/ subculture in which the family exists; for example, social early years setting, cultural early years setting, political context.

Influences on families are complex and interrelated, and the impact within families is cyclical.

Case Study 1

Influences on family and their effect on children

When 4-year-old Jasmine's parents separated, she was very upset that her father moved out of the marital home. The house was then sold and Jasmine moved to a flat with her mother. This meant changing to a new nursery and separation from friends and neighbours. Jasmine's mother started to have financial problems and became less tolerant and more short-tempered with Jasmine, often crying, shouting and making negative comments about Jasmine's father. Jasmine started to bed-wet, found it difficult to mix with other children at nursery and had angry outbursts at home and in the early years setting. Her mother found this behaviour very difficult to cope with on top of her other concerns, and she frequently shouted at Jasmine, locked herself in the bathroom and cried for long periods.

As Pugh (1994) argues, parenting cannot be seen in isolation from the social context within which it takes place, and work and unemployment, health, poverty and housing are all significant in determining the child's experience directly or through other family members.

Parenting styles and child-rearing

This section explores the extent to which parents can influence children's development and the evidence to support the view that different approaches to parenting have different developmental outcomes for the child. In discussing this, it is important to recognise that there is no one single concept of 'childhood.' Both 'childhood' and 'child-rearing practices' vary between different cultures and over time, depending on dominant social and cultural norms and values (Woods, 1998). The history of childhood reveals a range of different approaches to child rearing that reflect the economic and social conditions of different classes at different times and in different cultural contexts (Aries, 1982).

Child-rearing practices

Think about child-rearing practices that were common in your childhood, those of an older relative or friend, or those that are no longer considered acceptable. For example, caning in schools was once widespread, children were sent to bed without food, and some were beaten with slippers or belts. What do you think has happened to 'outlaw' these practices? Discuss your thoughts with your group.

Models of parenting styles

Models of parenting styles are used to analyse the relationship between parental behaviour and developmental outcomes for the child. However, as discussed above, parents do not just pluck a parenting style from nowhere. Parenting approaches tend to be shaped by a range of social, cultural and personal factors and experiences that combine to determine how an individual perceives and implements the task of parenting. Belsky's (1984) model of parental functioning identifies three main influences on the quality of parenting:

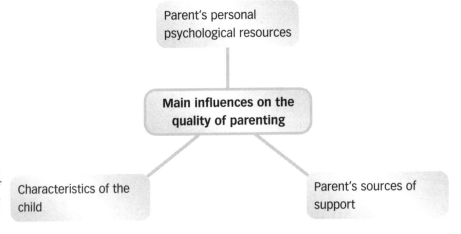

Figure 7.1
Main influences on the quality of parenting (Belensky, 1984)

These factors and the interplay between them will influence the parenting approach used by that person. The factors that have shaped an individual's experiences and lifestyle will also shape their approach to parenting. The interactions between these factors are also determinants of how a person will parent. For example, a parent who has experienced poor attachment and lack of support in his or her own childhood may find it more difficult to sustain relationships with partners or friends. This will have an impact on the social support he or she receives while parenting, which may in turn make the parenting task more stressful.

With reference to the three influences on parental functioning discussed in Figure 7.1, analyse your own parenting or that of someone you know well in terms of these influences. Note the interrelationships between the factors, and the impact on parenting style. Remember to maintain sensitivity and confidentiality when completing this exercise.

Baumrind developed a model of parenting styles that was adapted by Maccoby and Martin (1983) to establish a four-fold classification based on how demanding or undemanding parents are about a child's behaviour and how responsive or unresponsive the parents are to the child (see Figure 7.2).

Figure 7.2 *Parents' demands and their levels of response to a child's behaviour (adapted by Maccoby and Martin, 1983)*

	Responsive	Unresponsive
Demanding	Authoritative	Authoritarian
Undemanding	Permissive	Uninvolved

Maccoby and Martin classified the following parenting styles:

- ⊃ **Permissive parents** value the child's freedom of expression, provide few and inconsistent controls, and accept lower standards of cognitive and behavioural performance from the child.
- ⊃ **Authoritarian parents** are controlling and punitive, showing low levels of affection towards the child.
- ⊃ **Authoritative parents** set high standards for behaviour and self-reliance, encouraging independence and providing controls; they reason and explain, and are committed to all areas of the child's development.
- ⊃ **Uninvolved** or **neglecting parents** are 'psychologically' unavailable to their children, displaying little warmth and providing few controls.

Parenting style and implications for child development

Authoritative parenting has the best indicators for the child's development. Authoritative parents tend to provide children with clear, firm behavioural boundaries; explanations for rules and disciplinary measures; good communication; and warmth and responsiveness. Such children are regarded positively, given praise and affection and expected to behave maturely. Children raised in families where an authoritative parenting style predominates are likely to be more confident and independent, to socialise more effectively with peers and to conform more readily to controls and disciplinary measures. The long-term outcomes for such children in terms of success in education and beyond are better than for children raised in families where the other parenting styles predominate.

However, it is important to remember that:

- most parents use a range of styles at different times and stages of the child's development
- the child is not passive in this relationship and will influence the parenting style.

Limitations of parenting models

Models of parenting are limited in that none of them really reflects what actually goes on in families. Maccoby and Martin's (1983) classification has been criticised for reflecting the parenting of white families rather than those from a range of cultural groups. However, the classification does give us a starting point from which to analyse the impact of parenting behaviour on the child's development.

The extent to which parents can influence their child's development is disputed. Scarr (1992) referred to twin and adoption studies, which apparently demonstrated that family environment has little influence on the child's development. Scarr concluded that genetic factors are primary in determining the child's development and that parenting, beyond the minimum requirements, has little influence.

The factors that determine how an individual behaves as a parent are too many and complex to claim a cause-and-effect relationship between parenting style and child development. However, evidence shows that certain characteristics associated with authoratitive parenting styles are positive in their influences on the child's development (Bee, 2000). These are:

- **warmth** – warm families are linked with good attachment, and cognitive and social development in children (Maccoby, 1980: Ainsworth et al., 1974)
- **responsiveness** – parents who are sensitive to their children's needs are likely to have children who do well in cognitive, social and language development and who have secure attachments
- **control** – consistency of rules and high expectations of mature behaviour are linked with confident, competent children with good self-esteem and social skills
- **communication** – quality of communication depends on parents talking to, and listening to, their children. Children have a role in family decision-making and can disagree with parents, who expect to have to explain things to their children.

The opposite also applies. In a study commissioned by the Department of Health (1995) into the long-term effects of child abuse, the impact of low warmth/ high criticism parenting was determined to have a much longer-lasting and significant negative impact on the child's developmental outcomes than inflicted physical injuries.

It is also important to remember that siblings, grandparents and other close relatives and friends may all have their own influence on a child's development. There have been far fewer studies about the impact of behaviour of other relatives on young children, but there is evidence that, for many children, relationships develop early on with a range of significant others and not just parents.

Play aged 0 to 3 and the role of adults

The significance of the role of play in children's development is well established, based on research, the experience of practitioners, and the fact that children continue to play regardless of the current social and political status of play as a medium for learning and development. Theorists such as Vygotsky and Bruner have embedded the social context of play in our concept and understanding of the role of adults in supporting development through play. More recently, the implementation of the Foundation Stage has put play firmly back on the map for 3- to 5 year olds in early educare settings. In this section, we will look at children's play and its role in development in the 0 to 3 age group and the role of parents and other adults within this.

Play and development in young children

Tamis-Lemonda, Katz and Bornstein (2002:229) discuss the role of play in five areas of development. These are shown in Figure 7.3.

Figure 7.3 *The role of play in five areas of development Tamis-Lemonda, Katz and Bornstein (2002:229)*

Psychological	Regulation of arousal, expressing emotions, resolution of conflicts
Mastery	Attention span and task-directed behaviour
Cognitive	Acquisition of information and skills, creative and divergent thinking, representational abilities
Social	Giving and receiving, taking account of other's thoughts and intentions in decision-making
Culture	Means of transmitting social roles and cultural values

These five areas of development are crucial for a child to successfully access the community and curriculum of more formal educare settings. Tamis-Lemonda, Katz and Bornstein (2002) also suggest that an infant's development through play depends on a range of interactions with different types of others. For example:

> *After the first year, play interactions with peers and siblings increase in prevalence and may be more intense and affectively charged than those with mother.* Tamis-Lemonda, Katz and Bornstein (2002:231)

The implication is that different aspects of young children's development is supported through play with different types of people. For example, play with parents tends to be about 'conventional object use and convergent thinking' (Tamis-Lemonda, Katz and Bornstein, 2002:234) based on conveying information about the real world, rather than fantasy or imaginative play, which is more likely to be found in play with siblings.

How do 0 to 3-year-olds play?

It is generally agreed that children's play develops through stages that are loosely linked to the child's age and stage of development. Stages of play are far from rigid. Younger children will play at more advanced levels if they are with older children or adults; older children will return to previous stages of play if they are with younger children, or during times of stress, or just because they feel like it. Observe a family group of different-aged children and often they will cooperate in play across the stages. An older sister may play 'pretend play' using small world figures with a younger brother, and then help him to count or understand the rules of a board game. Piaget distinguished between 'practice play', 'symbolic play' and 'games with rules' as the stages of play young children go through. Developing the concept of stages further, Smilansky (1990) identified five basic forms of play, which are shown in Figure 7.4.

Form of play	Examples
Functional or exploratory play	A baby chewing, throwing and shaking a rattle.
Constructive play	A baby or toddler building with plastic bricks; a 4 year old making models with play dough.
Dramatic play	A 3 year old pretending to parent a doll; a 4 year old dressing up as Spiderman and acting in role.
Socio-dramatic play	A 5- and 6 year old dressing up and acting out scenes from a favourite film; a group of 6- and 7 year olds making up and putting on a play.
Games with rules	A group of 7- and 8 year olds playing Tiggy-off-the-ground in the playground; a family group of children aged 5, 7 and 8 playing a board game.

Figure 7.4
Smilansky's five basic forms of play

Children aged 0 to 3 tend to be involved mainly in the first three categories of play, although many 3 year olds will be learning about socio-dramatic play from siblings and other older children. Babies are most involved in functional or exploratory play, in which they develop manipulative skills and explore their environment through their senses. This may involve throwing, banging or chewing objects; manipulating objects to give a response, for example, shaking a rattle. Effectively, children of this age play largely as a medium of exploring their world and gaining knowledge and pleasure from it.

Goldschmied and Jackson (1994) discuss the concept of 'heuristic' play, suggesting that babies and young toddlers are absorbed in determining through experimentation what objects will 'do' or 'not do' through actions such as putting in and taking out (Holland, 1997).

Constructive play develops from earlier manipulation of objects and involves combining objects into structures, for example, building with bricks. In dramatic play, the child is developing 'pretend play' by adopting roles and using objects or imagination to support this process. Curtis and O'Hagan (2003) suggest that pretend play starts as a solitary activity at about 12 months old and is played in parallel with other children at about 2 years old:

> By the time the children are three or older they can engage in complicated dramatic play sequences, which become more and more involved with increasing age.
> (Curtis and O'Hagan, 2003:119)

Babies playing

Initially, babies play as part of their early interactions with their carers. Everyday routines such as feeding, bathing, changing nappies are opportunities for play through interactions such as reciprocal noise-making, eye contact and facial expressions. This type of play starts from birth and develops rapidly.

Case Study 2

Babies' play in early interaction with carers

Elaine is holding her 6-week-old baby son, Sol, on her lap in a café. She smiles at him and talks to him, while holding him to face her and making eye contact. He focuses on her face and follows the movements and sounds she makes with great attention. Elaine makes nonsense sounds at him and when he responds with attention and movement of his arms and head, she makes more noises.

This reciprocal attention and giving of responses is central to play with very young babies and is an important part of the development of attachment between child and carer.

Babies play using all their senses of touch, sight, smell, hearing and taste. As they physically develop they begin to look at things as well as people, reaching out for objects to explore and manipulate. Babies will reach and try and grasp objects and also push, throw, roll, suck and bite anything that catches their interest. Repetition is important as the baby explores the properties of the object. As babies get older and physically more competent they require opportunities for physical play in order to slide, jump, ride, swing and climb supported by parents and interested adults (Goldschmied in Robinson 2003:114, 115).

Toddlers playing

Through play, toddlers rehearse roles, pretend and imagine using a range of play props such as dressing-up clothes, cardboard boxes, everyday and natural objects. Toddlers use symbols within their play, which helps them to pretend in play situations they have created, and to act out real life behaviours in a safe environment.

Case Study 3

Acting out a life event

Sarah pushed a pram containing a soft toy cat with a blanket over the top for several days to and from the shops and to her grandmother's house. Her mother had recently had a baby and Sarah was acting out the significant life event of the arrival of her sister through this play scene.

Toddlers will increasingly play alongside, and in parallel with, others and will seek play with older children and adults. Tamis-Lemonda, Katz and Bornstein (2002) cite studies that support the view that different aspects of toddlers' development through play are influenced by who they play with, and that play with parents, siblings and peers is important to promote these different aspects of development. For example, language development is strongly associated with mothers who are verbally responsive in play (Tamis-Lemonda, Katz and Bornstein, 2002:237). By the age of 2 to 3, toddlers are seeking play with a range of others and this supports aspects of their development differentially to play with parents.

All of the child's experiences are potentially material for use in play. The toddler may increasingly use language in play to develop the 'action' or play theme. Children's play experiences will be influenced by their access to playmates, parents, older or younger siblings or friends.

Case Study 4

The benefits of playing together

When Dan was aged 2 and a half, he wanted a farm in the garden. With the help of his 5-year-old sister, he built enclosures from a range of materials, including sticks, stones, pieces of cardboard, some plastic food storage boxes and huge quantities of sticky tape. He filled the farm with snails and slugs, woodlice and earthworms. His sister's involvement was vital to realising his play plans, as there were tasks within the play that were beyond Dan's capabilities at the time (catching woodlice, for example.)

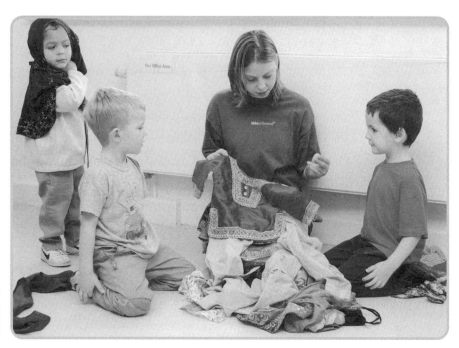

Toddlers use a range of props as material for play

Play in the home, for young children, is often spontaneous rather than planned. It may involve the child alone or the child and others, and it fits into the pattern of the day. Spontaneous play may result from the child encountering potential play materials or seeking play opportunities with a play theme in mind.

Activity 3) The playgroup

It is morning at the playgroup and parents are mainly sitting chatting in pairs and small groups. The room is light and warm and toys and play resources are set out in different areas, including a table with paints, crayons, paper and collage materials. Outside, one adult supervises several children playing on a small slide or on tricycles and ride-on cars. Inside, Adam, 18 months, is sitting on a blanket trying to get shapes into the shape sorter. He is watched by Emily, aged 2, who wants to intervene but is not sure how. Jasparl, aged 3, is sitting with a picture book looking at the pictures, although she would call this reading. She has the book the right way up and turns the pages one by one, looking at the left-hand page first. In a minute she will ask her father to read the words for her. Kyle, aged 2 and a half, is sitting with his mother's friend who is helping him to build a marble run. He watches her movements intently and then tries to put the connections together himself. When it is finished he repeatedly drops marbles into different openings in the run and watches them roll to the bottom. He is concentrating on the way in which the marbles emerge at different points, depending on where they are put in. In the home corner, Katie and Alisha, both 3 years of age, are 'making buns' using the play cooker and utensils and creating the action through shared language, until they squabble over who beats the mixture, at which point Katie's mother comes over and suggests that they have two bowls so they can both beat.

1 What sort of play is taking place here?

2 How might the play support the children's learning and development?

3 What role do the adults have in supporting the play?

The role of adults in play with babies and toddlers

Selleck (2001:81) discusses the knowledge we now have about young children's brain development and concludes that:

The main message from scientists seems to be that children need spontaneous playful interactions rather than any pre-planned or formal responses...

Selleck argues that young children are the 'creators of the curriculum' and the adult role is to observe and support that creativity. Vygotsky (1978) theorised that interaction with adults or peers at a higher stage of development than the child is central to children's learning development. Children can move from their actual level of development to the zone of potential development with adult support. Vygotsky argued that, in play, children demonstrated their skills at the highest level they could achieve at that point.

Wood, Bruner and Ross (1976) extended Vygotsky's ideas to introduce the concept of 'scaffolding' (see page 154). This theorised that adults can provide support in accordance with the child's level of development. This support can be removed gradually as the child accesses higher levels of ability and becomes more independent in play. Bruner also theorised that all play has rules and that children learn about the social and cultural norms of their society through acquisition of knowledge and understanding of these rules. Vygotsky and Bruner emphasise both child- and adult-initiated activities, with the adult taking a supportive role.

Facilitation and support

The adult role in play should focus on facilitation and support of the child, rather than intervention to introduce adult themes into the play. This means that intervention should be considered and based on observation of the play to ensure that it is appropriate, sensitive and designed to extend the play successfully (Heaslip, 1991).

It is important that adults are willing to join in play, but that they should not expect special privileges within the play. Adults can make suggestions to extend or enhance the play but should not assume these will be adopted. They can also contribute to discussions on play themes, remembering that children often have agendas that may not be explicit to adults. Adults have a role in providing materials and a suitable environment for play, but children should have choices in this also.

Children will choose their play materials to meet their own play agenda. These materials may not be 'toys' or objects that are designed specifically for play, but may be found objects, natural or manufactured materials, discarded items or household equipment.

Adult intervention in play, however, is not always child-centred. Lally (1989) found that adults generally believed that the activities they chose had a higher value than those chosen by the child, even where the adults were committed to the concept of play.

Play with parents

In this section we discuss the role of parents in play in the age group 0 to 3, and how this role differs between parents according to dominant cultural and child-rearing practices within the family. The impact on the child in terms of learning and development are discussed and, in the following section, related to the child's transition from home to early years setting and the wide range of diversity in developmental stage at this point. The term 'parents' will be used to refer to anyone with significant responsibility for a child.

The cultural context of play

Case Study 5

Wallowing in play

Calvin, aged 2, is observed walking through the park with his father when he sees a river of water running down the path from a recent cloudburst. He runs into the water, jumping, kicking and stamping, watching the silver spray patterns and experimenting with big and little jumps and kicks to see what the water does in response. His father watches and then joins in, creating even bigger splashes, to Calvin's delight. In the end they jump into the 'river' together holding hands, creating the biggest splash of all, whooping and yelling as they jump.

Bruce (1991:82) describes children 'wallowing in play' and this is a fine example. First-hand experiences are crucial to free flow play and allow children to wallow in ideas, feelings and relationships. In Case study 5, the child's parent is supporting the play by joining in, sharing the moment and communicating his own pleasure in the activity. However, this child's experiences may not apply to all children. Different approaches to parenting and beliefs about play may influence the extent to which children have opportunity to 'wallow' in new experiences. This observation in Case study 6 reflects another approach.

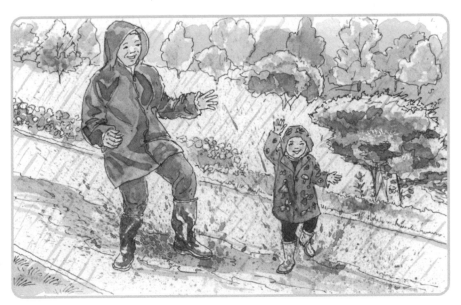

'Wallowing in play' may enable parent and child to enjoy playing on an equal basis

Case Study 6

Play provokes anxiety

The toddler arrived at the playground with her mother, wearing a neat, pretty, pastel summer dress, white ankle socks and dark-red patent shoes. As she ran towards the slide, her mother anxiously warned her not to get dirty. As the girl came off the end of the slide, she twisted round and checked the back of her dress, and then ran to her mother in some distress to report that it had been stained. Tissues were produced, the stain dabbed, and the slide banned. The child got onto the pedal roundabout with other children, and they started to work together to create speed, calling out and urging each other on. Inevitably, the patent shoes dragged on the floor and, just as the children achieved their aim, the roundabout was stopped and the child removed to be scolded. By this time, all the other children and parents in the playground were anxious.

Discussion Point 2

Parents' reaction to play

Discuss the ways in which each parent's reaction to the play may impact on the child in the scenarios above. What messages are the children getting about their play and how might this influence their future play?

A young child's family and community are significant in the type and quality of play experiences the child is provided with. The context in which children are brought up and the resources (personal, social and material) that a parent brings to the task of parenting will strongly influence the play that a child has access to. Different communities also have different expectations of children's play and may prioritise play differently. The cultural, linguistic, religious and social nature of a particular community will impact on how often children play, how this is valued by families, who children play with and where they play and what with. For example, in some communities, possibly those made up of British Asian families, older children may have responsibility for younger children and may play out with babies and toddlers in tow. More affluent communities with bigger gardens and widely separated houses may see less play on the streets than estates with cul-de-sacs and speed bumps. Toys may be selected according to income, so, for example, a child of an affluent household may use computer games by the age of two, while another child may not have access to a computer, according to Sayeed and Guerin (2000:18).

> *Whiting and Whiting (1975) view play and culture as a two-way process. In their opinion play is affected by cultural influences and acts as an expression of culture.*

Bruner argued that play reflects the cultural environment of the child and family and that children will play in ways that are determined by their cultural understandings. Tamis-Lemonda, Katz and Bornstein (2002:240) discuss the 'active socialisation' that takes place during role play and how this supports the acquisition of 'traditional thinking and behaviour'. Culturally specific play will influence what and how the child learns. In this way, play is an important factor in helping children learn in a culturally determined way. The cultural context, however, changes over time. For example, 'playing out' was common for toddlers as well as older children 30 or 40 years ago, but now it would be frowned on for such young children, and possibly for older children as well.

Differences in parental approaches to play are culturally determined. Studies showed that mothers in Mexico, Guatamala and Indonesia do not see value in, or the need for, play with their children, while middle-class American and Turkish parents actively play with their children (Tamis-Lemonda, Katz and Bornstein, 2002:240). The different content of role play between parents and children reflects and reinforces cultural values and influences different aspects of the child's development.

What parents know and understand about play

It is important to recognise that the knowledge and understanding that practitioners have about the role of play in development may not be shared by all parents. Parents may have diverse knowledge and understandings of play, and their personal experiences of play may also be very varied. Parents are often intuitive in their play with children, recognising that children enjoy and pass their time in play. However, not all adults value play in the same way, or recognise that promoting and supporting play is an important aspect of parenting.

Case Study 7

Analysis of play activity

Jake, aged 2 and a half, is sitting at the table with a pile of Duplo bricks. At the moment he is not building with these bricks by pressing them together as intended by the manufacturer, but instead he is trying to see how many he can balance, one on top of the other. After a while he introduces a colour pattern into the play, alternating red and yellow bricks and carefully putting aside blue bricks.

If we analyse this as a play activity, practitioners may see Jake's activities as experimental, as developing an understanding of the properties of the bricks, and as showing ability to recognise and make patterns, an important basis of mathematical understanding. However, an adult who lacks experience with young children may see that Jake is 'not using the bricks properly' because he is not putting them together.

Case Study 8

Attachment and babies' development through play

Play was the focus of a series of group work sessions with young mothers in low-demand housing, all suffering from social isolation and depression, and all a cause for concern in terms of actual or potential abuse or neglect of their children. In discussing play with babies, some of the young mothers told the facilitators that they had no idea of how to play with a child who was not mobile and verbal. One mother said that she 'felt silly' talking to a baby who could not talk back. Another asked how a baby could play as 'she can't pick up toys, can she?' One woman queried the need for play with babies, as they 'just need feeding and changing and bathing until they walk'.

The facilitators introduced the concept of attachment to the mothers, and also the concept of children learning and developing through play. They demonstrated the ways in which babies could enjoy play, and the times when this could take place. Some of the mothers started to enjoy talking to their babies, blowing raspberries on them to make them laugh, giving them objects to chew, throw and handle. Others found it hard to match their reactions to their babies and became frustrated when the child was unresponsive or cried. Many of the mothers continued to feel awkward and self-conscious in this 'playful' role for a long time.

For other parents, knowledge and understanding of children's needs may be more accessible and there may be positive social and economic circumstances to support time and energy for play. In the example of Elaine and her baby given on page 215, Sol was responding to his mother's behaviour almost from birth. Within a short time he was tracking her movements with his eyes, intent on her face. When she talked to him and made noises, Sol's arms and legs would wave vigorously and he would bounce up and down in response to her voice and movements. When the interaction ceased, Sol's face would crumple and he would start to cry or he would turn his head looking for his mother's face. By the age of 4 months he was making noises in response to the sounds Elaine made and this reciprocal noise-making took on the pattern of a conversation.

Parents may initiate play or support it as it develops. However, the involvement of parents in some form is an important factor in developing play for young children. According to Sayeed and Guerin's research (2000), parental involvement in play extends the length and enhances the quality of the child's play. They suggest that there is a continuum of involvement of parents in play from unaware parents who are not involved in play at one extreme, to very aware parents who have opted out of involvement to avoid interfering at the other extreme. Sayeed and Guerin (2000:20) conclude:

> Within any culture these extremes can exist but a parent's/carer's clear understanding of his/her role and a reasonable level of involvement can enrich the child's play in any given context.

During play with their parents, children absorb important information about the norms and values of their own culture and learn about culturally appropriate behaviour. First-hand experiences are significant in determining the play of younger children, and these are also culturally specific to families and communities. For example, cooking within one home may involve using the microwave to cook frozen food and serving it within a short space of time. In another household, the child may observe food being prepared in a much more lengthy and elaborate way. Children in some families may be taken on regular trips, holidays and days out, while others may be more home-based or use local facilities more often. The child's first-hand experiences are basic materials for role-play and socio-dramatic play, providing a rich source of remembered images to be used by the child. Access to first-hand experiences can vary significantly, depending on a wide range of social, health, cultural and economic factors influencing family functioning. For example, a child raised in an affluent family with two working parents may have access to a wide range of play materials, but there may be limited interaction between the child and parents if work is demanding and involves long hours. Poverty can affect the experiences a child has, which may be limited by lack of access to affordable transport, few local facilities and no money for holidays or trips. Health problems may also affect the parent's ability to interact with a child.

Approaches to play within the family

The types of play materials and objects and beliefs about the best types of play are also subject to cultural and family differences. For example, gender-specific behaviours are culture bound and may vary from culture to culture. Parents exert a strong influence on their children's play behaviour and choice of toys in the early years, and for the youngest children these choices may be made largely by parents. Thompson found parents influenced children's choice of toys by comments like 'only sissies play with dolls', 'girls don't climb trees' and 'boys like guns' (1986:19). Walters (2002) found that girls played with a wider range of toys because fathers, in particular, were against boys playing with 'girlie' toys.

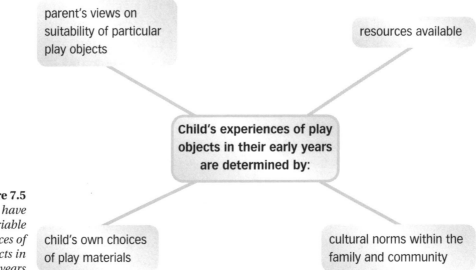

Figure 7.5
Children have variable experiences of play objects in their first years

Parenting style and the child's access to play

The dominant parenting style will have a significant influence on the child's access to play, the extent to which play is encouraged and resourced, and the range and quality of the parent's play with the child.

Ideally, the parent's role is to:

⊃ provide play opportunities for children

⊃ to extend and resource their play where necessary

⊃ most importantly, to allow time and space for children's free play so that they are able to innovate, create and imagine.

In Bruce's view, these three learning processes are important to babies and children's development and they occur in young children's free flow play (1991:2).

The extent to which parents are able to fulfill this role may depend on a number of interrelated factors. With reference to the discussion above on how parenting styles are developed, it is important to acknowledge that parenting is a unique experience for each parent and child. The factors that may influence the extent to which parents are able to support play are shown in Figure 7.6.

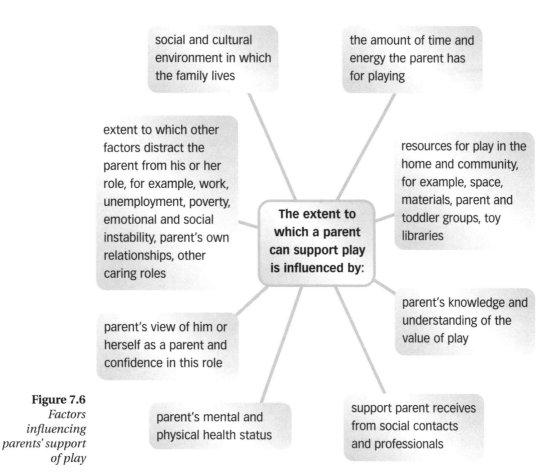

Figure 7.6
Factors influencing parents' support of play

The diagram shows: **The extent to which a parent can support play is influenced by:**

- social and cultural environment in which the family lives
- the amount of time and energy the parent has for playing
- extent to which other factors distract the parent from his or her role, for example, work, unemployment, poverty, emotional and social instability, parent's own relationships, other caring roles
- resources for play in the home and community, for example, space, materials, parent and toddler groups, toy libraries
- parent's view of him or herself as a parent and confidence in this role
- parent's knowledge and understanding of the value of play
- parent's mental and physical health status
- support parent receives from social contacts and professionals

Discussion Point 3

Julie, one of the young mothers in the example given in Case study 8 on page 222, lives alone with her 2-year-old son, John. Julie attaches great importance to keeping a tidy house and keeps John's toys boxed away behind the settee. He is not allowed messy play or to play with found objects. He has one toy out at a time during certain parts of the day. Julie does not play with him. She suffers from depression and has low self-esteem and a sense of failure about her life. She lives on benefits in low-demand housing. Julie's feelings as a parent are confused. She finds it difficult to express affection for John or to engage with him, but she is proud of his sturdiness and attractive looks. She feels that 'keeping on top of the housework' is one way of maintaining control in her life.

Make notes on the following questions and discuss with a colleague or mentor.

1 Consider the possible impact of Julie's approach on John's development and ability to access to nursery education in 9 months' time.

2 What sort of support might be available now to help Julie expand John's play experience and involve herself more in his play?

3 What support might be available at the point John takes up his nursery place?

Material resources can have a significant impact on parenting, but poverty in itself does not prevent parents playing with children. Rather, the impact of poverty on family life can have a negative influence on the time and energy that parents can give to their children. Often parents in poverty have to work long hours to maintain a viable income, or parents who are unemployed may spend long hours seeking work or may be depressed about lack of work and money. Parents are also subject to pressure to ensure that children have access to fashionable toys and expensive play equipment. These pressures can be ferocious even for parents of pre-school children and may add to the anxiety and stress that parents with financial problems may experience.

Poverty may not be the only limitation on parents.

Case Study 9

Play opportunities

Emma and Tom are a couple in their 20s, raised in working class families. They very much want their children to have a different upbringing to their own and to have the material benefits they missed out on. They both work, and in order to maintain promotion chances this means working long hours and bringing work home. Their first child, Daisy, who is nearly 3 years of age, is at a private day nursery where she enjoys a range of play activities. Emma and Tom often do not have the time and energy to play with Daisy. They believe that she has sufficient play opportunities at nursery and they avoid messy play and anything that will involve a lot of tidying up, such as cooking or elaborate role plays.

Although Daisy has play opportunities at nursery, she may be missing out on the spontaneous play that is so important to young children. Also, the proportion of time she spends at nursery is quite small compared to the time she spends at home. The unique play she could have access to in her family home is missing, as are some of the first-hand experiences from which role play is drawn. For example, Tom's African Caribbean family has a long tradition of story telling and recounting family history with their children.

Activity 4) Reflecting on home play

Reflecting on culturally specific and home play experiences can help practitioners to plan play and support children more effectively on entry to the early years setting. Recognising the wide range of experiences children have of play in the home, and the approaches to play children have already learned will help bridge the gap (where it exists) between home and early years setting.

1 What culturally specific and home play experiences have the babies or children you work with had?

2 Design a small questionnaire or interview to ask parents about play in the home.

3 How will this information help you in planning play experiences within your early years setting?

The availability and quality of play experiences for young children within the family therefore vary greatly, depending on many interrelated factors. The developmental outcomes for the child will depend on how play has been valued, supported and resourced within the home, as well as other factors affecting the child's ability to access play. These may include the child's level of ability, character and stage of development. Development will also depend on the cultural messages children learn through the types of play they have access to, and the involvement of parents within this.

Transitions to educare settings

In this section, we discuss the child's transition to an educare setting, focusing on play within the pre-school curriculum and the challenges and expectations it creates for both children and practitioners. In addition, strategies for supporting a diverse range of young children in their transition to formal learning situations are considered.

Play within the pre-school curriculum

Increasing numbers of children are entering educare settings at the age of 3. The government agenda within the National Childcare Strategy, to extend early learning to all 3- and 4 year olds, has produced many more places for children, although access to these remains highly variable, depending on geographical location and level of income (Pugh, 2001). Many parents seek places for children in order to return to work and to ensure their children have access to pre-school social and educational experiences. Although play regularly comes under attack as a medium for learning and development, it currently maintains a role in the formal pre-school curriculum. The Rumbold Report (DES, 1990) in reporting its findings about the quality of provision for four year olds recognised the value of play in young children's learning and development.

Play underlines a great deal of young children's learning. For its potential value to be realised a number of conditions need to be fulfilled:

    ⊃ *Sensitive, knowledgeable and informed adult involvement and intervention*

    ⊃ *Careful planning and organisation of play settings to provide for and extend learning*

    ⊃ *Enough time for children to develop their play*

    ⊃ *Careful observation of children's activities to facilitate assessment and planning for progression and continuity.*

These recommendations are incorporated within the play provision in the Curriculum Guidance for the Foundation Stage (QAA, 2000) for 3- to 5 year olds. At present there is no statutory curriculum for children under 3 years of age; however, the recently developed framework for learning and development *Birth to Three Matters* supports children's learning and development in their earliest years and play is central to this framework (Sure Start, 2003).

As children begin at an early years setting, they continue to need adults to help them to play, places to play and materials to play with. Their varied experiences of play within the family and other 0 to 3 play environments need to be built upon and developed. The Curriculum Guidance for the Foundation Stage (2000:25) requires a play-based curriculum of 'well-planned play' that is predominantly planned for children by practitioners. The role of the practitioner in children's play is defined:

> *The role of the practitioner is crucial in:*
>
> ➲ *Planning and resourcing a challenging environment;*
>
> ➲ *Supporting children's learning through planned play activity;*
>
> ➲ *Extending and supporting children's spontaneous play;*
>
> ➲ *Extending and developing children's language and communication in play.*
>
> *Through play, in a secure environment with effective adult support, children can:*
>
> ➲ *Explore, develop and represent learning experiences that help them make sense of the world;*
>
> ➲ *Practise and build up ideas, concepts and skills;*
>
> ➲ *Learn how to control impulses and understand the need for rules;*
>
> ➲ *Be alone, be alongside others or cooperate as they talk or rehearse their feelings;*
>
> ➲ *Take risks and make mistakes;*
>
> ➲ *Think creatively and imaginatively;*
>
> ➲ *Communicate with others as they investigate or solve problems;*
>
> ➲ *Express fears or relive anxious experiences in controlled and safe situations.*

Three-year-olds entering educare settings

The National Childcare Strategy, implemented in 1998, has resulted in greater numbers of 3-year-olds in group care settings. This in itself has created a challenge for meeting the needs of these young children. The wide range of early experiences, languages, cultural behaviours and levels of development that early years settings may encounter with their youngest children require a well-planned and considered response in order to meet the diverse needs of the children in their care. When early years settings fail to acknowledge and respond adequately to this range of needs, children may suffer in terms of their emotional and social development, as well as their learning development. There is evidence that ability to successfully access the curriculum in pre-school early years settings may have a strong positive influence on the child's long-term educational success. The reverse may also be true.

Case Study 10

Learning delay

Lauren was 3 and a half when she started nursery school at a large inner city primary school in a socio-economically deprived area that had a considerable number of children who did not speak English on entry. Lauren was fostered with a family in the area. She had few early first-hand experiences of her environment outside the home and her access to pre-school play had been limited by neglecting parents and an overburdened foster carer. When Lauren left the school just over a year later to live with her permanent family, the nursery teacher commented that 'she never spoke to anyone and she doesn't play with the others much. I think she's shy and doesn't want to join in'. When she started in reception class at her new school a month later, Lauren was hysterically terrified of being left, cried every day, and could not play either by herself or with others. Despite the support of parents and the school, it took two years for Lauren to develop the confidence to make friends and join in with others. She continued to lack confidence in play and her development of play skills was slow. Lauren's learning delays persisted and her low self-esteem continued to influence all aspects of her development.

Meeting the different needs of a group of children

The diverse nature of a group of children's experiences creates a challenge in itself. How do we meet the different needs of a group of children within

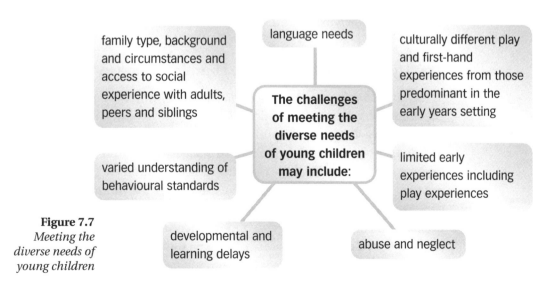

Figure 7.7
Meeting the diverse needs of young children

a single curriculum structure? How can each child's unique early experience be reflected in the curriculum and built upon?

The type and size of the early years setting will influence the individual child's response and the extent to which individual needs can be met. For example, a childminder may have the flexibility to feed children at different times of the day and work with the child's natural patterns in terms of play, sleep, rest and nourishment. A group early years setting such as an independent day nursery may not have this flexibility because of staff shift patterns and the constraints of managing group care with a range of staff.

The factors shown in Figure 7.8 will also be significant in determining the young child's experience:

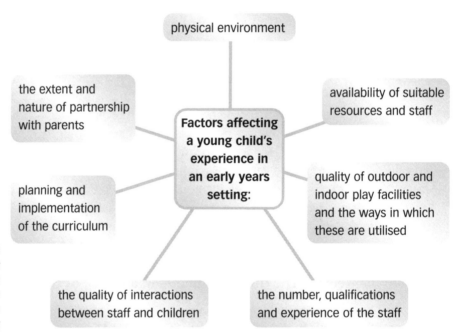

Figure 7.8
Factors that determine the child's experience in an early years setting

The factors shown in Figure 7.8 are discussed in more detail in Chapter 8.

Transitions from home to the Foundation Stage

Transitions from home to an early years setting involves challenges for practitioners, parents and children. The wide range of experiences that children have at 3 years of age is a challenge to early years settings and individual practitioners when planning the curriculum and developing relationships with each child. Children may find that their experiences do not have much in common with events, activities and routines within the early years setting. They may find that they have little to build on or that expectations of them are hard to understand. Children may find that the experiences valued in their home and own culture are ignored or given little value within the early years setting.

Parents may have complex feelings about their child going to an early years setting. These may focus on separation and loss of the special relationship, fear that the child may 'change' in ways that the parent has little influence over, or that the child will be unhappy. The parents' reasons for sending their child to an educare early years setting may vary. Parents may find talking to professionals difficult or feel hostile to early years practitioners, because of their own experiences of education. They may not understand the expectations placed on them in terms of partnership and involvement and there may be resistance to this. Parents also have varied understanding of child development and children's needs and this may influence the extent to which they support current practices in childcare and education. Cultural factors may result in mothers, in particular, not being able to relate to, or communicate with, the staff in an early years setting. There may be language differences or perhaps cultural practices that, for example, do not allow women to be with men outside their family group. One school provided a room for Muslim women to unveil for special needs reviews and other purposes.

It is not uncommon for parents to question early years settings about the role of play in the curriculum. The distinction between play and work may be made and there may be a lack of understanding of how children do their work through play. The role of play in development may be difficult to explain and practitioners need to be clear about their own position and the commitment of the early years setting to play. It is also important to recognise that planned activities chosen by adults may be described as play but not experienced as such by children.

Discussion Point 4

Play and development

1 How do you establish a dialogue with parents in your early years setting about the importance of play in their child's learning and development?

2 How do you build upon the child's home play experiences?

3 How do you include parents in children's play in the early years setting?

Issues for children

These relate to the match between their experiences and the dominant cultural practices within the early years setting with reference to:

- languages spoken and conversational themes
- play themes, resources and expected experiences of play
- expectations of behaviour and responses to misbehaviour
- expectations of gender roles

- attitudes
- relationship development
- clothes, appearance, hygienic practices and attitudes towards these
- food and drink
- exposure to an understanding of popular culture.

For some children this list will also include the early years setting's response to developmental delays across the range of indicators including the impact of abuse and neglect on all aspects of the child's development.

Issues for parents

These include all the issues identified for children and also the parents':

- own feelings about their parenting skills, abilities and the role of being a parent
- parenting style and child-rearing practices
- confidence in their ability to discuss their children's needs with professionals
- level of engagement with the parenting process
- attitudes towards and feelings about educational institutions and practitioners
- understanding of child development and their own child's needs.

The parent's ability to effectively engage with the early years setting and form partnerships with practitioners will depend on the individual's socio-economic, emotional and health status, among other factors.

Issues for practitioners and the early years setting

These include:

- acquiring knowledge and understanding of a range of different children's individual needs and the cultural and social underpinnings of these
- recognising the influence of the dominant culture within the early years setting on 'success' and 'failure' for some children
- developing skills to make relationships with a wide range of others
- planning the curriculum to meet the individual child's needs within a group context
- understanding a range of strategies to engage parents and how to use these effectively
- acknowledging diversity in a positive and responsive way that does not patronise or stereotype
- becoming a reflective practitioner.

Practitioners also need to consider their own views and assumptions about the parenting role and their responses to a range of parental approaches. Approaches that are judgemental, negative and critical of parents and children or cultures different to their own can be damaging to relationships and limit the child's experience.

Case Study 11

Judgmental approach limits a child's experience

Di was cautioned by the police and her 3-year-old son was placed on the Child Protection Register after she admitted bruising his face. When she next went to nursery, although nothing was said about the incident directly to her, the reaction of the practitioners was sufficient to ensure that she withdrew her child and he no longer had a nursery place.

Making the transition work

Effective strategies for helping children to access the early years setting begin well before the first day of attendance.

Practitioners need to have information about the child's needs and experiences to date, and have time to reflect on what these needs mean when planning the curriculum. Practitioners may also need time to research into the specific needs of a child, where existing knowledge is limited.

Case Study 12

Baby with specific needs

A private day nursery agreed to offer a place to a 6-month-old baby with Down's syndrome. Few of the staff had worked with Down's babies and lacked knowledge about the child's possible needs or developmental pattern. The practitioner who became the baby's key worker went on a short course to widen her knowledge and also contacted other practitioners who had more experience in this area. She attended the child's review meeting, organised by social services, to find out about the range of support services offered to the child and family and to make links with other practitioners involved with them. She also made a home visit and spent time talking to the parent's about their hopes and fears for their child.

Reflective practice is central to the process of ensuring that differential needs are met successfully, and this needs to be promoted through both the individual practitioner's own development and through management strategies and ethos.

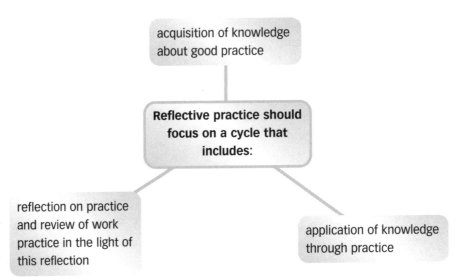

Figure 7.9
Reflective practice

acquisition of knowledge about good practice

Reflective practice should focus on a cycle that includes:

reflection on practice and review of work practice in the light of this reflection

application of knowledge through practice

Practitioners who perceive themselves within a cycle of learning and development will be able to respond more effectively to diverse needs. Early years settings need to regularly review their arrangements for the entry of young children in order to improve practice and meet a wider range of children and parents' needs. Reflective practice is discussed in detail in Chapter 2.

Strategies to help children settle: pre-entry

The following are some suggestions about the sort of approaches that may work to help early years settings to meet children's needs before a child enters an early years setting. The list is not exclusive, and 'what works' will depend on:

- ⊃ the experiences of the child
- ⊃ the type of early years setting

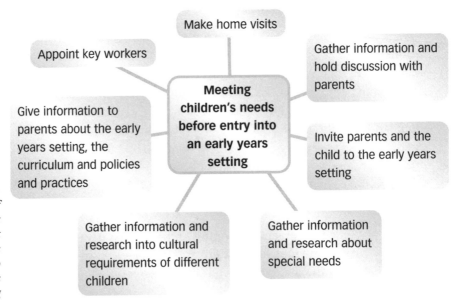

Figure 7.10
Examples of approaches that may help to meet children's needs before entry to an early years setting

Make home visits

Appoint key workers

Gather information and hold discussion with parents

Give information to parents about the early years setting, the curriculum and policies and practices

Meeting children's needs before entry into an early years setting

Invite parents and the child to the early years setting

Gather information and research into cultural requirements of different children

Gather information and research about special needs

- the cultural and socio-economic context
- the skills and knowledge of individual practitioners
- and the management ethos within the early years setting.

Strategies to forge a link between home and school need to be creative. For example, a nursery could take photos of the child playing with his or her favourite toy to display in the nursery, ready for the child's first day.

The aim of working with parents and children prior to entry is not just to assess the child and give information to the parent, but also to establish a relationship with both parents and child and to set up a dialogue about the ways in which the child's needs can be met. Practitioners need to consider the use of interpersonal skills to engage with adults as well as the child, and to establish a positive relationship. This involves actively listening to the parent and establishing an understanding of the parent's approach, the child's early experiences and ongoing factors influencing the child's development.

Strategies to help children settle: on entry

Factors to consider on entry to the early years setting may include:

- establishing a play-based curriculum that reflects the previous real life and play experiences of all the children
- recognising the stages of play that different children are at and ensuring differential needs are met
- understanding the emotional and social developmental aspects of differential early experience and responding to these
- recognising and responding to language needs in all children, including those who have different types of English to the practitioners
- recognising that the use of controls may differ greatly in families depending on child-rearing practices and this may influence behaviour within the early years setting
- avoiding either assumptions or stereotypes about children's experiences and parenting.

Case Study 13

Traveller children

Traveller children who attended nursery school during a winter layover found that staff did not understand their accent and that other children made fun of them and avoided their company when playing. The traveller children had a different understanding of play and had little experience of indoor play. Their behaviour was described as 'unruly'. The traveller support worker was heavily involved in bridging the cultural, social and linguistic gap between these children and the rural school early years setting.

Play for all

A number of children are at a playgroup where parents bring their children and stay with them for the morning to enable both parents and children to socialise and play.

1 Fazan, 2 and a half years of age, leans against his mother's knee, staring at the other children playing. He has not moved to play or use toys or play materials. When the other children come near him he shrinks back further against his mother's knee. His mother has not spoken to anyone yet and she is the only British Asian parent there.

2 Jack, aged 2 and three quarters, is racing around in a play car. He comes only to play on the car, as there is no room for big toys in his home or garden. He has patiently queued for the car and will play on it for as long as possible. He does not play with other children.

3 Safura, nearly 3 years of age, and her friend who lives next door to her, Britney, aged 3, are playing in the home corner with the cooker, pretending to bake cakes for birthdays. They are partially playing alongside and partially playing cooperatively, using language to develop their play themes and ideas. They pretend to read a 'cook book' because this is what Britney's mother does at home. Declan, aged 2 and three quarters, is hovering close by and watching their play with great interest.

4 At the table, two other 3 year olds are painting, gluing and talking about what they are doing with one of the volunteer workers.

In 6 months' time all these children will be in the same nursery school class.

The challenge of meeting diverse play needs has to be met for all children in order to ensure that they can access a play-based curriculum successfully. If children are not able to extend and develop their learning through play, this may have an impact on their ability to tackle more structured learning activities at a later stage. In meeting their diverse needs, a range of play opportunities need to be provided, including socio-dramatic play, free flow, planned play, group and individual play activities.

Smilansky (1968) studied children in socio-dramatic play and concluded that it supported cognitive, social and emotional development. Children who were inexperienced, or unable to access socio-dramatic play, were supported by play trainers in order to help them learn to both plan and play in this way, and reflect on the play. This type of play became more common in these children after the play training. Practitioners need to be aware that some children will need support in learning to play in different ways. Ways in which play can be supported include those shown in Figure 7.11.

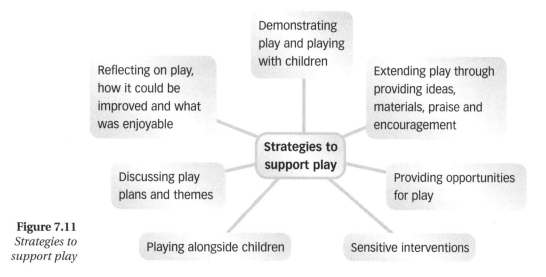

Demonstrating play and playing with children

Reflecting on play, how it could be improved and what was enjoyable

Extending play through providing ideas, materials, praise and encouragement

Strategies to support play

Discussing play plans and themes

Providing opportunities for play

Playing alongside children

Sensitive interventions

Figure 7.11
Strategies to support play

Individual children will need different levels of support to access play; therefore a broad range of play opportunities needs to be provided.

> **Activity 5** **Providing support in an early years setting**

Look back at Case study 14 on the previous page. Fazan is on the waiting list for your nursery school and he will be offered a place to start two months after his third birthday. Fazan's first language is Punjabi and he lives with his mother, father and two older sisters, now 5 and 7 years old. Fazan's sisters had quite a lot of difficulty on entry to school because they did not attend nursery or pre-school and did not speak English very well. They are both settled into the school but still struggle with some aspects of the curriculum. Fazan's mother wants Fazan to have a better start to school, which is why she has joined the playgroup and put Fazan's name down for the nursery at his sister's school, where you work. However, she is worried that Fazan does not play or join in with the others at playgroup. Fazan's mother speaks some English and her husband is fluent, but he works long hours as a bus driver and is not around very much.

1 What sort of support could be offered to Fazan and his mother before he enters nursery?
2 What sort of support would help Fazan settle into nursery?
3 What strategies would you use to make a relationship with this family in order to better support all the children?

⟩ Conclusion

There are no easy answers to meeting diverse needs within an early years setting. Recognising that children differ greatly in their real life and parenting experiences is an important starting point, as is absorbing the complex factors that influence the child's development to date. Responding to a range of needs means working hard at understanding and valuing what the child has done, rather than what the child has not yet achieved. Giving equal weight to different experiences and valuing cultural behaviour that is unlike your own requires the ability to learn, apply knowledge and reflect on one's own practice. Play is a medium through which children can express emotions and develop social skills, as well as learn. However, children may have very different experiences of play on entry to an early years setting and supporting the development of play behaviour is a crucial part of the practitioner's role in providing each child with a worthwhile experience in an early years setting.

Early years practitioners also have a role in promoting and supporting play between children and parents where this is limited or absent. Not all parents understand the role of a play-based curriculum and settings have a responsibility to explain this to them and to encourage play at home. Developing partnerships with parents is crucial to success in helping the development of play at home and in the setting. However, helping parents to understand the need for play with their children in the early years may lay the foundations of parent and child play throughout childhood.

References and further reading

Aries, P. (1982), *Centuries of Childhood: A Social History of Family Life*. London: Cape and Sears

Bee, H. (2000), *The Developing Child'*, 9th Ed. Boston, MA: Allyn and Bacon

Bruce, T. (1991), *Time to Play in Early Childhood Education*. London: Hodder and Stoughton

Bruce, T. (1996), *Quality of Play in Early Childhood Education*. London: Hodder and Stoughton

Bruce, T. (2001), *Helping Young Children to Learn Through Play*. London: Hodder and Stoughton

David, T. (1996), 'Their Right to Play', in Nutbrown, C. (Ed.), *Respectful Educators – Responsible Learners: Children's Rights and Early Education*. London: Paul Chapman Publishing

DES (1990), 'The Rumbold Report': *Starting with Quality*. London: DES

Giddens, A. (1989), *Introduction to Sociology*. Cambridge: Polity Press

Goldschmied, E. and Jackson, S. (1997), *People Under 3: Young Children in Day Care*. London: Routledge

Hurst, V. and Joseph, J. (1998), *Supporting Early Learning: The Way Forward*. Maidenhead: Open University Press

Kindersley A. and Kindersley B. (1997), *Celebrations!* (*Children Just Like Me*). London: Dorling Kindersley

Messer, D. and Millar, S. (1999), *Exploring Developmental Psychology: From Infancy to Adolescence*. London: Hodder Arnold

Moyles, J. (ed.) (1994), *The Excellence of Play*. Maidenhead: OU Press

Pugh, G. et al (1994), *Confident Parents, Confident Children: Policy and Practice in Parent Education and Support*. London: National Children's Bureau

QCA (2000), *Curriculum Guidance for the Foundation Stage*. London: DfEE

Robinson, M. (2003), *From Birth to One: The Year of Opportunity*. Maidenhead: Open University Press

Rutherford, D. (1998), 'Children's Relationships', in Taylor, J. and Woods, M. (eds), *Early Childhood Studies: An Holistic Introduction*. London: Hodder Arnold

Smilansky, S. (1968), *Effects of Sociodramatic Play on Disadvantaged Preschool Children*. New York: John Wiley

Smilansky, S. (1990), 'Socio-Dramatic Play: its relevance to behaviour and achievement in school' in Klugman, E. and Smilansky, S. (eds) *Children's Play and Learning: Perspectives and Policy Implications*. New York: Teachers' College Press

Summerfield, C. and Babb, P. (2003), *Social Trends, No. 33 National Statistics*. London: HMSO

Sure Start (2003), *Birth to Three Matters*. London: DfEE/Sure Start

Tamis-Lemonda, C., Katz, J. and Bornstein, M. (2002), 'Infant Play: functions and partners' in Slater, A. and Lewis, M. (eds.) *Introduction to Infant Development*. Oxford: Oxford University Press

Thompson, J.(1986), *All Right for Some! The problem of sexism*. Cheltenham: Nelson Thornes

Thurtle, V. (1998), 'Child In Society' in Taylor, J. and Woods, M. (eds), *Early Childhood Studies: An Holistic Introduction*. London: Hodder Arnold

Woods, M. (1998), 'Early Childhood Studies – first principles' in Taylor, J. and Woods, M. (eds), *Early Childhood Studies: An Holistic Introduction*. London: Hodder Arnold

Useful websites

www.qca.org.uk
For information provided by the Qualifications and Curriculum Authority, follow the links to the Foundation Stage section. Includes downloads and curriculum guidance.

www.foundationstage.net
Discussion and advice on the Foundation Stage.

www.surestart.gov.uk
Covers all the aims and achievements of the government's SureStart programme.

www.parenting.org
Offers advice and answers questions about play.

www.bbc.co.uk/parenting/play
Play resources, toys and activities for parents to try with their children.

Planning for early learning: Foundation Stage and Key Stage 1

8

Elaine Hallet and Iain MacLeod-Brudenell

This chapter aims to explore a range of generic issues to be considered when planning learning experiences for young children. Its secondary purpose is to encourage reflective approaches to planning that best meet children's individual learning needs.

This chapter addresses the following areas:

- ⊃ the curriculum as a framework for assessment
- ⊃ theories of children's learning
- ⊃ the importance of planning for learning
- ⊃ the role of the practitioner in planning for learning
- ⊃ building a relevant curriculum for children's learning.

By undertaking the suggested study within this chapter it is hoped that you will be able to:

1 understand the importance of 'match' between the child's ability and planned activity in order to meet the prescribed curriculum

2 be able to plan activities that acknowledge children's individual needs and support them in their personal, social and emotional development

3 effectively evaluate your own experiences of planning within the workplace.

The curriculum as a framework for assessment

Understanding the curriculum

In order to consider the purposes of planning, it is important to have a clear understanding of the curriculum. Important factors include:

- ⊃ What is a curriculum?
- ⊃ Who is it for?
- ⊃ Why does the curriculum include what it does?
- ⊃ How does the curriculum differ to other curricula?

Addressing these questions determines how the curriculum is approached.

What is a curriculum?

Education is usually viewed as a body of knowledge to be acquired by children, the content of which is linked to stages or ages. Many people liken this to a curriculum. However, in addition to elements of knowledge and understanding, the curriculum can also include aspects of social and personal development.

A curriculum represents the values of the society in which it is used. The content is often determined by government at national level, as is the case in the countries comprising the United Kingdom, or at local or regional level, such as the cantonal governments in Switzerland, the German Lander or the Canadian provinces. Curricula may also reflect the values of parents, who may opt to support their children's education by paying for private education; this most frequently occurs in countries where the private education system has a different curriculum to that provided within mainstream education. International examples of this are Montessori, Steiner or Froebel educational settings.

The role of the curriculum in early years learning

Early years learning takes place within a curriculum. This may be 'formal' learning within a school or nursery, or 'informal' learning within a home setting with parents and carers, or a blend of both. Childminders often provide a curriculum that draws on both formal and informal activities. A comparison of the early years curricula provided in different countries clearly shows that there is no consensus as to the most effective means of teaching children.

Different curriculum approaches

A key way in which curriculum approaches differ is that some emphasise knowledge content while others emphasise the process of learning. Different approaches to curriculum delivery are shown in Figure 8.1.

In England, the Foundation Stage and National Curriculum place greater emphasis on knowledge content than the process of delivery. However, this

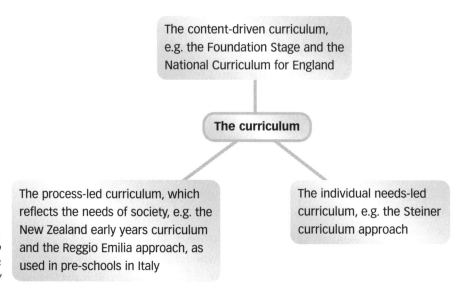

The content-driven curriculum, e.g. the Foundation Stage and the National Curriculum for England

The curriculum

The process-led curriculum, which reflects the needs of society, e.g. the New Zealand early years curriculum and the Reggio Emilia approach, as used in pre-schools in Italy

The individual needs-led curriculum, e.g. the Steiner curriculum approach

Figure 8.1
Approaches to curriculum delivery

is not to say that the different approaches are mutually exclusive; in England, the development of the individual child is recognised when working with children with special educational needs. It should also be remembered that curricula are not set in stone; they may be changed and developed to meet the needs of the individual child and the early years setting. Indeed, in the past twenty years in England, there have been massive changes in the curriculum: in how it is taught, in the expectations of those who teach it, and in its focus on the end users (children).

The emphasis on the individual recording of children's achievements, which forms such a major part of the workload for practitioners in England, is not the norm in other education systems. This method may be seen as one way of reconciling a content-focused curriculum with the need to acknowledge the importance of the individual.

The National Curriculum

The National Curriculum was introduced by the government in 1988 for use in England and Wales (DfEE/QCA, 1999) for children of statutory school age. Following a number of revisions and changes in emphasis upon curriculum areas, a 'slimmed down' version of the curriculum is now in place for schools in England. For example, the development of literacy and numeracy skills in the early years is now a priority, and the methods prescribed within the Literacy and Numeracy Strategies provide a template for curriculum delivery. Thus, in English schools the original emphasis on a broad and balanced curriculum providing opportunities for creative thinking and an holistic approach to curriculum delivery has been overtaken by a narrow skills-based curriculum.

The curriculum in Scotland has always been distinctly different and has provided guidance for teachers rather than prescriptive targets. In addition, recent political developments in Wales have promoted a more regionally focused curriculum that is more attentive to local needs and more broadly based than the English curriculum.

Raising standards

The National Curriculum lies at the heart of policies in England to raise standards. It sets out a clear, full and statutory entitlement to learning for all pupils. It determines the content of what will be taught, and sets out attainment targets for learning. It also determines how performance will be assessed and reported. An effective National Curriculum, therefore, gives teachers, pupils, parents, employers and their wider community a clear and shared understanding of the skills and knowledge that young people will gain at school (QCA, 1999:3).

In England, there are now statutory and non-statutory curriculum guidance materials for children from birth to sixteen years. The quality of delivery of the curriculum is checked through inspection and the response of children is measured through rigorous age-related testing against national criteria. It should be noted that children are not legally required to attend a school or nursery and that alternative educational provision within the home is a legal right. However, most children in England will begin school at the age of five years and leave at the age of sixteen, the statutory age range for full-time education. Children in England now have an entitlement curriculum in which planning is integrated with assessment.

The historical context of the early years curriculum in England

The National Curriculum was implemented several years before an early years curriculum was established in England via the Desirable Learning Outcomes (DLOs), (SCAA, 1996). Thus the development of the early years curriculum and its planning was largely influenced by the National Curriculum. This influence was not entirely beneficial, resulting in a high-content, goal-centred and adult-led curriculum rather than a curriculum that was process- and child-led. The appropriateness of using a curriculum intended for 5–7 year olds with 3–5 year olds is questionable; indeed, the National Curriculum should more logically have emerged from an early years curriculum, as Bruce indicates:

> *building on the unique early childhood principles and practice that could then grow through the primary curriculum.*   *(Bruce, 1987 in 1991:7).*

Prior to the introduction of the Desirable Learning Outcomes (DLOs) in England (SCAA, 1996), there was no uniform approach to the early years curriculum. Previously, local education authorities (LEAs) and individual nurseries and schools had generally developed their own approaches to planning; nursery schools devised their own curriculum often following advice from the LEA Advisory Service. In many cases, nursery units and classes attached to primary schools had used the National Curriculum for Key Stage 1 as guidance when preparing children for progression to the reception class.

The Desirable Learning Outcomes were the first prescribed curriculum outlines provided to enable planning for four year olds. These guidelines indicated which areas were to be covered within a curriculum, and the settings delivering the curriculum were inspected by Ofsted.

The Rumbold Report

The Rumbold Report (DES, 1990:9) investigated the provision for under-fives in England. It found patchy, often unplanned curricula provision and proposed a curriculum for the under-fives that would:

> *provide experiences which support, stimulate and structure a child's learning and bring about a progression of understanding appropriate to the child's needs and abilities.*

The Rumbold Report defined the curriculum as comprising:

> *concepts, knowledge, understanding, attitudes and skills that a child*
> *needs to develop*   *(DES, 1990:9).*

For the educare practitioner, the report highlighted the importance of considering not only the content of delivery but the process of learning – the opportunities and experiences offered by adults to give each child relevant and appropriate learning contexts.

> *How children are encouraged to learn is as important as, and inseparable*
> *from, the content – what they learn*   *(DES, 1990:9).*

The Foundation Stage: an early years curriculum

An attempt to provide a developmentally appropriate curriculum for three to five year olds evolved from the Rumbold Report and resulted in the introduction of the Foundation Stage (DfES/QCA, 2001). The Foundation Stage Curriculum Guidance (2000:8) explains that three, four and five year olds:

> *need a well-planned and resourced curriculum to take their learning*
> *forward and to provide opportunities for all children to succeed in an*
> *atmosphere of care and feeling valued.*

This is the first time that educating children of this age has been recognised as a distinct and separate phase of learning within the maintained, state sector. The 'Stepping Stones', which form an integral part of this educational programme, feed into the National Curriculum Key Stage 1 programme but allow for development at a pace appropriate to the needs of the individual child. The Foundation Stage approach recognises that learning occurs constantly, whether intentional or incidental.

A framework for planning

Planning for Learning in the Foundation Stage (DfES, 2001) may be seen as a landmark in that it provides a framework to ensure a common approach to planning in the early years curriculum. The approach that is promoted

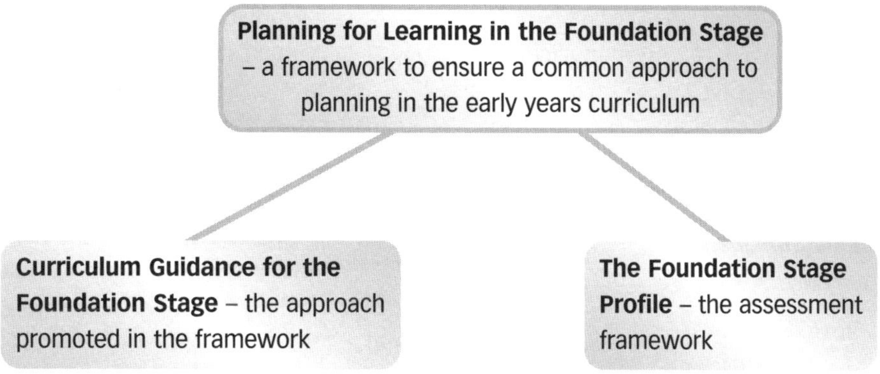

Planning for Learning in the Foundation Stage
– a framework to ensure a common approach to planning in the early years curriculum

Curriculum Guidance for the Foundation Stage – the approach promoted in the framework

The Foundation Stage Profile – the assessment framework

Figure 8.2
The Foundation Stage: a complete package for planning, teaching and assessing the early years curriculum

in the framework is Curriculum Guidance for the Foundation Stage (DfEE, 2000) and this, together with the assessment framework The Foundation Stage Profile (DfES, 2002), provides a complete package for planning, teaching and assessing the early years curriculum. There is no doubt that the framework provides useful assistance, particularly for those practitioners who have received little formal training in how to plan.

Birth to Three Matters

In 2003, Sure Start published *Birth to Three Matters*, a framework for learning to support practitioners working with babies and young children. Its aims are:

⊃ to raise the quality of learning and development opportunities for babies and children from birth to five years

⊃ to provide training and professional development for practitioners to implement curricula frameworks.

The opportunities for learning emphasised within the framework form the basis of a holistic curriculum for very young children, which focuses on individual development. The publication of *Birth to Three Matters* prompted a re-examination of the expectations of those working with under-threes and out-of-home settings.

Early years learning: the curriculum from birth to seven years

Practitioners and parents now have a clearer picture than previously of an average seven year-old child at the end of his or her Key Stage 1

BIRTH TO THREE MATTERS	FOUNDATION STAGE	NATIONAL CURRICULUM
0–3 years; non statutory framework for learning	*3–5 years; curriculum guidance*	*5–7 years; Key Stage 1 statutory curriculum*
Four areas of development:	**Six areas of learning:**	**Ten subjects:**
1) A Strong Child	1) Personal, social, emotional development	1) English
2) A Skilful Communicator	2) Communication, language and literacy	2) ICT and communication technology
3) A Competent Learner	3) Creative development	3) Art and design
4) A Healthy Child	4) Mathematical development	4) Design technology
	5) Knowledge and understanding of the world	5) Music
	6) Physical development	6) Maths
		7) Geography
		8) History
		9) Science
		10) Physical Education

Figure 8.3 *Non-statutory and statutory curriculum for babies and children from birth to seven years*

programme of learning. This more detailed picture has required practitioners to spend additional time in long-term, medium-term and short-term planning.

Figure 8.3 illustrates the non-statutory and statutory curriculum for babies and children from birth to seven years. It shows how each curriculum develops and builds upon the previous one to form a cohesive curriculum framework.

Limitations of the Foundation Stage

There are various drawbacks arising from the approach outlined in the Foundation Stage Curriculum:

- ➲ Difficulties have arisen for some early years settings with a long established curriculum that differs from that promoted by the current government. For example, some Foundation Stage practitioners follow methods supported by organisations such as the Pre-School Learning Alliance, Montessori or Steiner; others may have implemented methods used within a maintained school to which their nursery class is attached. Early years settings that subscribe to these philosophical traditions need to achieve a compromise with the government-driven curriculum in order to receive funding.

- ➲ In the initial and ongoing in-service training of teachers, planning as a professional tool features prominently. However, there may be less emphasis within such training on the philosophical underpinnings of planning, partly due to time constraints but also because emphasis is on compliance with forms of planning promoted by the government.

- ➲ In Key Stage 1 classrooms, National Curriculum requirements form the basis of planning. As would be expected given the emphasis on literacy and numeracy within the curriculum, more materials are available to support these areas than others.

Play and the practitioner's role

Play is fundamental to an under-five's way of life, yet the play provision found in the Foundation Stage is planned play only. This play is adult-led, with the adult's role clearly identified:

> *Well planned play, both indoors and outdoors, is a key way in which young children learn with enjoyment and challenge.*   (QCA (2000:25))

Figure 8.4 shows the government's recommendations on the practitioner's role in play during the Foundation Stage.

The emphasis on planned play in the Foundation Stage would appear to provide little opportunity for child-initiated free-flow play. As practitioners, we need to provide opportunities for children to take risks and explore their environment in a playful way. It is also important to recognise that at

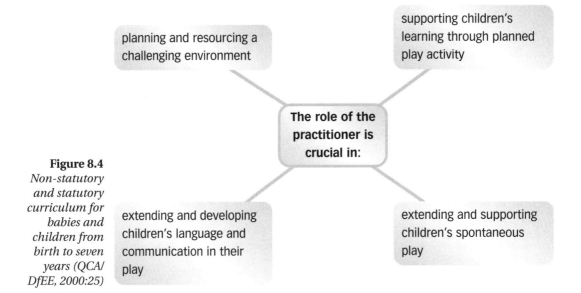

Figure 8.4
Non-statutory and statutory curriculum for babies and children from birth to seven years (QCA/DfEE, 2000:25)

each child's stage of development there may be differences between aspects of their learning. As Bissex (1980) suggests (in Bruce, 1991:13):

we need to trust the teacher that is in the child.

Planning time that allows for free-flow play is possible and desirable for younger children.

However, planned play is not without its benefits: the help of a more experienced person is essential for children's learning. In addition, a key benefit is that planned play provides adults with the opportunity to observe children. These observations may be used to assess children's developmental progress and determine how best to support and extend their learning.

Theories of children's learning

What is learning?

The curriculum is about learning that achieves the development of cognitive, social, emotional and physical skills, as well as knowledge and understanding. 'Learning' is a word we all use frequently and often without really considering what it means. It is a word we use to describe an enormous range of experiences and events. To illustrate this, consider Figure 8.5.

If you analyse each of the statements in Figure 8.5, you will find that we sometimes use the word 'learning' in the context of how we acquire skills; for example, learning to drive, walk or use a knife and fork. We also use the word 'learning' to describe how we acquire attitudes; for example, learning to enjoy books or appreciate the taste of olives. We use the word 'learning' in our development of social dispositions, including how we relate to other people. In short, 'learning' is a broad term that defines what happens to us

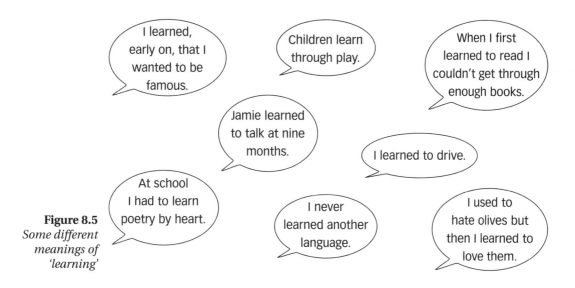

Figure 8.5
Some different meanings of 'learning'

in a range of circumstances and over an indefinite period. Children learn at home, in the playground, at school, in the streets; learning happens all the time.

Key learning theories

There are many formal theories of learning that address the question as to what learning involves; you will have studied these in your previous training. There are also many informal theories that practitioners come to through their involvement with children. In this sense, views of the ways in which children learn are the natural consequence of working with children; they arise from both practice and observation. Often ideas expressed in theory may be presented as something unique and different; however, newly presented ideas are often very similar to those that have gone before (see also Chapter 1, page 18).

Piaget and Vygotsky

Approaches to learning that acknowledge socio-cultural influences on children are generally built on the theories expounded by Piaget and, especially, Vygotsky. Planning for learning in accordance with these theories means that learning is seen to arise from the child's active participation in the learning process. Constructivist theory thus closely involves children in planning and constructing their own learning. Practitioners who adopt this approach will also acknowledge that children's learning is achieved via constructing and then building on increasingly more challenging tasks, thereby to develop and extend understanding. These ideas currently permeate the curriculum in England.

In addition, Vygotskian approaches emphasise the part played by the adult in helping children to remedy misconceptions about the world and make sense of their culture and environment. The psychological aspects of this are discussed in Chapter 11, but in terms of planning children's understanding is fickle and changeable! For example, language carries meanings that may differ according to levels of previous understanding.

Physiological aspects of learning

What is actually happening when we learn is that connections between cells in the brain are laid down and strengthened. Thus, 'learning' also has a very precise meaning in physiological terms. At birth, the human infant has all the brain cells needed for human development. In order for the human being to function, however, connections, or pathways, need to be formed between these cells. Learning during the first five years of life is more rapid than at any other time; thus the early years of life are crucial in terms of learning. Research has shown that these neural pathways are formed most effectively through experience. Each time a child encounters something new and interesting he or she explores the new object or situation and so connections between brain cells are laid down.

Learning styles

Children and adults learn in different ways; however, it is very useful to remind ourselves of the difficulties we may face when presented with new learning. People have different preferences of learning style. Children as well as adults will not learn effectively if they are expected to be passive recipients of a curriculum (David, Curtis and Siraj-Blatchford, 1992); most people prefer active approaches to learning.

You may have been presented with such a challenge when faced with a self-assembly flat-pack item of furniture: a group of adults presented with a 'flat-pack' kit to assemble will quickly demonstrate a very wide range of approaches. Some people will contemplate the diagrams and logically tackle the assembly in the correct sequence. Others may gather together the pieces and go straight into assembly. Most of us do not grasp things easily, particularly when mechanical or technological tasks are involved. Many if not most people need time to practise and make mistakes in order to consolidate their learning. Even when confident, we will often seek advice or reassurance that we are doing things correctly from another, more experienced person. When we have developed competence through trial and error, and by using skills in different contexts, we can approach these tasks in a more creative and playful way.

There may not be an exactly right way of tackling a problem and many methods may be equally effective in producing the desired result. As adults we often forget the importance of hands-on experience – solving problems by playing with materials or ideas, although we use this skill, or are forced to use it, at different points in our lives. Some may tackle this as a chore, others as a playful experience. If the latter approach is taken, learning may be not only more enjoyable but more effective and long-lasting.

The importance of planning for learning

Practitioners or potential practitioners in childcare and education need to have a clear grasp of why we are planning for learning and, more importantly, who we are planning for. The role of the practitioner in both supporting and extending children's learning is a complex one. We will not provide a range of experiences for learning that are well matched to the needs of the child unless we make the effort to understand *how* children learn. Skilled practitioners should approach planning that:

- interprets the curriculum
- is grounded in the natural qualities which children possess – their capacity to learn and their individual needs.

There is a sound track record of evidence to support the success with which this has been achieved through Her Majesty's Inspectorate reports (DES, 1989a) and through Ofsted reports.

Planning for learning: some key points

The primary purpose of planning is to meet the learning needs of children. Some ways in which this may be achieved are to:

- be aware of children's existing skills in order to extend their learning
- work collaboratively with other professionals in the setting to ensure:
  - cohesion of the learning experience for children
  - consistency in approach to avoid confusion for children
  - continuity of provision
- consider time factors: children need different periods in which to learn, and learn at different rates; activities and extension activities should reflect these needs. It is important when planning to include periods when children are able to explore ideas, develop skills and solve problems
- provide adequate space: appropriate indoor or outdoor space needs to be planned for the successful implementation of activities
- plan for extending learning and the careful introduction of a new aspect: the bridge between this new aspect should be carefully considered so that it extends learning in measured steps. The gap between the existing knowledge and the new learning must be carefully matched in small steps and short-term achievable goals
- plan for the role of the practitioner – how will she or he support learning?
- extend learning and develop learning experiences and opportunities through talking, questioning and listening. How will these provide resources for learning?

Planning for learning

It may be useful to consider the following factors:

1 **Where does learning take place?**

   ➲ How may the context in which learning takes place affect a child's ability to learn?

   ➲ Should planning take account of where learning takes place, e.g. indoors, outside, in a quiet area, as a collaborative activity?

2 **Does the way in which we learn affect our ability to learn?**

   ➲ Do individual children have different preferred methods of learning? Can these be included in the way that we present new learning opportunities?

   ➲ Individual learners may have different interests and dispositions that affect the way they learn. (The term 'disposition' is here used to explain the way in which children approach learning, particularly in their openness of response to learning opportunities.)

3 **How do we learn from others?**

   ➲ For many children, learning opportunities are enhanced through interaction with others, both experienced children and adults. How can planning take account of this?

   ➲ Learning may be promoted through language and imitation, replication and modelling. We copy and imitate to acquire skills in making best use of tools to achieve a purpose, e.g. writing, drawing, spreading and fastening. Imitation is particularly important for children's acquisition of skills in using materials and tools. We also learn to use equipment in particular ways, e.g. holding a pencil for purposes of writing may differ between cultures.

The role of the practitioner in planning for learning

Defining childhood and creating an image of the child

In planning for early learning, it is important to define childhood and create your own image of a child. This can be achieved by using the Foundation Stage and National Curriculum content requirements as pegs on which to hang relevant contexts and experiences for children's learning and development. At the same time, practitioners should value and build upon the knowledge, skills and understanding that children bring with them from their home and local community.

Childhood is seen as valid in itself, as part of life and not simply as preparation for adulthood. Thus education is seen similarly as something of the present and not just preparation and training for later.

(Bruce 1987 in 1991:7)

As early years education is clearly linked with society's view of early childhood and citizenship, it is important for practitioners to reflect upon their own image of a child and early childhood. They should also reflect on the extent to which their curriculum provision develops not only competent thinkers and learners, but future citizens.

> *Once we become aware of the ways in which childhood itself is constructed in different societies or at different times, we also begin to ask ourselves why children are treated in certain ways, what is considered an appropriate education for children at different stages in their lives and what does all this tell us about that society.*   *(David in Abbott and Moylett, 1999:82)*

Activity 1   What is your image of a child?

1 Write down key words, sentences or draw pictures to illustrate your child.
2 Write or draw the curriculum you would like your child to experience. Include approaches, activities, opportunities and learning experiences that you would plan.
3 Describe the adults' role in supporting children's learning in this curriculum.

European images of the child

Practitioners in the Reggio Emilia region of Italy use a specific image of a child as having 'a hundred languages'; each child may express him or herself in any one of these. The curriculum provided in the pre-schools within the district of Reggio Emilia is based upon this multi-dimensional view. The children lead a process-based curriculum rather than a content-based curriculum (as in the UK), in which adults support and extend children's learning through careful observation, documentation and dialogue with children and their significant adults:

> *All children have preparedness, potential, curiosity, and interest in engaging in social interaction, establishing relationships, constructing their learning, and negotiating with everything the environment brings to them. Teachers are deeply aware of the children's potentials and construct all their work and the environment of the children's experience to respond appropriately.*   *(Hendrick, 1997:16)*

It is interesting to compare children's experiences under the English curriculum with those of children who follow European curricula and early childhood policies. In general, children from other European countries start formal education at a later age with an emphasis on the development of children's language, personal, social and emotional skills. For example, early childhood policy and curriculum provision in Denmark is formed around community-based day centres, as described by Jensen:

A children's culture is emerging which values listening to and involving children, including them in the life of the centres.

(In Moss and Pence, 1994:154.)

Planning according to your image of the child

In defining an image of a child, it is useful for staff teams to discuss their whole school or nursery approach to learning and then develop a policy based upon this image, to be implemented throughout the setting. This policy for learning could be an alternative to subject policies or used to support them. The setting's image of a child and philosophy to learning can be used as a basis for planning the curriculum.

The following 'Framework to support the planning of the curriculum' (Figure 8.6) is based upon Bruce's view of the early year's curriculum:

A curriculum for the early years should be constructed from the child, the processes and structures within the child; the knowledge the child already has; and knowledge the child will acquire competently but with imagination.   *(Bruce 1987 in Pugh 2001:56)*

Planning the curriculum	
THE CHILD	⊃ Identify what a child can do ⊃ Carry out regular observations and assessments
KNOWLEDGE	⊃ Recognise the child's existing knowledge ⊃ Identify the child's future knowledge
CONTEXT	⊃ First-hand and direct play experiences ⊃ A wide and appropriately matched range of experiences ⊃ Appropriate material provision and organisation ⊃ Good relationships between the child and significant adults ⊃ Sensitive response and intervention from adults ⊃ Adults extending and supporting the child's learning ⊃ Human, physical and consumable resources that match, support and extend the child's development

Figure 8.6
A framework to support the planning of the curriculum

Recognising assumptions

Knowledge of the child's skills will provide evidence on which to base planning. This knowledge base will differ – a practitioner's views may be influenced by his or her training, values and experience. In addition, the practitioner's understanding of and relationship to the expectations of society will influence the behaviour he or she looks for and encourages. Thus, people working with young children in different types of setting may have different expectations of children. In planning a curriculum it is therefore valuable to reflect upon where and how your views have originated.

Extending children's existing learning

A curriculum is a framework for learning. Before a child enters nursery, he or she will begin to learn through an informal, often unplanned curriculum based on events and happenings within his or her home, family, local community and local environment. This is provided by interaction with significant adults, and the environment and culture in which the child lives. Each child acquires knowledge, skills and understanding through this learning process. It is important that nursery and pre-school settings build upon the learning and experiences that a child has had in their home and local environment.

Learning through interaction

Babies learn from their interactions with people and their immediate environment. Most babies learn a great deal very rapidly about the world that surrounds them; this is acknowledged in *Birth to Three Matters* (DfES, 2002). Planning for working with very young children builds on these skills.

By the time of entry to out-of-home settings, children have begun to develop many of the skills they need to operate in the wider world. The practitioner who provides the first experiences of out-of-home education will build on this past experience. Recognising, valuing and extending what children already know and can do is crucial in order to extend their learning and development.

Planning for these first out-of-home learning experiences requires that children have a wide range of learning opportunities. They need to be actively and physically engaged in meaningful and purposeful activities. These should be intellectually stimulating and involve first-hand exploratory and imaginative experiences that fully develop the use of their senses. Learning experiences should be matched to the child's level of ability and concentration, building on his or her home experience.

For some children, their home experience will not have provided opportunity for practising social skills; for others, early pre-school experience will offer opportunities to refine their existing social skills. Planning should include opportunities that will enable children to be nurtured and supported in their efforts to become confident and independent learners. Interested and informed practitioners can plan for and provide opportunities for children to solve their own problems, and talk about and share these experiences.

Figure 8.7 considers the learning styles of three and four year-old children, and the implications of this for planning.

How three and four year-old children learn	Implications for planning
They are active learners and like hands-on activities	⊃ Vary activities and have plenty of different resources, experiences and contexts. ⊃ Introduce new equipment gradually and over a period of time. ⊃ Consolidate skills by offering opportunities to practise, use and evaluate skills in different contexts.
They are keen to use all their senses	⊃ Provide a range of sensory experiences to support their exploration.
They are often very 'physical' learners	⊃ Provide staged but physically challenging opportunities. ⊃ Use outdoor opportunities to build confidence in using and developing physical skills.
They have a short span of concentration	⊃ Do not use the same form of learning activity – provide a variety of experiences.
They experiment with materials in different ways	⊃ Find new ways of using resources. ⊃ Help children to make connections between their home and pre-school experiences. ⊃ Provide adults to interact with them.
They are social beings	⊃ Plan for opportunities to practise and refine their social skills within other activities. ⊃ Encourage focused conversation – allow children to talk about their experiences.

Figure 8.7
Understanding how three and four year-old children learn and the implications for planning

Equality and diversity issues

As practitioners, our aim is to enhance children's learning and development. To achieve this, learning must be appropriately matched to the child's stage of development, and the activities we present to children must be relevant to their needs. It is therefore essential within our planning to take account of a child's cultural and religious life. Recent research by the Commission for Racial Equality (CRE), which has examined Ofsted inspection reports, reveals that the reports contain little reference to cultural diversity. Clearly this is an area of utmost importance and the absence of this aspect when planning teaching and learning in schools and settings is a concern.

Children have differing needs at particular points within their stages of development; for some children developmental differences will necessitate specific and highly structured provision. The Special Needs Code of Practice (DfEE, 1994) provides detailed advice for appropriate planning. For other children, a specific need may be of a temporary nature. The Curriculum Guidance for the Foundation Stage (DfEE, 2000:17–18) acknowledges this need and provides guidance for providing equal opportunities for all children.

Planning for the needs of all children

Equal opportunities may be taken for granted; familiarity often presents dangers of omission. Therefore, there is always a danger that conscious awareness for vigilance in equal opportunities may be forgotten. Planning for equal opportunities includes planning to meet the needs of all children, both boys and girls. This will include addressing and challenging gender stereotypes. It involves taking account of children with special educational needs (SEN), children who are more able and children with specific disabilities. We need to be aware of the needs of children from all of the groups that comprise society; that is, children from different social, cultural and religious backgrounds. Stereotypical views of racial and religious difference must be challenged. For some practitioners, planning for equality will also require recognition of the needs of children from different minority ethnic groups and children from diverse linguistic backgrounds. This will also mean providing a safe environment for travellers, refugees and asylum seekers, free from harassment and discrimination. In every sense and in every area, children's contributions should be recognised.

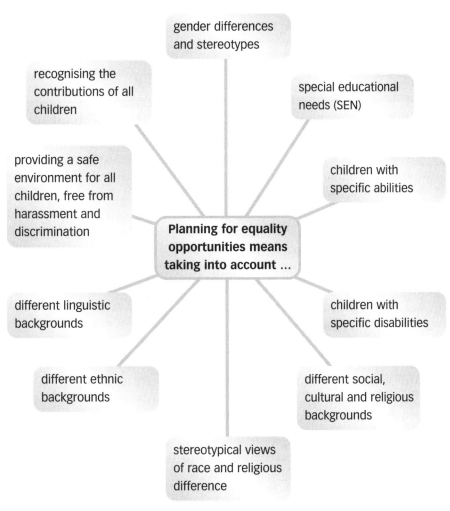

Figure 8.8
Planning for the needs of all children

Planning for children with special educational needs and disabilities

The Curriculum Guidance for the Foundation Stage (DfEE, 2000:18–19) provides advice to support planning for children with SEN or disabilities. Although the guidance is concise it does point to some important issues. Practitioners new to planning for children with special educational needs will have the support of a Special Educational Needs Coordinator (SENCO). All settings, including childminder networks, have an identified SENCO who can assist staff in recognising and responding to the needs of children with SEN within their setting. They will also assist staff in progressing policy to practice. In this way, practitioners are supported in planning for individual children's needs. The basis for planning is the Code of Practice on the Identification and Assessment of Pupils with Special Educational Needs (DfEE, 2002). Help with implementation of planning is also available in the SEN Tool Kit.

Planning for inclusion is important. All children have a right to have access to the curriculum, but it may need to be adapted to meet their specific and different needs. It would be useful to look at the planning sheets included in this chapter and to adapt these to meet the needs of a child with a special educational need. Learning may be different through approach but it should aim to achieve the same goal.

Prescriptive versus flexible approaches to planning

Some practitioners argue that we should not be over-prescriptive in planning the learning activities presented to young children. Others argue that this is a requirement of a skills-focused curriculum that develops children as citizens. Whatever the chosen approach, learning activities and opportunities must have a clear purpose. There is, however, a significant difference between a planned activity that is sufficiently flexible in its response to children's interaction, and a prescriptive and inflexible plan. All planned activities must have a valid learning goal in mind but be sufficiently flexible to respond to children's interests. This is because very young children will, if provided with opportunities, develop and extend an activity in a direction that was not part of the original plan. The skilled practitioner should be able to capitalise on this interest and draw effective learning from it.

> ## Activity 2   Prescriptive versus flexible
>
> Where are you on this continuum?
>
> Child-directed ◄─────────────────────────────► Practitioner-directed
>
> **Figure 8.9**
> *Continuum of child-directed (flexible) and practitioner-directed (prescriptive) approaches to learning*

To help you decide, think about the following points:

- ⊃ Do you vary your approach when planning different areas of learning?
- ⊃ Do you observe and listen to the child's responses and then propose actions?
- ⊃ Do you plan in advance for possible interactions?
- ⊃ Who has control – the child or the adult?
- ⊃ To what extent is the learning experience controlled, moulded and paced by the child; or is the child simply responding to the adult's needs?

When planning a curriculum, the practitioner may follow a child-directed or an adult-directed approach. However, it is unlikely that for either approach a polarised position will be adopted. It is more likely that many early years practitioners will position themselves at different points on the continuum.

The locus of control

The term 'locus of control' is at the very heart of early years education. It raises questions about who has control of the learning experience – the child or the practitioner. Identifying the locus of control requires consideration of the roles played by children and adults, and interactions between them. Do the children or the practitioner extend and determine the outcome of the activity? Consideration of what is happening in these interactions is crucial when planning for effective learning.

Recognising opportunities for learning

Practitioners will acquire skills in recognising opportunities for learning that relate to specific experiences. For example, when regularly observing an activity where children explore floating and sinking using the water tray, the practitioner will note patterns of behaviour. Children will respond in particular ways, similar questions will be asked and similar discoveries made. Capturing young children's imagination provides a starting point, and an incentive and impetus for an interest in learning. As practitioners become more familiar with the curriculum and, through their observations of individual children, concerning how children respond to planned experiences, they will be able to match activities to children's capabilities. When activities are planned on the basis of what has been observed, the appropriateness and match of learning goals to children's needs will be secure.

Making judgements

One of the key skills of an effective practitioner is helping children to make connections between areas of learning. In order to do this, the practitioner must be confident in making judgements that identify connections in their planning. Providing 'match' and extension of the learning will only occur when there is a sound grasp of the curriculum and the opportunities for the child to support experience of one area of learning with another.

Modelling

Modelling by an adult is often incorporated into planning as a means of encouraging a child's participation in an activity. Modelling may be seen simply as a 'show and copy' approach; however, this fails to recognise the immense potential of modelling. The adult's role is not simply as a director of learning or a role model; rather, for effective learning, modelling should be considered and carefully constructed. The balance between observation, intervention, direction and stimulation is thus crucial, as is effective conversation with the child.

Discussion Point 2

Supporting children's learning

Look at the following list and reflect on how you achieve these goals.

1 Help children to build on existing knowledge.
2 Provide opportunities for children to concentrate on an activity.
3 Provide opportunities for extending thinking.
4 Become involved in what children are doing but do not 'take over'.
5 Observe and provide appropriate intervention/ extension when required.

Activity 3) Observing children's activities

1 Undertake an observation of an activity in your workplace, for example, children playing with malleable materials.
2 Make a reflective evaluation of this activity:
   ⊃ Look at the roles played by children and adults. How do they interact?
   ⊃ Who has control of the learning experience? The child or the practitioner?
   ⊃ What evidence do you have to support your view?
   ⊃ Do the children extend or determine the outcome of the activity in any way?
   ⊃ Does the practitioner extend or determine the outcome of the activity in any way?

The role of observations in planning and assessment

Observations form an integral part of planning and assessment. Although this chapter does not discuss assessment, it is important to acknowledge its integral role in the planning process.

Having conversations with children and observing them in action acknowledges the competences with which children come to school, not only at the beginning but throughout their school careers. Observations and conversations are tools for assessment that recognise children's individual competences as the baseline against which their future learning needs should be identified. (Fisher, 2002:37)

Practitioners who have a grounding in understanding child development and who can relate theory to practice are better equipped to observe children and to act on these observations in their planning.

Time management

Organisation of the day is a crucial element of effective planning. If the day is blocked entirely into short periods, this prevents the extension and exploration of skills. Children need to explore learning activities not just over one day, but over several days. Consolidation requires children being offered opportunities for revisiting experiences in different contexts, in different ways and at different paces of learning. When children are engaged in exploratory play, for example, they frequently add an additional 'prop'. Planning that involves support for exploratory play should include making available a range of opportunities for adding new props or taking them away. This will provide additional challenges and aid further exploration. This builds in many ways on the ideas of Vygotsky and his zone of proximal development (see page 153), and on Bruner's theory of scaffolding (see page 154).

If children are offered something new and additional in a context of learning, this will aid their learning development. Particular emphasis is placed on measuring and judging the appropriateness of the gap between existing and new knowledge. The theory of 'match' is closely linked to a Vygotskian approach and is very useful to consider when planning activities.

ICT as a learning tool

The importance of information and communications technology (ICT) and the role played by computers over the past decade is remarkable in its permeation of all areas of the curriculum, both within schools and in nursery provision in the maintained sector. Foundation Stage settings in the voluntary and private sector have been slower to develop ICT provision. Programmable toys, control technology and software are now used in a wide range of settings with children. The potential benefits of ICT have been recognised for use with children who have particular and special needs, to enhance their learning and provide equality of access to the entitlement curriculum. Practitioners who observe children with special needs using technology at home or in other informal settings, and pay close attention to how children use and manipulate technology such as videos, DVD players and computer games, will learn much about their abilities.

Many children have an interest in ICT that develops in the home. A curriculum that responds to these interests and needs will be more current, relevant and proactive than an officially prescribed curriculum, which may take some time to catch up with the most recent developments in ICT. This is evident in the use of popular culture and media in delivering the curriculum, as indicated in the case study below.

Case Study 1

Integrating ICT in early years learning

Research by Jackie Marsh (1998, in Marsh and Hallet, 1999:158) integrated the use of cameras and computers in her 'Teletubbies' custard' project. The aim of this project was to introduce nursery children to non-narrative texts. Children read the recipe about how to make 'Teletubbies' custard' and then made the custard. They wrote their own 'Teletubbies' recipe' independently at the writing table or by using word-processing software. Some children downloaded the recipe from the Teletubbies website. Discussions about the children's viewing of the Teletubbies television programme were threaded in with some focused key terms; for example, 'dissolve' and 'temperature'. The activity of making the custard was recorded by the children using a digital camera.

Building a relevant curriculum for children's learning

Each setting will provide a curriculum based around its understanding of childhood and its approach to learning. The curriculum approach, for

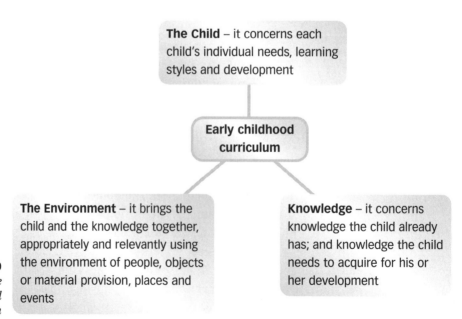

Figure 8.10
Elements of the early childhood curriculum

The Child – it concerns each child's individual needs, learning styles and development

Early childhood curriculum

The Environment – it brings the child and the knowledge together, appropriately and relevantly using the environment of people, objects or material provision, places and events

Knowledge – it concerns knowledge the child already has; and knowledge the child needs to acquire for his or her development

example, Steiner, Highscope or play-based, will be evident in the setting's long-, medium- and short-term planning.

The key to the early childhood curriculum is to observe, support and extend, and it is the quality of practitioner's interactions that do this. The early childhood curriculum is constructed from three different elements (Bruce 1987 in Pugh 2001:56), as shown in Figure 8.10.

Many practitioners have been influenced by the process-led approach to curricula as evident in the Reggio Emilia pre-schools, although the approach to learning in Reggio Emilia is specific to that region of Italy and cannot be replicated in its entirety in the UK. However, the pedagogy and approach is influencing practice here, as the following Case Study shows.

Case Study 2

Informed planning, based on Italian models

At the Brearley Nursery School, Birmingham (2001), the head teacher had visited some pre-schools in Italy and as a result had changed her nursery school's planning. The long-term planning was maintained, the medium-term planning was eliminated but daily observations of children's learning and development was increased through documentation and photographs. At the end of each day, the practitioners met and discussed their documented observations of children's progress. These were used to inform the planning for the next day, according to the opportunities and experiences for children's progression. This change had been implemented for only one term when, in the head teacher's own words, 'the dreaded brown envelope appeared – Ofsted were coming!'

The head teacher and staff decided not to alter practice and informed the inspector at her pre-visit of their change in planning. The inspector responded with, 'Fine – prove it to me.' The nursery school received an excellent inspection report. At the end of the inspection, the inspector commented that she knew more about the children's progress and achievement through the detailed observations and documentation that informed the daily planning than any medium-term planning documents could provide. This illustrates that quality planning that meets children's individual learning needs is important and preferable to the production of a quantity of planning sheets. Observations, talking and listening to children, parents and other practitioners are the key to informed planning and should be embedded within the daily practice.

Changes in the English teaching curriculum

Approaches to teaching the curriculum in England have changed from a spontaneous child-centred form of curriculum delivery to a content- and assessment-led approach. Case Studies 3 and 4 describe classroom experiences in the 1980s in English maintained infant schools.

Case Study 3

Spontaneous planning

Teaching in the 1980s was very different from teaching now in the twenty-first century. As an infant teacher, I had autonomy within my classroom and control of the curriculum. Planning was sometimes evident and sometimes not: it was spontaneous – sometimes planned a week in advance or sometimes on the bus journey to work! Topics were developed from my own interests and from the children's own interests. In my class, the children became very experienced spinners and weavers due to my interest in textile crafts. A whole term's work was developed from a day trip into the Derbyshire hills where the children collected sheep's wool. They dyed the wool with bilberries and onion skins; they collected sticks and made them into weaving looms; the leaves, grasses and flowers they picked became entwined in their cloth. Back at school, the classroom became a mill with children spinning and weaving their own creative pieces of natural cloth.

If a child brought in a jam jar containing a stick insect, some rotting leaves and a legless spider, these examples of natural history would be used as the focus of learning for that day. The children's interests and experiences were used as the basis for the curriculum and their early learning.

Student teacher at Rivelin Infant School, Sheffield, 1982

Case Study 4

Responding to natural phenomena

When a child spotted a rainbow outside the classroom window, in typical 'child-centred curriculum style,' I took the whole class out to gaze at this colourful natural wonder. How did it get there? How long will it last? The impact of its appearance permeated the day's classroom activities and children's learning. Change and refraction of light was explored by the children through their play. Washing-up liquid and pipes were put in the water tray; children were encouraged to make bubbles and to look at the rainbow colours. The washing-up liquid was taken outdoors and the children blew multicoloured bubbles up into the air to chase the rainbow. Mirrors and coloured cellophane paper was put out for children to experiment with and to explore colour and control change in colour. Children painted and drew rainbows; they read and wrote poems, songs and stories about rainbows. The day's planned activities were subsumed by this unexpected event, which formed the basis of a relevant curriculum for children's learning that day.

Deputy headteacher at Halfway Infant School, 1993

Case Study 5

A focused approach

The morning session in the Year 1 class was planned around the big book 'Smarty Pants', a story about a clever clown. This was read at the beginning of the Literacy

Hour. The children then split into groups and worked on phonic and word activities, based around the theme of circus. At the end of the session, the plenary time was spent with children showing their work and explaining what they had learnt about.

> **Activity 4** **Similarities and differences**

Read Case Studies 3, 4 and 5.

1 Note any similarities and differences between the approaches described in the case studies and your setting.

2 How could children's learning opportunities be enriched or extended in each of the case studies?

Who is the curriculum for?

We have indicated that those who devise national curricula strive to respond to the needs of society. The stakeholders, those people who have an active and sometimes influential interest in the curriculum, are many and varied. Employers, local organisations, children, faith groups, adult family members and carers are just some of the stakeholders who will have a part to play in shaping the curriculum.

The curriculum is, therefore, often viewed as a means of inducting children into society's expectations about norms of behaviour and values. There may be conflicts of opinion between different stakeholders and a consensus may never be possible, given the diverse nature of society. Attitudes to gender, to the role of education and moral values may differ markedly between groups of stakeholders and this must be borne in mind when planning for curriculum delivery. For example, a faith group may have expectations of the practitioner's role regarding moral education, which may not be a contractual obligation. Tension may arise in planning and delivering particular aspects of the curriculum that involve expectations about cultural traditions: for example, food, dress or physical activity. Sensitivity to local rural and urban cultural traditions is also important, and an equitable approach is required that acknowledges and responds to difference in a positive way. Children have different needs and require a differentiated approach to teaching and learning; equal opportunity requires differentiated action in order that all children can access the curriculum.

⟩ Conclusion

This chapter has discussed how the curriculum is a framework for learning, the historical and current context of the curricula with reference to other European curricula, and the role of the practitioner in the planning and implementation of curriculum planning. By participating in the different activities you have been able to reflect upon and review your own involvement in curriculum planning.

> **Activity 5** **Reflect upon the planning process within your early years setting**

Planning the curriculum is a complex process. The following activity will help you to reflect upon your own understanding of planning as well as your involvement in it. Write down your responses to the questions below. When you have finished, make recommendations for improvement based upon your personal reflection.

1 What type of planning is used?

2 How are you involved in the planning process?

3 Is the planning amended and adapted as it is being implemented?

4 Who sees the planning?

5 How is planning monitored to ascertain implementation?

6 How is assessment integrated into planning?

7 How is planning part of your setting's policy and approach to learning?

8 How are parents involved in the planning process?

9 How are governors involved in the planning process?

10 How are children involved in the planning process?

Comment on Activity 5

An effective long-term plan for the Foundation Stage is likely to include:

⊃ an indication of when you plan to teach aspects/ areas of learning

⊃ an indication of how regularly and frequently you plan to teach aspects/ areas of learning

⊃ an indication of how you will link aspects/ areas of learning in a relevant and interesting way for children, i.e. via special events and activities that provide a meaningful context and enhance learning, e.g. a visit to a city farm, a cultural or religious festival.

To make sure that you have planned a balanced curriculum, check that:

⊃ you have included all aspects of learning

⊃ there is a balance between and within the six areas of learning

⊃ there are sufficient opportunities for children to revisit all aspects of learning regularly and frequently.

References and further reading

Abbott, L. Moylett (ed) (1999), *Early Education Transformed*. London: Routledge Falmer

Bearley Nursery School (2001), *Sightlines*. Conference of Reggio Emilia Pre-schools, Northumberland

Bruce, T. (1991), *Time to Play*. London: Hodder and Stoughton

Bruner, J. (1980), *Under Five in Britain*. London: Grant Mclntyre

DES (1990), 'Starting with Quality' in *The Rumbold Report*. London: HMSO

DfEE/QCA (1999), *The National Curriculum: Handbook for Primary Teachers in England*. London: DFEE

Donaldson, M. (1978), *Children's Minds*. Glasgow: Fontana

Fisher, J. (2002), *Starting from the Child* (2nd edn). Buckingham: Open University Press

Hall, N. and Robinson, A. (1995), *Exploring Writing and Play in the Early Years*. London: David Fulton

Hendrick J. (ed) (1997), *First Steps Toward Teaching the Reggio Way*. New Jersey, USA: Prentice Hall

Maxwell, S. (1996), 'Meaningful Interaction' in Robson, S. and Smedley, S (eds) *Education in Early Childhood*. London: David Fulton Publishers

Moss, P. and Pence, M. (eds) (1994), *Valuing Quality in Early Childhood Services*. London: Paul Chapman

Pugh, G. (2001), *Contemporary Issues in the Early Years*. London: Paul Chapman

Robson, S. and Smedley, S (eds) (1996), *Education in Early Childhood*. London: David Fulton Publishers

Schools Curriculum and Assessment Authority (1996), *Nursery Education: Desirable Outcomes for Children's Learning*. London: SCAA

QCA/DfEE (2000), 'Curriculum Guidance for the Foundation Stage', London: HMSO

Stenhouse, L. (1976), *An Introduction to Curriculum Development and Research*. Oxford: Heinemann

Sure Start (2003), *Birth to Three Matters: A Framework to Support Children in their Earliest Years*. London: DfES

Wells, G. (1986), *The Meaning Makers*. London: Hodder and Stoughton

Useful websites

⊃ www.ofsted.gov.uk
   Ofsted reports which are available for scrutiny on the Ofsted website.
⊃ www.dfes.gov.uk
   The DfES website provides resources to support the Key Stage 1 National Curriculum.

Appendix 1: Example of a planning sheet

Week 1	Monday	Tuesday	Wednesday	Thursday	Friday
Initial Activity	Walk to baker's shop or bakery department of a supermarket. Note features of journey for a map of the route to the shop	Making map of the route to the shop Looking at a selection of maps	Children draw pictures of their own house to put on the map ———→	Looking at a selection of maps Making symbols for maps	Children draw maps collaboratively
Language	Story: 'The Gingerbread Man'	Story: 'The Gingerbread Man': link with creating map (adult led)	Bookmaking activity: individual or group book	Make a poster for the puppet show (adult as scribe) ————————→	
PSED Activity	Circle activity: Things we see on the way to nursery	Circle activity: Describe route followed by the Gingerbread Man	Circle activity: Feely bag: describe what you feel in the bag (items related to the story)	Children engaged in explaining it to other children	Circle activity: 'I would give my gingerbread biscuit to…because they are ……'
Maths	Identify and talk about numbers in the environment as seen on the walk.	Sequencing actions relating to 'The Gingerbread Man' (link to Monday's activities)	Sorting shapes and sizes of gingerbread figures	Matching activity (size): Make figures using construction kits: order them in size. ————→	
Science	Slopes and inclines	Exploring slopes using tractors, lorries and cars (link to hills)	Looking at baking ingredients through a magnifying glass	Link to baking activity: how do the ingredients change? What caused the change?	
ICT and Computers	Draw a map using mouse (link to story) ————————→		Roamer on a car mat or map: following/giving directions (link to story)	Recording sounds using a tape recorder (link to story) ————————→	

Week 1	Monday	Tuesday	Wednesday	Thursday	Friday
Sand Tray	Using sand and found materials to create a model of the route to the shop	Using sand and found materials to create a model of the route to the shop.	Provide additional materials to make roads and features	Adding vehicles with sand ⟶	Differentiating textures: Adding water to mould tunnels, bridges etc.
Water Tray	Land and water: characters and animals from 'The Gingerbread Man'	Animals made from different materials: floating and sinking	Providing a way for the the Gingerbread Man to get across the water, using rafts and boats	Building bridges	Rafts, boats and bridges
Physical Activity (Indoors/ Outdoors)	Movements based around the characters and animals from 'The Gingerbread Man'	Making a course based on land and water (adult leads movement): different pace.	Building and navigating an obstacle course: different pace	Music and movement: Dancing to fast and slow music	Movement: dramatising the story
Creative Area	Making puppets for the characters from 'The Gingerbread Man'	Experiencing fixings and fastenings in puppet construction ⟶		Making a puppet theatre, large box ⟶	
Sensory Area	Manipulating play dough with cutters and rollers Making a gingerbread figure	Smelling and touching ingredients used to make a gingerbread biscuit. Making gingerbread biscuits and eating them ⟶			Using different materials, e.g. sandpaper, pvc etc to make gingerbread figures for a feely board
Role Play	Provide costumes for the children to act out the story of 'The Gingerbread Man'	Bakery: pots, pans: overalls, scales etc	Bakers' shop: till, paper bags etc	Adding/removing props ⟶	

Observation and assessment

9

Vicky Cortvriend and Iain MacLeod-Brudenell

This chapter is designed to encourage you to extend your skills in the complex process of observing children. It will help you to develop skills in reflection on the purposes and practice of observation as a pedagogic process. In addition, it will enable you to achieve the analytical and reflective skills required for work at degree level, as well as the range of competencies required for the award of senior practitioner.

This chapter does not look in depth at every aspect of observation within early years practice. It does, however, provide you with suggestions for developing observational skills. It is hoped that by using the approaches suggested you will be sufficiently encouraged to undertake further reading.

This chapter addresses the following areas:

- ➲ the reason for observation and understanding its purpose
- ➲ children's developmental needs
- ➲ developing your skills in using observations and different techniques
- ➲ making informed reflections upon your own role.

After reading this chapter you should be able to:

1 reflect on the purposes of observation
2 link children's developmental needs more closely to your planning
3 use observation skills more effectively as a tool and choose a technique to suit your purpose
4 reflect upon your own practice.

Typically, students who undertake a foundation degree are aspiring to achieve senior practitioner status and will have completed training in undertaking observations of children in childcare courses in further education. Such observations will usually have focused on sequential recordings of the developmental progress of an individual child. For those students who have progressed to work in educational settings – pre-schools, nursery or school classrooms – the skills they have acquired in recognising and recording children's physical, emotional and physical development may have been superseded by other professional requirements. Classroom teaching assistants may, for example, be required to monitor children's cognitive development or to record specific educational targets. Practitioners working with children under 3 years of age will be using the observational skills acquired in their course of further education to observe, record, monitor and assess children's emotional, social and physical development, as well as their levels of understanding.

Observation of children should be used to inform and strengthen our support for all aspects of child development in every care and educational context. The skill of a practitioner in an early years setting is in recognising and acting upon all aspects of children's developmental progress through a holistic and integrated approach.

Our aim in this chapter is to extend and to consolidate your existing skills in oder to achieve those analytical and reflective skills required for work at degree level, as well as the range of competencies required for the award of senior practitioner.

The reason for observation and understanding its purpose

Observation is often introduced to students new to childcare and education courses as a means of eliciting information about a child. This is a useful starting point; general unfocused observations provide opportunities for seeing how children interact in different contexts and react to different stimuli. Focused observations encourage the observer, for example, to look at a specific behaviour and to note conditions or factors, which relate to actions during the space of the observation.

Why observe?

In childcare courses at level 2 and level 3, students are required to follow formal patterns of observation; these are often referred to as observation methods or techniques. However, students are often not sure about:

- how they can use their observations
- what to do with the data
- why they are required to carry out so many observations on the children in their care.

This has been known to lead to frustration and negative reactions towards the process of observation.

Observational methods or techniques are of little value in themselves; they are often simply a descriptive record of what the observer sees. A primary purpose of observation is to record in order to inform our response to the needs of children. Observation is therefore more than looking and seeing – it is a means of recording linked to considered reflection and analysis. Sound reflection on the observations we make not only enhances professional practice, but also aids our understanding of children.

Objectivity is key

Observations must be undertaken in as objective a way as possible. It may be difficult to make a completely objective observation of children with whom we are familiar. It is essential that value judgements do not influence the accuracy of **description** in our observation. However, the crucial value of the observation lies in how the complex data contained in such description is evaluated. That is how we unravel and interpret the findings. This is because the key to developing our understanding of children is in the **interpretation** of what we see. Interpretation involves careful consideration of all of the detail recorded in an observation, with an informed eye for detail and a wide understanding of the purposes of the activity or events observed. **Analysis** of the information, the data, draws on our understandings of the child, the area of development we are considering, (for example the 'norm' levels of capability), the response offered by the child to particular stimuli or, the development stage achieved by the child compared with other children in similar cultural contexts.

Purposes of observation

It is clear that observations on children and the conclusions that practitioners in early years settings draw from them are among the most important and rewarding aspects of their work. The knowledge of the child that practitioners gain from their observations should underpin all the work they do with children. This knowledge can then be shared with the parents or main carer, and other professionals on a need-to-know basis to ensure the best possible care and education for each individual child. The principal reasons for observation are to:

- ⊃ determine if the baby/child is developing according to recognised norms
- ⊃ share information with parents or main carer
- ⊃ enable the practitioner in an early years setting to plan effectively for the baby's/child's continuing care and development
- ⊃ share informed, accurate and objective information with other professionals on a need-to-know basis.

Personal development

Observation has far more potential value to practitioners than simply recording actions in order to see how well the child is progressing. Observational records are useful data by which to measure and monitor our own effectiveness in predicting progress, and as a means of assessing our skills in making accurate and useful observations. Analysis of our observations can be very revealing. Reflection on our assumptions and predictions can raise doubts in our ability to make valid interpretations. What must be remembered is that not only are children's behavioural patterns difficult to predict, but also our behaviour as observers can be subject to mood, time and other conditions.

Recording and interpretation

Observation is a diagnostic tool, confirming capability or progress at a point in time. It is a means of unobtrusively collecting potentially rich information about children's development. Most children will usually be observed in naturalistic conditions, at play either inside or outside, although there will be occasions where children are more formally assessed, using observations in contrived and regulated situations. An example of this is when carrying out baseline assessments in reception class. The data from either of these situations may be used to obtain factual information, often recording physical development or a child's capability to perform an action. Or, an observation may focus on providing data for interpretation, on unravelling factors, and providing evidence for analysis. This is likely to be related to observation of emotional, social or cognitive development.

All observations must be recorded, and then evaluated using recognised milestones (see Figure 9.1).

Milestones of development	
The Stycar Sequences	Described by Mary Sheridan in the 1950s and demonstrated very clearly by Meggit and Sunderland (2001). These milestones of development are to be found in the majority of childcare textbooks and are described briefly in Chapters 3, 4 and 6.
The goals described in the Curriculum Guidance for the Foundation Stage	Can be used as an extra source of information when the child reaches the age of 3. Published by the Department for Education and Employment in May 2000.
The works of theorists such as Piaget, Erikson, Chomsky and Kohlberg	These theories are described in detail in Chapters 5 and 6.
The National Curriculum Key Stages 1 and 2	Can be used once the child reaches the ages of 6 and 7.

Figure 9.1
Recognised milestones of development

Observations may present the unexpected, that is, information that had not been predicted, and such data will inform our understanding of the observed child. As practitioners we may be unaware of subtle changes in children's development. We all recognise that there will be times when we are required to observe the changing patterns of behaviour of a child, or the way in which he or she relates to other people, both children and adults. Observation can provide the opportunity to note and record these changes. We could say that this data is the best means to record our sensitivity to the variations and changes that occur in children over a period of time. It provides evidence of our professional approach to assessment, showing that we know the children in our care.

This important aspect of observation is often undervalued in an assessment process where recording targets is the primary purpose. As practitioners, we should approach undertaking observations with a fresh enquiring mind, rather than seeing the activity simply as a required task. It is useful to retain observations, not to simply discard them after they have served an immediate use. This data can be used to monitor progress and to provide evidence of development.

It is important to remember that observations can be subject not only to children's changing behaviour and mood, but also the observer's. Periods of stress and pressure may impact on our ability to make objective judgements.

Research

It is often not fully recognised that observation can be used as a form of research, but the use of observation as a research tool in early childhood studies is invaluable and central to our personal understanding of children as well as for our own professional development. Young children may not be able to convey verbally what they are thinking. The key to unlocking our understanding of young children's development is through careful reflection on the observations we make.

Observation may be used in conjunction with other methods and approaches such as interviews or questionnaires in more formalised research projects.

Planning

A further important use of observations is their use in planning the curriculum for the setting. When planning, in the short, medium or long term, it is essential to be able to demonstrate how you are meeting the children's individual needs. The theorists Vygotsky and Bruner both expounded the belief that children will develop to their full potential only with the assistance of adults or more experienced peers (Vygotsky's Zone of Proximal Development and Bruner's Scaffolding theory – see Chapter 4). Using the detailed evaluation from each observation it should be possible to plan or moderate activities so that each child benefits according to his or her own unique needs. Differentiation is a key word that practitioners in early years settings need to keep in the forefront of their mind when planning the curriculum. The judicious use of observations will provide you with the information needed to enable you to plan for individual children's needs by either moderating, or extending, planned activities. Some children may benefit from an individual learning programme, which could be devised using the information gleaned from the evaluations. Following the activity, observations will then tell you if your adaptations were successful. This differentiation ensures the practitioner is committed to equality of opportunity as he or she is meeting the needs of all the children in the setting.

Sharing information

Confidentiality must be foremost in the practitioner's mind when deciding who needs to know about specific observations. There may be times when he or she will be required to write reports on the children in the early years setting. These may be routine reports to share with parents or main carers, or reports to be sent to other professionals such as educational psychologists, pediatricians, speech therapists and social workers. Reports might also be sent to a child's new setting. It is of vital importance that these reports are accurate and only contain relevant objective information.

Demonstrating professional responsibility and integrity is essential when building and maintaining a partnership with parents. The Children Act of 1989 makes it very clear that this partnership with parents is expected of all practitioners in early years settings and the series of Parents Charters during the 1990s described parents' rights in relation to their expectations for their children's care and education.

Reflection

Reflection can change our practice for the better. When reflecting on our own practice, records of observations provide the data by which we may measure and monitor our own effectiveness as practitioners. Such reflection cannot only provide opportunities for self- assessment but also help to set targets for professional development. It is important to assess personal skills in an objective and honest way. The use of accurate observations is a useful tool in helping to assess these skills. Careful analysis of professional observations can reveal aspects of practice that may otherwise go unnoticed. It is not uncommon for practitioners to undertake observational tasks as part of regular routine without fully realising the detailed knowledge that is brought to these activities. Reflection and justification of the assumptions we may make in our judgements on children may promote a reassessment of the validity of some of the ways in which observation is tackled.

Action research

One method of continuing development is by using action research, which is carried out in the workplace in order to reflect upon and inform practice. Observations that include details of a practitioner's own practice in an early years setting, or that of other practitioners, can be a very useful tool. They can assist you to become aware of yourself as a practitioner and can be used as part of the cycle of enquiry, helping you to reflect upon, and then plan, how to modify your practice. Finally, they can be used to compare your previous practice with your present practice.

Ethics in observation

Observation is usually associated with recording what is seen for a variety of purposes and for different professionals concerned with children. Increasingly, they are also used as evidence for inspection purposes. As with all records, there are issues relating to ethics in terms of objectivity of the observer, storage of the data, accessibility, and the purposes to which the data is applied.

As a student and a practitioner you must consider two contexts for your own observational records: your university or college, and your workplace. An ethics checklist is shown in Figure 9.2.

Ethics checklist

Before the observation
Permission
☐ Obtain permission from supervisor of setting
☐ Obtain permission from parents of child

After the observation
Anonymity
☐ Change all names of children
☐ Change all names of places
☐ Change all names of staff

Objectivity
☐ Check that all statements are accurate and not discriminatory
☐ Check that all statements are supported by evidence

Confidentiality
☐ Ensure records are kept in a secure place

Figure 9.2
An ethics checklist

Maintain anonymity

It is essential that you maintain the anonymity of those you observe and the contexts in which they are observed. The identity of those observed and the setting in which the observation takes place may be recognised by people reading your notes. It is therefore important that you neither identify the children you observe, nor the early years setting in which the observations took place. You can refer to the early years setting by describing it as a nursery setting, or a school, or a playgroup. Refer to the child purely in factual terms, for example, 'a female child aged 3 years 5 months'.

Obtain permission

When planning to do an observation in a setting, you will need to obtain permission from the supervisor and from the child's parents or carers. It is preferable to obtain this permission in writing. Various techniques suitable for carrying out observations are described on page 280, but it is important to maintain a professional attitude and carry out observations in a discreet manner at a time that does not disrupt the routine. Sharing of information should be discreet and limited to your supervisor at the setting, the child's parents or carers and your college tutor, unless otherwise directed.

Confidentiality

Maintaining confidentiality is vital. Keep all your records secure, and make sure that you treat the children's files in a confidential manner. Do not share information with anyone.

Bias

Another ethical consideration relates to bias. We all bring a personal bias to bear on our observations and the reflection and analysis of the data derived from such observations. We must be aware of our own personal values, particularly where they may compromise our impartiality as neutral observers. Initially, we may be unaware of bias and for some practitioners this continues to be an issue.

Children's developmental needs

Observations are the key to helping adults plan their support for children's ongoing development. So where does this process begin? Different professionals carry out observations on babies and children throughout their early years. Health care observations of babies and young children take place before birth, directly after birth and through the early years of a child's life.

Pre-birth medical observations

Probably the very first pre-birth medical observation for most babies is an ultrasound scan, carried out at around 12 to 18 weeks of pregnancy to determine:

- ⊃ position of foetus
- ⊃ size of foetus
- ⊃ normality of development
- ⊃ number of foetuses
- ⊃ the probable delivery date

and to detect any problems with the foetus, placenta, uterus or chord. This screening observation is carried out by a suitably qualified health professional and measures the foetus's long bones, circumference of skull and pelvic girdle. It checks the spine, internal organs and the primitive heart and blood supply.

The results of the scan are recorded on the mother's chart and it is common practice that she is given the opportunity to obtain a copy of the scan picture. Even at this early stage, before the foetus could be deemed viable, the professional is beginning to develop a partnership with the prospective parent. This partnership is necessary so that both can work together to ensure the best possible care for the baby.

Birth medical observations

The next series of observations (unless any problems were detected on the first scan, in which case the foetus would be monitored and observed closely throughout the pregnancy) take place directly after the birth. The midwife, pediatrician, obstetrician or doctor will carry out a full head-to-toe check on the baby, including observing its reflexes and recording its Apgar rating. The results of these observations are again recorded and shared with the parents. The mother is given a Personal Child Health Record book in which health care professionals record the results of all the developmental and health checks and observations they carry out on the child. (For examples of child health surveillance and centile charts, see Chapter 3.)

Should any deviation from the norm be noted then the health care professional may refer the child to a specialist.

Early years medical observations

During the first year of the child's life the health visitor will monitor the child's development and health. This is done in the child's home and at the local clinic. Screening tests will be carried out to determine if there are any problems relating to hearing, sight, growth or developmental skills. The child will in all probability undergo an immunisation programme to protect him or her against some childhood diseases (see Chapter 14).

Once the child attends a childcare or educational setting then the observations that health care workers continue to record will be augmented by the observations that the staff in the setting carry out. These regular observations will continue throughout the child's life, becoming less frequent towards the end of primary education, dependent of course on the child's particular needs. The observations that practitioners in early years settings carry out will measure the child's holistic development and will be used in the planning of activities aimed at consolidating and extending each area of development.

Developing skills in observation and techniques

This section discusses the range of techniques that you may choose to use when conducting your observations.

Skills and abilities required for observation

Observation requires a disciplined approach. This disciplined and systematic approach can be acquired through practice. There is a danger that established practitioners may undervalue the importance of observation as a means of professional understanding and development because they are so familiar with the activity within the workplace. However, for work at university level, more is required than a disciplined approach; the ability to record accurately is of equal importance. The process of observation if done well is not easy; it requires concentration, an open mind and an ability to make skilled and informed analysis based not only on practice, but also on reading and discussion. A skilled observer who is also a reflective practitioner has an understanding of the advantages and disadvantages of a range of techniques, and can apply an appropriate method to a specific need then use the data for focused reflective analysis.

Means of recording

The ways in which you will record your observations will differ according to the method you use. It is certain, however, that as a practitioner you will not often be able to take time out to make lengthy observations – so how do you manage the process?

If a 'key worker' system operates in your early years setting (that is, one practitioner has responsibility for a particular group of children), you may have the responsibility for observing the children in your group only. But in practice it is highly likely that children will not be restricted in their movements and you may be required to make informal observations of other children as well. It is common for a practitioner to observe not only the children in his or her group but others who happen to be in proximity but are not part of the key group. In settings that use the key worker approach, the organisation of reporting and recording of observation is usually undertaken as group activity.

There is no 'right' way, but some ways are more efficient than others.

Case Study 1

Techniques?

In one nursery school, each of the eight staff has a group of children for whom they are responsible. During the week staff are expected to undertake observations, which are usually recorded on clipboards in their areas or in their diaries. At the end of each session, staff talk about anything particular that they have noticed and these are recorded in the main log. This is useful as children do wander between the two rooms and sometimes another key worker will notice something that is important and which can be followed up. On Fridays, staff write up notes about each child.

Techniques – taking turns

At a second nursery school, staff take turns for a week and observe the children in different areas of the pre-school. Observational notes are recorded in notebooks. Because staff do not have time to make the long observations they were trained to do, they jot down the things they think are important. They talk about the children at lunch time and home time and share their observations. This ensures that they all see the overall picture of the children in different activities and get to know them better. Staff have also started to share these observations in their daily dairies, which they write for parents.

Activity 1 · Personal needs analysis

Considering the above case studies and thinking about your own particular setting, it would be a good idea to complete a personal needs analysis before beginning your observation portfolio. Make a personal analysis of your own needs in observation.

- ⊃ List your skills
- ⊃ List your development needs
- ⊃ How can you address these needs?
- ⊃ Make a plan of action

The format shown in Figure 9.3 may be helpful for you when carrying out this Activity.

	Skills I currently have	Development needs	Actions to take
Date			

Figure 9.3 *Personal needs analysis*

Monitor this plan of action – place dates next to the action when you have started and then note when you have developed skills in the area.

Participatory observation

Participatory observation occurs when you are observing children whilst engaged in an activity with them, or involved in part of your daily routine of caring for and educating the children in your care.

Parents or carers watch and note the actions, reactions and responses of the children in their care. They observe, note and often comment on their children. It would be highly unlikely that such observations would be recorded. This is, however, valuable information if it is recorded.

Practitioners in early years settings and some teachers may write a diary of observed details relating to a child in their care. This is often to inform parents or carers of their child's daily activity. Most people who work with young children use participatory observation as part of their everyday practice. It is an almost instinctive part of caring for children.

But this does not always lead to written entries in the child's record. Participant observation may initially seem difficult to manage, in that notes must be made either at points during work with the children, or immediately afterwards if the knowledge and evidence is not to be lost. Often practitioners think that they will remember something and will be able to note it down later. Given the pace at which events can develop in the nursery, however, these observations can easily be lost or inaccurately remembered.

Hints for recording observations

⊃ Placing sticky notes, clipboards with paper or note pads strategically around the room. This will help provide both the incentive and the means with which to record the incident, briefly, as it happens.

⊃ Ensure that you always carry a notepad with you, from place to place.

⊃ Notepads often become the focus for children's attention, too, with them leaving messages and writing their own 'notes' down.

Observations made in this way may often be incidental and unplanned, but they can, like planned observations, be incorporated into the general system of observations, which add to the developing picture of a child.

The habit of recording observations almost automatically comes with practice and notes often become shorter but more telling in their content as your experience increases. One teacher in the PROCESS Research Project (Stierer et al., 1993) said that as she became more experienced at observing she wrote less but it told her more!

Non-participatory observation

Non-participatory observation means that the observer stays outside the activity in order to concentrate on the child or aspect being watched. If a single child is the focus it allows the observer to watch that child both as an individual and in the context of an activity. Similarly, a focus on an aspect of provision, or on a particular activity, allows the observer to concentrate on that aspect of the nursery alone, without having to watch for anything else.

If the observation is to be non-participatory, children need to know which adults are available for help while that person is busy observing. One teacher in the PROCESS project (Stierer et al., 1993) wore a hat when observing, and the children knew that they had to go to the other adults while this hat was being worn. Where to sit while observing in this way is also important, but becomes less of an issue as children become used to seeing adults watch them. Sitting too near or far from an activity may affect the quality of what is seen or heard by the observer. What is most important is that where an adult sits does not have a limiting effect on the children's activity.

Understand the purpose of the technique you are using

Health professionals and practitioners in early years settings often use different names for the same technique. This is not important; but it is essential that you are clear about the purpose of the technique.

In selecting a method of observation to apply to a particular situation you will focus on choosing a technique that will best serve your purpose, matching the appropriate technique to the aim of the observation. You may choose to use a number of different and complementary techniques to provide the information required to test for accuracy of your findings.

Confirming your conclusion may lead naturally to more rigorous forms of observation as research. Your ideas and hunches may be formulated as a hypothesis – your theory. You can test your hypothesis by collecting observations and examining them. For example, by using sociometric observation (see page 289) of a child you may identify a particular friendship, which encourages sustained concentration on a particular task or activity. Focused tracking observation (see below) or duration recording (see page 289) in this area would highlight any other factors that contribute to sustained concentration. By using these techniques, you will gather specific data which can help you to predict behaviour, support learning, and ultimately to test and verify the accuracy with which you can predict the child's behaviour. Hypothesis testing in this way will provide very good experience for using observation as a research tool.

Tracking

This method of observing a child is usually non participative and involves having a floor map of the setting with the various activities marked on it. A child is then tracked during the course of a morning or afternoon session in order to observe:

- concentration levels
- social interactions
- interest
- behaviour.

The time spent at each activity is recorded, and the sequence of activities. Other relevant information may also be recorded.

Case Study 3

Observing behaviour – tracking

Joe, age 4, is due to start reception class in September. He has problems socialising with peers and concentrating on activities. The educational psychologist is working with him and the staff of the nursery to help to prepare him for the transition to Key Stage 1. He is going through the statementing process in order that he can obtain the necessary support at school.

This observation tracks Joe's choices of activity throughout a morning session with a view to evaluating his level of concentration for particular activities and his behaviour exhibited.

The observation		
Time (am)	**Activity**	**Joe's behaviour**
9.10	**Group Time**	Joe sitting quietly listening; suddenly he knelt up, pointed to a picture on the wall and shouted, 'What they doing?'. He then began to move to the front of the group, pushing through the other children.
9.20	**Free Play**	Joe leapt to his feet and dashed over to the sand tray, where three children were playing. He began to frantically gather wet sand, piling it up at the side of the tray. Picking up a bulldozer, he started to use it to push the sand back and forth so that some fell onto the floor. During this time, he carried on a conversation with an educare worker.
9.25	**Speech Therapist**	The speech therapist came over to the sand tray and asked Joe if he would like to come and have a chat with her. Joe began jumping up and down, shouting, 'Look at my yellow shoes'. Then he took her hand and said, 'Yes'.
10.14		Joe arrived back in the playroom, holding the speech therapist's hand. Letting go of her hand, he looked around the room.
10.15		Joe rushed over to the sand again; there were already four children playing there. 'How many children are allowed at the sand tray, Joe?' an educare worker asked him. 'No, no, no,' he shouted.

		'Joe, would you like to come and paint?' she then asked. He turned and ran to the aprons, asking 'Can I paint, can I paint?'. He painted quietly for 5 minutes, lips pursed, gazing intently at his work.
10.21		After hanging up his apron, he dashed back to the sand and began grabbing fistfuls of wet sand, throwing it into the sink. 'Joe, please don't do that,' an educare worker said, taking him by the hand and leading him to the play dough table. 'No, no, no,' he shouted, struggling in her grasp.
10.22		Joe cuddled a teddy and sat close to the worker, listening to the story and looking at the illustrations.
10.30	**Snack Time**	Joe picked up his milk carton and threw it over the table.

Interpretation and analysis of case study

Joe did not move quietly around the room; he rushed everywhere, unless an adult held his hand. He was aware of the rules of the setting as demonstrated by his shouting 'no' when the carer asked how many children were allowed at the sand tray. He was aware that he had to wait for one child to leave before he could join in the activity, but he did not want to. He seemed to behave in a way designed to attract adult attention by messing in the sand tray, throwing sand around, and finally spilling his milk over the table. When he gained the attention he then wanted adult touch, holding the adult's hand or cuddling up beside her, clutching a teddy. He was in fact capable of maintaining concentration during an activity as shown when painting; however, this lasted only 5 minutes. During the entire observation there was no interaction with his peers.

Norms of development

Joe is almost 5 years old. At this age, according to norms of development, he 'should be able to understand the needs of others and be able to share and take turns'.

He should also be aware of what is right and wrong in behaviour. He should enjoy being with other children, show some sensitivity and be developing a sense of humour (Meggit and Sunderland, 2000). At the age of 4, he should enjoy companionship with other children and adults. He may have bouts of quarrelsome behaviour as well as close cooperation. At the age of 5, he should pick his friends and play companionably, understanding rules and find them acceptable. He should want to please, cooperate and help (Holt, 1991). Holt also writes that much of the period between 1 and 5 years of age is spent exploring and moving through stages of transition, which is often a cause of rebellion, but most of these problems are usually resolved as children approach 5 years of age.

It is clear that Joe is still expressing these rebellious feelings and has not yet reached the developmental norms in relation to his emotional and social development that would be expected of a 4-year-old child.

This observation was one of a series on Joe. It is not possible to build up an accurate picture of a child based on one observation, as so many different factors can influence the findings. Diet, illness, allergies, emotional distress, personal likes and dislikes, and even mood and temperament are significant in this context.

This observation and evaluation was shared with Joe's parents, the educational psychologist and his teacher to be. The purpose was to continue to build up a picture of Joe in order to plan for his particular individual needs.

Observation can provide starting points, assessment can be used to plan and review. (Nutbrown, 2001:69)

> ### Activity 2) Tracking

As part of your usual assessment routine you may use tracking as an observation tool.

1 Carry out a tracking observation on one of the children in your setting, and then list the advantages of tracking.

2 Every form of observation has disadvantages as well as advantages. List any disadvantages of tracking, which may occur in your setting. How could these be addressed?

Free description or snapshot

There will be many opportunities for teachers and other adults to observe children while they are working alongside them. This is not quite the same as a participatory observation. By supporting a child in a task, or facilitating their activity, the adult is able to observe and, if appropriate, to record what the child says and what the child does as evidence of their growing conceptual awareness or skill development. They can also observe how the child approaches tasks, what strategies they use for solving problems, their persistence and motivation and their attitudes in general. This can then be recorded using the free description technique, which involves recording the event as it happened over a period of perhaps 10 or 20 minutes. If the event lasted for less than 5 minutes it is known as a snapshot observation.

Frequency sampling

Frequency sampling is a way of tracking incidences of particular aspects of behaviour in a child or group of children. In this, the observer identifies a

- ⊃ feature of behaviour and notes whenever this occurs. For example, a child may appear always to play alone in the nursery. Observations would focus on whether or not this was indeed the case, and would include:
- ⊃ looking at whether he or she approached another child, children or adults
- ⊃ whether he or she initiated any interaction
- ⊃ how any interaction was initiated
- ⊃ where in the nursery this occurred.

As its name suggests, frequency sampling can be useful in giving an accurate picture of the frequency of aspects of behaviour, and can be used to monitor both progress and concerns.

Time sampling

Time sampling is similar to frequency sampling except that the observer records behaviour over a set period of time, typically recording behaviour, social interactions and language over a 2-minute period every 10 minutes for a total period of one hour. It involves, therefore, observing children at the end of a predetermined period and recording exactly what is happening.

The recording format in this case would be a chart, as shown in Figure 9.4.

Time sampling chart			
Time	Behaviour	Language	Social Group

Figure 9.4
Format for a time sampling chart

Yule (1987) suggests that precise timing is needed in order to avoid biased results. He gives the example of a nurse on a busy ward who is observing a patient every 5 minutes to see whether he or she is rocking or is engaged in some other self-stimulatory behaviour: 'Unless the nurse does look at exactly the end of the five minute interval, then she may find herself remembering to record only when she sees the patient engaged in the undesirable activity' (Yule, 1987:19-20). In this case, the technique was useful in revealing whether the behaviour was as problematic as was first thought. If the nurse recorded that the patient was rocking on the hour, six or seven consecutive times, she would need to investigate the problem further. If, however, the rocking only occurred once during the six or seven occasions on which she recorded, perhaps it was not such a problem after all! Repeated (compared with random) observations will reveal the extent to which the behaviour is consistent.

Wragg (1994) uses time sampling (which he refers to as 'static sampling') rather differently in that observers build up a series of snapshots of a situation at regular intervals. Using the technique in this way, it is possible to take a small number of pupils and to build up a comprehensive picture of their activities over a period of time.

Event recording and diary observations

This method is often used to record a sequence of events and its frequency and occurrence. It may be used to track the number of times an action occurs within a given time. Typically, it will be used as a means of recording the effectiveness of an intervention programme for modifying a child's behaviour.

It can be used to provide data for an identified problem where there is a need to record the frequency of a particular response given by a child or group of children. Event recording is a useful method for observing a child's emotional development as you can record responses to a range of different events over a period of one or two days. Any longer and the type of observation becomes a diary observation. This is essentially the same as an event sample but is longitudinal, carried out over a period of time.

An extension to event recording is referred to by Wragg (1994) as a 'critical event approach', in which the observer looks for specific instances of classroom behaviour that are judged to be illuminative of some aspect of the teacher's style or strategies. This might be an element of class management, for example, perhaps a rule being established, observed or broken, something which reflects interpersonal relationships or some other indicative event.

Recording can be carried out on an adapted ABC Chart, which can then be discussed with the children in order to obtain their perceptions. (A means Antecedents of the behaviour, B is the Behaviour itself and C is the context in which the behaviour took place.)

Although event recording is an appropriate observational technique for a wide range of behaviours, it has obvious limitations. Hall, Hawkins and Axelrod (1975) emphasise that it is most appropriate for responses of a short duration, which can be readily divided into single units. They give examples of its use in measuring the frequency of a shy pupil speaking, or an aggressive student making positive (rather than negative) comments, but they stress that the technique can have limitations when a behaviour cannot be defined precisely.

Tick list or check list

This is a simple method of recording whether or not a child is capable of achieving specific age-related tasks. The observer designs a chart using either norms of development (see Chapter 3) or Foundation Stage Goals or Key Stage 1 attainment targets, depending upon the child's age; he or she then observes during set activities whether or not the child can achieve the task with or without assistance, or cannot it manage at all.

The professional in an early years setting can then use this information to plan appropriate activities to extend the child's development, and inform other interested professionals of the child's ability. The information can also be used to write a factual report for parents. It can be recorded in a form like that shown in Figure 9.5.

Child A: 3-years-old. Physical development.

Skill	Can do	Can't do	Requires assistance
Build a tower of nine bricks			
Cut paper with scissors			
Thread large beads onto a thread			
Jump from a low step			
Climb upstairs with one foot on each step			

Figure 9.5
Example of a tick list to record a child's physical development

Duration observation

Duration observation is a way of accurately tracking how long children spend at particular activities or using certain equipment. It may seem sometimes as though a child or group of children spend all of their time in the construction area or riding the bikes: duration observation is a good way of establishing just how much time they do spend in these areas, and can help to ensure that the observations we record are accurate. 'Kuldip spends all of his time on the bikes' may, in reality, be that Kuldip chooses the bikes first, generally spends half an hour on them and then moves on to other activities.

Sociometric observation

This is usually used when observing children to research their friendship groups and integration into groups. The findings are often demonstrated using a pie chart or graph.

Making informed reflections upon your own role

This section discusses how to use observations to reflect upon and develop your own practice. In addition it considers both the short- and long-term management of any observations carried out.

Using observations to reflect upon and develop your own practice

A vital skill to develop when writing up observations is how to evaluate or analyse the observation and then decide what to do next. (Refer to the case study of a tracking observation on Joe on page 284.) The evaluation depends upon the aim of the observation. If the observation took place in order to determine if the child was developing according to expected norms in development, then the evaluation would compare the skills observed with those described in developmental charts. (See Chapters 3, 4 and 6 for developmental norms.) If the observation was made to determine if the behaviour exhibited by the child is socially acceptable for his age, then the evaluation would focus on acceptable behaviour, comparing the child's behaviour with expected norms. Observations may also be carried out to determine if a child is settling into the setting, or, socialising with peers. If so, the analysis or evaluation would focus on that aspect of the child's behaviour. We are analysing what we know about that particular child, and also what we know about how young children learn. So we use what we see and hear as the information we record and then interpret this in light of our knowledge. Close observation allows us to make guesses about what children already know and about what their current interests are. We make our guesses in light of what we already know to help us plan what we will offer next to take learning forward.

Recommendations that are related to the aims of the observation

Once you have determined, by analysing the observation, whether the child is developing according to expected norms or not, you can make informed recommendations, again related to the aim of the observation. Typically, these recommendations would be:

- activities to consolidate or extend the child's skills
- a plan to manage the child's behaviour
- plans to inform parents and/or other professionals about the child's progress
- a referral to other professionals for a second opinion.

Observing children and evaluating the findings in this manner inform practice by enabling the practitioner in an early years setting to plan effectively for individual children's needs and then, by carrying out further observations, determine whether or not the plans have been successful. By using the observations to reflect upon your own practice (see Chapters 7, 8 and 10) or to carry out your own action research (Chapter 10) you are able to constantly be aware of your effectiveness as a practitioner in an early years setting and to modify your practice accordingly.

What to do with your observations

The first and most obvious thing you do with your observations is to use them to plan what to offer next. In this way, you are basing your planned programme on the interests and needs of the children as you have observed them. So observation informs planning. Planning based on the observed interests and needs of individual children ensures that the programme provided offers genuine equality of access and opportunity to all children.

Once you have used your observations to plan what to offer next, you can also think about how to use them to build a record of the child's progress over time. Inevitably, if all members of staff are keeping notes on what they notice, you will gather a veritable mountain of paper over the days and weeks. It is here that you need to use your judgement about what is significant. Each key worker could be responsible for collecting together the bits of paper relating to his or her key children, then sift through them, extracting what is significant and discarding the rest. There is absolutely no point in keeping every observation note made. You need to track each child's progress and the best way of doing this is to chart leaps in learning.

In addition, each key worker needs to ensure that he or she has observation notes covering all aspects of the curriculum. When you have been worried about a child's emotional development it is natural that your

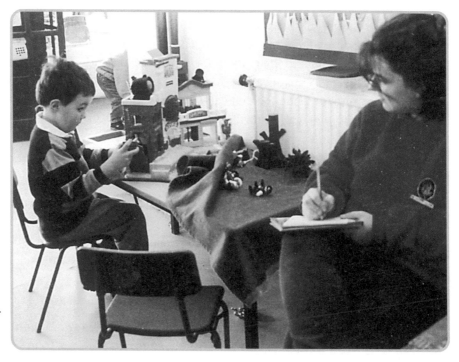

Observations are a basis for planning and a helpful record of a child's behaviour

observation notes will reflect this. But the child's overall development needs to be charted and you need to ensure that you have noticed something about the child's learning across the curriculum.

Your skills in using observation as a reflection on your practice and the practice of others may lead to situations in which you may feel uncomfortable. In early years practice the tensions between curriculum demands and the needs of individual children may sometimes appear to be at odds. Criticism of established as well as more recent patterns of teaching and learning strategies or comments about what should be happening in classrooms may not be pleasant to hear.

Management and storage of observations

As the notes and paperwork accumulate it is important to have some way of managing the volume, both in the short and long term. These pieces of paper initially provide support and information for the planning of future work with the children: they have a formative purpose. They are also needed for formative, and then summative, report-writing, when statements are made about the child's progress, often for communication to others, in particular to parents or carers, and other practitioners.

Develop a manageable filing system

In the long term, developing a manageable form of filing system for the observations is important if all of these observations are to be useful, and are not to be lost. A pocket file for each child, ring binders and a section in a filing cabinet are all possibilities, but solutions will be individual, dependent upon available space and storage facilities and the time to support them. Keeping these samples of evidence is, however, very important both in order to inform planning, and for when it comes to the summative stage(s) in a child's time in the nursery or class. They give insights into the child that can inform the understanding of parents, head teachers, inspectors, educational psychologists and other agencies, and provide evidence that can support statements made of the child's competence, in a wide range of contexts and areas of experience.

Short-term management

The short-term management of observations includes the sharing of these with other staff at the end of day or at team meetings so that everyone is aware of the successes, efforts and concerns about individuals, areas and resources. Gaps in professionals' knowledge about particular children can be identified, and plans can be made to fill these gaps.

Sharing observations with parents/carers

How these observations and records are shared with parents and carers is an important aspect to consider, and ways of doing so need to be developed. Not all parents are able to collect their children at the end of a day or session. This does not, of course, mean they are not interested in their child or do not care about supporting them. In order for all parents to have the opportunity to share such observations on a regular basis, the school may have to examine ways of making time available for teachers to do so – time which may involve extra resourcing, and therefore have staffing implications. Having another adult come in to take a story session at the end of the morning or afternoon for half-an-hour a week, or putting groups of children together for a period at the end of the day, may free up some time, but a range of options need to be considered if as many parents as possible are to have the opportunity to participate. Bartholomew and Bruce (1993) describe how parents who cannot come in actually contribute observations to the records via a parent observation sheet, which feeds in to the nursery's records. Recording in a home and setting diary is another idea that different settings use.

At summative stages, at the end of the school year, not all of the observations themselves will go forward to the next teacher or setting. They do, however, form the basis for formal records and report writing. Evidence for the statements you make will be drawn from the observational records. The summative statement or report then goes forward, the observations that fed it are stored or discarded, and the process begins again with the next intake.

Involving parents

It is a cliché to say that parents know more about their own child than anyone else but, like most clichés, it is true. Workers and teachers do, of course, get to know children well, but it is important to recognise that their knowledge of the child is limited. The person who sees the child in every situation at every time of the day and year is the parent. Parents are, indeed, experts when it comes to their own child. Despite this fact, many parents are made to feel that they know nothing and that their understanding of the child may be flawed or limited. This applies particularly to parents whose first language is not English or to parents who feel threatened by the education system and by authority. These parents find it difficult to have their voices heard and tend to adopt the stance that 'Teacher/playgroup workers know best!'.

Parents send young children to a nursery, crèche or playgroup for many reasons; some do so because:

- ⊃ they feel their children will benefit from contact with other children
- ⊃ they want their children to have a head start in the education stakes
- ⊃ they need to work or study.

But all parents want the best for their children and all parents deserve to be kept informed about how their children are making progress.

Case Study 4

Keeping parents informed

In the Italian nurseries, described in Chapter 8, a great deal of work goes into keeping parents informed about their children's progress. Each child has a plastic wallet up on the wall and staff put brief comments into this about what the child has done that day. This makes parents of very young children feel involved in their children's progress. No parent wants to miss his or her own child's first step or first word. Parents of older children are equally entitled to learn of their children's progress. Furthermore, they will notice changes in their child's behaviour and learning at home and can add these to the child's profile.

Involving parents in this process is sometimes difficult and always requires that workers be sensitive and supportive in their approach. Most nurseries and playgroups collect information from parents when the child starts in the nursery. This will often include practical details, but some nurseries now invite parents to say something about their child's interests, fears, passions, likes and dislikes. This gives practitioners a starting point on which to base their assessment of progress. All children starting in the nursery or playgroup arrive with a history. You can only assess progress against a starting point.

Many nurseries and playgroups now invite parents to become involved in contributing to the child's profile. Parents are invited to read through the profile and add their comments. You will, of course, need to think carefully about how you can manage this.

Conclusion

Observation provides the only true test of the quality of the practitioner's work and offers the most reliable information about each child's progress. Using it turns the practitioner into a learner and often brings about a transformation of perspective, since the open-minded stance necessary makes practitioners question previously held assumptions and rethink their practice.

Activity 3) Self-analysis

1 What aspects of observation do you enjoy most?
2 Which aspects of observational research have been of most professional interest to you?
3 Indicate how data gathered in an observation has influenced your understanding of a child.
4 Have your views been changed purely as a result of this observation or have other things influenced you? For example, has your response to the child changed because you have focused more on the child as an individual?
5 Have your perceptions changed because you have talked to others?
6 Is all this evidence reliable?

References and further reading

Cockburn, A. D. (2001), *Teaching Children 3–11: A Student's Guide*. London: Paul Chapman

Fisher, J. (2002), *Starting from the Child*. Maidenhead: Open University Press

Harding, J. and Smith-Meldon, L. (2000), *How to Make Observations and Assessments*. London: Hodder and Stoughton

Hobart, C.and Frankel, J.(1999), *A Practical Guide to Child Observation*. Cheltenham: Stanley Thornes

Laishley, J.(1999), *Working with Young Children*. London: Hodder and Stoughton

MacNaughton, G., Rolfe, S. and Siraj-Blatchford, I. (2001), *Doing Early Childhood Research: Theory and Practice*. Maidenhead: Open University Press

Meggitt, C. and Sunderland, G. (2000), *Child Development: An Illustrated Guide*. Oxford: Heinemann

QCA (2000), 'Curriculum Guidance for the Foundation Stage'. London: QCA

Taylor, J. and Woods, M. (1998), *Early Childhood Studies: An Holistic Introduction*. London: Arnold

Research methods

10

Iain MacLeod-Brudenell

This chapter is designed to develop your skills in understanding the relationship between theory and practice in the field of educare through focused research. It will encourage you to develop the insights gained in your practice experience and your own personal interests in education and care.

Recognising and utilising your existing skills in observation and extending these into more formal research skills requires a commitment to being a researcher. What does research entail? What is a researcher? Firstly, research does require an openness of mind. Ideas and values that we hold may be challenged by our research findings. Secondly, a researcher in educare is usually a practitioner and it would be likely that research would, therefore, form a basis for professional and personal reflection. This would be followed through with action to enhance practice.

There is a process to effective research, whether it is on a small scale and conducted with one child, or a larger scale survey. Careful organisation, clarity of purpose and recording will help to ensure that your efforts are tangible rather than transitory, or confused in outcome. Ensure that you read through the whole of this chapter before you start working on your research project!

This chapter addresses the following areas:

⊃ research: an overview

⊃ devising a research question

⊃ the literature search: accessing information

⊃ planning your research study

⊃ research methods

⊃ using a research diary

⊃ ethical considerations

⊃ approaches to small-scale enquiry

⊃ analysis of data.

By undertaking the suggested study within this chapter you should be able to:

1 make informed reflections upon an area you have selected to research

2 tackle an in-depth enquiry of relevant issues with confidence

3 understand how to secure an appropriate body of substantive and relevant knowledge

4 feel confident in formulating the questions you wish to address and implement appropriate means of securing answers to those questions

5 present and evaluate those answers as a means to identifying further questions to pose

6 evaluate the quality of your achievement.

Introduction

Research projects are commonly required of students in the second stage of a Foundation Degree course. They may be given any one of a number of different names, including:

- ⊃ extended project
- ⊃ special study
- ⊃ focus study
- ⊃ work-based project
- ⊃ independent study.

Although such projects have different names, they perform the same purpose – to test your ability to conduct a small-scale research project. A focused research project helps you to pursue in greater depth issues that relate to your existing knowledge of younger children.

Some students will have prior experience of undertaking research as part of their courses leading to a Higher National Diploma or an Advanced Diploma in Childcare and Education; for others, this will be an entirely new experience.

Research: an overview

Why research?

Research study within an educare course is designed to enable you to learn, practise and develop a range of research techniques in order to aid your understanding of children.

Opportunities for focused study are usually selected from a personally chosen field of study. This may be an issue of professional interest that has been selected in order to help you to become a better or more effective practitioner, or it may be an area of personal interest that relates to a current and critical issue in early childhood studies.

What will tutors expect of you?

It is usual for students undertaking research studies to be supported but not directed by tutorial staff. They will expect you to be independent and to manage your time effectively. You will be expected to:

- ⊃ have a clear idea of the topic you are researching
- ⊃ develop lines of argument and justify your judgements by demonstrating your ability to present, evaluate, and interpret your research findings
- ⊃ read widely
- ⊃ incorporate references from your reading in your research study.

Glossary of terms

There are many terms used within research, which may be unfamiliar to you. They may appear to be 'jargon' and be unnecessarily complicated. To simplify your first steps in research it may be useful for you to refer to the following glossary of terms. As you gain confidence and extend your reading you will become familiar with the terms and realise just how basic the following explanations are!

Data The information gathered through research.

Epistemology Theorising about knowledge and how we can access it.

Ethics Consideration of possible effects of the research on those you are researching. Research ethics involves being clear about how you research, for example getting informed consent from those you interview, question and research.

Experimental approach A research approach that involves introducing changes.

Experimental design Designing an experiment. This will usually allow you to make at least one change to assess its effects on those you are researching; to control anything that may influence those you are researching; to organise and control the conditions of the experiment.

Field notes The data you gather formally and informally, such as the notes you make when you go out and research.

Interpretation The process of drawing meanings from your research.

Interviews Asking questions of those you are researching. These may be structured, using a prescribed list of questions, or unstructured, a more loosely conducted interview where you allow the person you are interviewing to extend their thoughts as they wish.

Longitudinal research This form of research investigates change over a substantial period of time. It allows analysis based on the monitoring and recording of change.

Method The tools of data collection and the techniques used (such as interviews and observations).

Methodology The theoretical approach used to get knowledge through research. The methodology sets out the way of systematically getting knowledge.

Observational approach is one that is conducted with the researcher as an 'outsider'. Observational in this sense means that you do not intervene in the process.

Observation as a research method for eliciting data, finding out information. It can be participatory or non-participatory.

Participant observer Researcher can intervene and in this sense it can be experimental.

Praxis Practice informed by theory and theory informed by practice.

Questionnaire A means of gathering data from research subjects by using written questions, which should be unbiased, focused and carefully chosen.

Reliability The accuracy and consistency of research. Researchers strive to make the research as error free as possible by using various means to check for accuracy and eliminate possible bias.

Replicating Repeating the experiment. This may happen for various reasons, for example as a means of checking for reliability of evidence or for comparative purposes.

Research methods The techniques you use to gain knowledge.

Sample This usually refers to a group of people who are the subject of research. The sample is taken to represent part of the whole. For example a group of children in a year 1 class may be used as the sample in a research project. Your findings may provide data which informs you in a more general way about other children in year 1.

Triangulation Using, combining and comparing different forms of research method and/or different sources of information to arrive at a fuller understanding of an event.

Validity The endeavour to arrive at an accurate and 'truthful' outcome to the research.

Most practitioners would agree that there must be a purpose to research. We all have our own view of a researcher. Initially, this may be of a person who spends time studying a specialised, even narrow, aspect of childhood that has little relevance to everyday practice. What we would all probably agree on is that the researcher is systematic in his or her study and that the end result of such study is new knowledge. All active and interested practitioners working with young children are 'researchers', but we may not be engaged in systematically recording and remembering what it is that we find out about children through our daily interactions with them.

Many of us take knowledge for granted; we know what we know without questioning how we know it. If questioned we may be unsure that we really know what we know and it is sometimes hard to justify our arguments.

When our research deals with people, gaining accurate information is often more complex than would first appear. How children relate to each other, to adults and to you may provide insights that were not anticipated. Children react to situations and construct meanings in different ways at different times. Noting how the reactions may differ, given the same opportunity at different times, provides insight into children's behaviours and emotional and cognitive development.

As we are researching children, careful consideration must be given to ethics. In schools and nurseries we are now used to taking care to observe confidentiality of information. In research that is written up names must be changed to maintain confidentiality (children, adult and the name of the research setting). Written permission to undertake the research must be obtained from an appropriate person before research is started; this may be a parent or carer, a manager or head teacher. In research, it is important to be objective in your interpretation. Statements must be supported by evidence.

Devising a research question

For some people, thinking of a topic to research may be easy. You may have an issue that has occupied your interest for some time. This may be a family interest or concern; you may have a member of your family, a young child whom you have supported in a particular way. Examples of research topics based on personal experiences include bereavement or the daily support of children with a health condition or disability. Some students may wish to closely examine an issue about which they have particularly strong views: putting the issue 'under the microscope'. There is a danger here that personal values may interfere with an objectivity of approach to the research. Ideas for research may arise from your lecture notes; possibly too many questions come to mind and you will need to prioritise your ideas. There are some students who appear to have difficulty in finding a subject to research. Some ideas for research are more appropriate than others in relation to your professional development. You may have ideas related to your own practical experience in the workplace but which you feel unable to tackle because there may be difficulties for you in your professional role. Such issues may be tackled using another setting or range of settings and gathering data by interview or questionnaire. You need to have in mind that whatever you choose can be subjected to very focused research and that it will have a clear and 'achievable' outcome. You will be researching with a real purpose. The time in which you undertake your study will be limited and you will wish to make best use of this.

Choosing an area for your research study

When you initially consider an area for research study your reasons for choosing one may include a range of factors. Some of these are illustrated below.

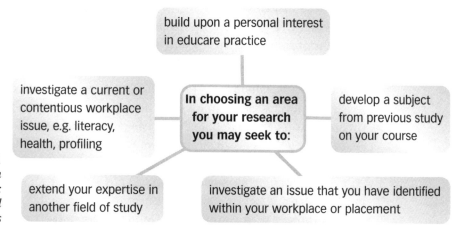

Figure 10.1
Choosing an area for research: initial considerations

The chosen area may have the potential to demonstrate your awareness of current and critical issues in educare. It should most definitely be related to your own personal interest; you should enjoy the research! It should also inform and extend your professional knowledge and understanding and the professional practices associated with children.

The most interesting research reports are those that start with a clearly formulated question. Examples of starting points for research questions are shown below.

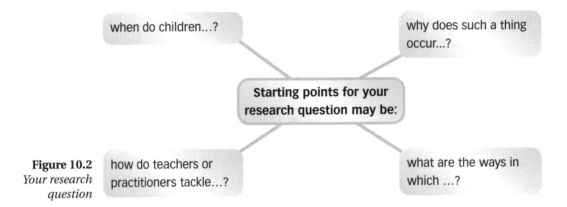

Figure 10.2
Your research question

Clarifying your research question

It is essential that you approach research with an open mind. You are not simply finding a means of justifying an opinion. The research question should indicate that you are approaching the study with impartiality and objectivity. Your research question is very important, as it forms the key to the research design and each part of the research process. If it is too broad in approach you will find difficulty in focusing and although you may find some interesting strands of research you will become very frustrated when you are trying to make a clear and concise analysis of your study.

Key in your question onto your computer; print it out and keep it nearby as a reminder to help you to focus on the real issue. It will help you to remain on task. If your notes are written on disc you can add to and edit your text, formulate and modify your ideas, and plan more systematically. This will help you to draw out the main issues and it is a far more efficient use of your time than writing and rewriting notes by hand.

Keep your question clear and simple. The value of your study, for yourself and for others, depends on how well your formulate your question. The research study is easier to focus if the question is clear and unambiguous. Some people find it easier to talk about their ideas rather than writing them down straight away and it is often useful at this point to identify a critical friend to help you with your study. This could be another student, someone you can trust to answer your questions in a straightforward way. It may be that you would find it helpful to work collaboratively with your critical friend to offer mutual support. Although

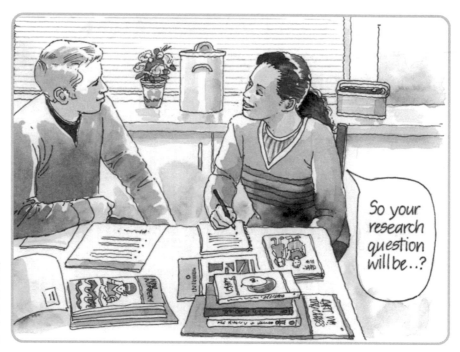

Discussing research issues with a critical friend can help to clarify your ideas

you may be researching different areas, the recording process using research diaries will be similar. You do not have to share all your thoughts – but you may find talking through the issues raised by your research easier to record if you talk to someone about it. If you select a critical friend who demonstrates enthusiasm and an interest in your work they can prompt you into providing more detailed description of your findings – and vice versa!

Talking your ideas through with someone else should help you to clarify your ideas before you commit them to print. You could provide your critical friend with some questions as prompts to get you started. Some students find it useful to use a tape recorder for conversations with their critical friend or just to record their own thoughts. It can be played back and notes made on your computer.

Dos and don'ts

⊃ Do focus on a research question

⊃ Do plan your time – be realistic

⊃ Do monitor and manage your time effectively

⊃ Do keep two copies of your work – one on disc and one on the computer

⊃ Don't delay the start of your work

⊃ Don't try to work in long stretches – work little and often (you will spot mistakes or lack of clarity more readily)

⊃ Don't be too ambitious – choose a topic that can be completed within the time scale you have been allocated

Figure 10.3
Research: some dos and don'ts

Activity 1 Your research question

1 Formulate your research question.

2 Find a critical friend.

3 Discuss your idea for the research question with your critical friend.

The literature search: accessing information

Once you have defined your research question you can then plan your reading and begin your literature search. This requires a systematic and disciplined approach. A very common mistake is for students to become diverted from their initial course and extend their reading beyond the confines of the research question. It is all too easy to find unanticipated areas of interest. Looking at other people's research reports is a valuable way of finding out about which aspects of your research question have been answered by others and what has been discovered and discussed. A thorough search of the literature will provide you with other leads for investigative reading. Often there may not be a direct reference to a research question in a book or article, but there may be references to follow up within the bibliography.

When you write up your research, you will need to show that you have made an effort to find out what has already been done in the area, and that you have taken account of it in your planning and carrying out the work. This is commonly written up in a section headed 'literature search'. Writing up the results of your search is often a really useful way of further clarifying your thoughts and moving your research question on. Doing this is a good way of leading up to making a clear statement of the research question and giving some theoretical backing to it. When making notes of your readings, make critical comments. This does not mean negative comments! You are striving to analyse and to draw out the key points from your reading, which you will then compare and contrast.

You should avoid writing your literature review as a series of paragraphs, where a synopsis of each author's work is presented. If you follow this approach it appears as though you have just made notes on each author without reflecting on how views differ or relate to one another and how they help to answer the research question. It takes some time for a book to be published and to demonstrate your awareness of more recent developments in the field you must make use of journals and publications, newspapers, television, magazines and the Internet. You may find that there is little available material on your chosen topic in academic literature, but that there is a wealth of material published on the Internet through, for example, government websites.

As you undertake your reading you may find that someone else has already answered your question. Do not despair; you could use this existing research as a basis for your own. Examine the research report and modify it to meet your professional interests or needs. You could use a different research method or conduct it using a sample with very different characteristics.

Carrying out a literature search

You may make effective use of the literature if you draw from the full range of sources to answer your question.

1 What do academic authors think of the issue?
2 What is the latest research presented at conferences or published in academic journals? How is this impacting on practice and how is this described in professional magazines and journals?
3 What reports on the issue are presented to the public in newspapers or on television and radio?
4 What is on the Internet that relates to your question?

You will need to sift through the materials available with care. The key to this section of your project is to demonstrate your familiarity with the subject. Draw out the important issues and relevant points from your reading. Consider why they are important. Do they convey specific knowledge or ideas? Is this supported by evidence? Is this evidence secured from primary or from secondary sources? Is it original data from research reports or is it reflection upon practice?

Set aside a regular time to do your reading – when you are not tired. Keep track of your references.

Citing references

You must check with your tutors for your university's approved referencing format. As you undertake your reading, copy your references and quotations and ensure that you take all bibliographical details. Figure 10.4 illustrates which information you should note, if you are going to quote from Coady's discussion of ethics, for example, which appears on page 68 in *Doing Early Childhood Research*.

Publication	Points to note for reference purposes	
Rolfe, G., MacNaughton., S. and Siraj-Blatchford, I. (2001), *Doing Early Childhood Research*. Maidenhead: Open University Press	Author: Date: Title: (The work is a chapter in an edited book)	Coady, M. (2001) 'Ethics in early childhood research' in MacNaughton, S., Rolfe, G. and Siraj-Blatchford, I. (Editors)
	Book Title:	*Doing Early Childhood Research.*
	Place of Publication: Publisher: Page number:	Maidenhead: Open University Press p68

Figure 10.4
Example of points to note when citing references

Add all the details to your bibliography as you go along. Do not leave it until you have completed all of your reading. You can quote a page reference to particular study like this (2001:68), where '2001' refers to the year the reference was published, and '68' refers to the page reference. This format is used in this book.

> ### Activity 3) Web search – using web-based resources

One of the things that it is really helpful to do early on in a research study is to find out what other people have already done in the area you are interested in.

1 There are a number of electronic journals of early childhood studies; download electronic copies of journal articles that relate to your study.

2 Use keywords to search bibliographic catalogues for appropriate references to your topic.

Planning your research study

Planning your research is often referred to as 'designing'. Designing, when used in an art or design technology context, implies careful thought for the nature of what is produced, for the audience as well as the maker. Research design is similar to this. Careful consideration is given to how well the product meets the purpose; there is a measured response to the planning of time to craft the product. There is care in checking and monitoring that the product meets the defined need and, finally, that it is useful for others as well as you.

An early decision that you must make is whether you are going to design a project that will depend upon observation or be experimental in design. An observational approach will usually be conducted with the researcher as an 'outsider'. Observational in this sense means that you do not intervene in the process.

If the research is designed with care it will produce results that have validity. Without care in the design stage you will undoubtedly find that there are gaps in the process. Try to predict as much as possible in terms of the process. Research in educare involves working with children, and working with them can be very unpredictable. Children's behaviour can change if they know that they are being studied. Absence, weather conditions and age or development-related responses may have a bearing on what is, or is not, possible within a given time span – as anyone working with 3-year-olds can verify!

Make use of your computer in planning

Use your computer to help you to design your study. If your design is well organised it will help you to keep on track and ultimately that you finish with a product of which you are proud. If you rush the design you will encounter more problems than you should – and you may take longer to complete the study because you have overlooked something of importance.

Each section of the research question can be looked at separately. You will find that methods of tackling the research will spring to mind – note these on the computer as these may help you to form ideas for your methodology. You will focus on the target group; this should be noted on the computer as the possible sample. Cut and paste the answers on separate pages on the computer and put these into appropriately titled folders: Sample and Methodology.

Making a submission

Your tutors will define this in a submission that will be presented for approval. The format of the submission may differ from one university to another but will usually include the elements illustrated in Figure 10.5.

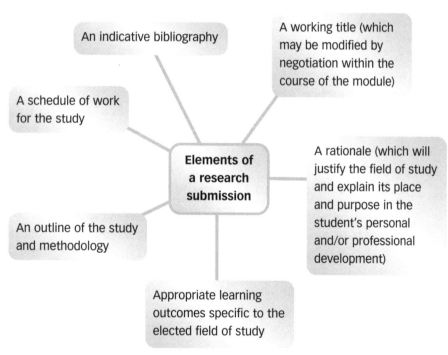

Figure 10.5
Elements of the research submission

An indicative bibliography

A working title (which may be modified by negotiation within the course of the module)

A schedule of work for the study

Elements of a research submission

A rationale (which will justify the field of study and explain its place and purpose in the student's personal and/or professional development)

An outline of the study and methodology

Appropriate learning outcomes specific to the elected field of study

Research methods

Guides on how to research may appear daunting for first-time researchers. The following sections address aspects of research methods in terms that are accessible to students in the second stage of a Foundation Degree. These are starting points and once you gain confidence you should make reference to the more formal guides to research indicated in the reading list at the end of this chapter.

The sample

It is hoped that your research will be useful to others: your colleagues at work, your fellow students or others who have an interest in your area of study. It is important that the sample (the group studied) represents a typical range of children or adults so that your findings could help to make general statements applicable to other similar groups. The size of the group will also have a bearing on the results. If you have a very small group then data must be very detailed to allow comparisons to be made with other groups. Your sample, its size and location will influence the research approach you will select.

Case Study 1

Using a small sample

Liz made a study of the provision of play for reception children in small rural schools. The study used responses from practitioners gained through use of questionnaires and telephone interviews to analyse data. Liz reflected upon provision generally and was able to identify factors that may affect the ability of small schools to provide play provision for reception-age children. Such factors related to size of groups, the location of school and the training of staff. Although a varied range of schools across the country were contacted and staff made a good response, the findings were limited. A small-scale piece of research, such as that undertaken by Liz, where there is little existing research literature available, is very valuable as a springboard for further personal research.

Qualitative and quantitative research methods

There are two approaches that students of care and education are likely to use: qualitative or quantitative research methods. The latter is the most frequently used as it enables students to have direct contact with the group that is the focus of the study, using a variety of research methods to gather data. In your reading of other literature on research you will find that each research approach has its supporters and critics. Try to make your own mind up and match the method with what you hope to achieve. We do not all get it right first time! Qualitative researchers are more likely to be concerned with interpreting observed behaviours. Quantitative researchers tend to be more interested in interpreting data gained by measurement.

Quantitative methods

These involve the collection of data that can be analysed statistically.

Supporters of this method argue that its key advantage is that data is objective. There is not necessarily a direct interaction with the group being researched; it is more likely that contact will be fairly formal and regulated.

This distance does help to maintain objectivity. As educare students are likely to be researching children rather than parents or carers this method is used infrequently. In studies of parents or practitioners, statistical data gathered by questionnaire may be very useful. Examples of students' work using this method are shown in Figure 10.6. All of the studies could be verified by undertaking replication of the research.

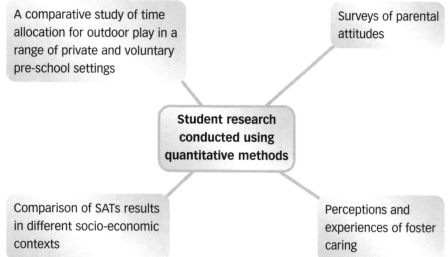

A comparative study of time allocation for outdoor play in a range of private and voluntary pre-school settings

Surveys of parental attitudes

Student research conducted using quantitative methods

Comparison of SATs results in different socio-economic contexts

Perceptions and experiences of foster caring

Figure 10.6
Examples of student research conducted using quantitative methods

Quantitative methods often use survey and questionnaire as a means of gathering data. The statistics are analysed and the results may provide a broad snapshot of the issue. When dealing with large groups of people this is the most cost-effective method of research in terms of time; it may be more expensive because there are other related costs such as postage, printing and telephone calls. If the sample is large and the study replicated it may be possible to identify patterns: of values, views, perceptions, actions and behaviour. Although surveys may be seen as an ideal way of ensuring objectivity in your research, this very much depends on the neutrality and objectivity of your survey questions. Questionnaires and interview schedules are not easy to construct and there is always a danger of bias. This will be expanded on further in this chapter in the section on questionnaires and interviews.

Case Study 2

Quantitative research approaches

Rashida has an interest in adoption and for her study selected to focus on an aspect of particular personal interest: attitudes towards adoption of children by lesbian couples. Rashida wished to gather accurate data and was concerned that honest responses would be more easily elicited if she could maintain anonymity.

There were particular concerns about cultural and religious pressures. Quantitative research was undertaken using questionnaires, which were circulated to students on a number of other courses and at other universities. The courses selected were unrelated to childhood studies so that a more general impression of attitudes could be gained from a representative sample of the population. Rashida was more interested in this point of her studies in finding out general opinion than specific detail. The sample was restricted to students, mostly 'younger' students and her selection of participants was based on pragmatic factors such as time, accessibility to groups of students and consideration of reliability, who would return the completed questionnaires.

Measures

Measure is a term used to describe what you regard as being particularly important aspects of the research, a research measurement. What you choose to measure is of crucial importance. It could be an impression of children's reactions to particular stimuli, interaction between adult and child which would be subjective, your impression. It could be more objective if it is a measure of time; for example, when tracking children engaged in particular activities over a period of time. A measure should be consistent in approach. Whatever measures are used you must strive to ensure validity. In other words can your measures provide the same or similar results if they are undertaken at another time or by a different person?

Qualitative research

This focuses on asking questions about observed behaviour. It is likely that if you are following this approach to research you will be looking at a particular context, a setting for the research and at how those you are studying react or interact in that setting. Data in qualitative research are used to help understand situations without necessarily arriving at a definitive explanation.

Because this approach seeks to understand a particular context or situation, a variety of methods are used in order to provide a broad and rich picture. Questionnaires, interviews and observations are often used to tease out understandings. These may be structured with a particular design such as case study or action research.

Gomm and Woods (1993) illustrate more fully the differences between qualitative and quantitative research. This text provides useful examples of qualitative and quantitative approaches to educational research.

Qualitative research approaches

Sam and her husband had recently successfully applied and been accepted to foster a young child. Their experience of this process had raised many questions for Sam. The links between the agencies involved, the preparation for parenthood and the self-examination and questioning relating to conflict of values in child-rearing practice had been contentious issues within the early stages of the process. Sam made contact with other families who were fostering and, through means of a diary, noted and reflected on the key developments. The research design was purposely left fairly open so that issues raised could be pursued in more detail. The methods used to gather data included informal and semi-structured interviews, observations and questionnaires. Sam's purpose was to find out if families engaged in this process encountered similar problems and issues and how they were tackled. The research journey was one of personal understanding as well as professional development.

Methods can be combined in research

In your research project you can combine methods. Quantitative data can be used in conjunction with data collected by qualitative methods. In the Case study above, for example, Sam could have used statistical data relating to numbers of successful long-term fostering as a benchmark, larger numbers of foster carers could have been contacted and statistical data used to analyse geographical differences in provision. Sam decided to concentrate on a pragmatic approach and use face-to-face contact.

Often students new to research identify very quickly with one particular approach. Early childhood studies tend to veer towards the qualitative approach because this approach involves familiar methods such as observation and interview in order to find out about a specific group of people. These students are often less comfortable with statistics and generalisability.

The methods are different but each can support the other. In order to extend research findings into practice in more than one context, generalisability must be taken into account.

Some students have used the research project at stage two of a degree course as a pilot for their independent study in the honours year of their degree programme. For some, a qualitative approach was found to be useful as a starting point to examine live issues in their pilot. A quantitative approach was used in the final year when the research question had been answered, the theory was clear and could be tested with a wider-ranging sample.

It may be useful at this point to illustrate how a similar topic may be tackled from either perspective.

Case Study 4

Use of equipment in outdoor play

A quantitative approach may focus on the frequency of use of specific items of equipment. This may be conducted as a longitudinal study over a period of time to ascertain if there are patterns to usage. It may be a comparative study or a survey of use in a number of settings.

A qualitative approach may focus on the use made of the equipment by individuals over a period of time to note any linkage with social development.

Activity 4) Accessing a research project

Aim High Stay Real: Outcomes for children and young people: the views of children, parents and practitioners (Sinclair, R., Cronin, K., Lanyon, C., et al., 2002) is a recent research publication that is very easy to read and demonstrates very effective use of qualitative research which incorporates elements of quantitative research methods in areas of early childhood. It would be useful to extend your understanding of this form of research by accessing a real research project through the Internet or as a paper-based report.

Observation as a research method

Observation as a research method can be participatory or non-participatory. As a participant observer you can intervene and in this sense it can be experimental. The experimental approach will involve introducing changes.

Case Study 5

An experimental study

Iram's experimental study was conducted in the home corner of a reception classroom. She began by looking at language and particularly the quality of spontaneous talk that was taking place. The home corner was, in Iram's words, 'the only place children could play without teacher control'. In designing her study, Iram considered varying and extending the 'props' that were available to children and to observe, record, monitor and evaluate the children's responses through language. The study was conducted over a year and was thus a longitudinal study of the context as well as of individual children.

Influence and control

As your research develops you will encounter a number of issues that relate to influence and control. For example, when you are working with children, either observing them from afar, or as a participant observer engaged with them more closely, your presence may influence them. You will know that when a video camera or a tape recorder is introduced to the class or group of children there is a reaction. Your presence as an observer may have a similar initial reaction: behaviour is different. You will also realise that after children have become accustomed to a video camera or a tape recorder behaviour reverts to more usual patterns. Build in time for children to become used to your new or different role. Be aware of the impact you may have on behaviour. Plan time to allow for settling down.

Case Study 6

Awareness of observer on behaviour

John's research project was undertaken in a small nursery school with children from a wide range of social and cultural backgrounds. Twenty languages were used within the nursery and the use and reticence or hesitancy in the use of spoken English was the focus of the project. John was given permission by parents and staff to tape-record children speaking. Initially, there were many problems: children were excited or curious when the tape recorder appeared; some were more hesitant; others were more than usually ebullient. Once children became accustomed to the tape recorder they reverted to usual behaviours – although some children did point out when the tape was running out! Over the next few weeks, John found that transcribing tapes was very time consuming and that the quality of the recordings was affected by lots of unexpected extraneous noise. We tend to focus on other people's speech when listening to them and ignore much peripheral noise. Tape recorders do not do this! John had to find quieter areas in which to research and record. His presence in these new areas, where such activity had not previously taken place, raised more questions from children and another settling-down period was implemented.

Validity

There are a number of ways of ensuring reliability and validity so that others may benefit from your research. You could collaborate with your critical friend and exchange roles, using each other's measures to test their reliability. You could ask another colleague in your workplace to use your measures. In practical terms, this is not often possible. In qualitative research, however, a valuable means of ensuring validity is through use of triangulation.

Triangulation involves getting another person's views or perceptions of an event being observed. Typically, in an early years setting this may involve asking another professional or a parent for their perspective on an event. You may also ask children. An observer makes an interpretation of what is observed, no matter how objective we strive to be.

Tape recording can be used for purposes of triangulation when analysing language; however, visual cues and body language are, of course, unrecorded and interpretation is focused solely on verbal communications. Video is more useful for purposes of analysis and confirmation of validity. The video can be analysed by others and findings confirmed or questioned.

Longitudinal research

You may possibly be expected to conduct your research over the full academic year. This provides for longer-term involvement in an early years context and for detailed research into the development of a child or a group of people. Longitudinal research has advantages in that it provides opportunity for a broad picture of an issue over time. The subtle complexities can be recorded and monitored with a degree of richness.

Long-term involvement in an early years' context, which is constantly changing, requires the use of a variety of approaches to confirm data. Involving others in confirming your data, offering different perspectives, helps to provide a more rounded picture and to confirm reliability of your interpretation of events. When working with other adults in longitudinal studies, a problem that may emerge in that participants change in their response to and involvement with the research, and misunderstandings may result. Keep people informed, fully involve them at all stages, not to the extent that they may feel that they are bombarded with information, but simply to update them about progress. Your 'contract' between yourself as the researcher and the other adults needs to remain open for negotiation.

People do change their minds; time and experience alters perception of events. In short-term research projects this is less of a problem than in longitudinal studies. Check your diary for any inconsistencies in people's responses or changes in perception. Be objective in your analysis of such issues and remember all notes should retain anonymity of the research subjects.

> ### Activity 5) Choosing research methods
>
> 1 Match your research question to a research method.
> 2 Write a short justification as to why you have selected these methods rather than others.
> 3 Discuss your ideas for the research methods with your critical friend.

Using a research diary

One of the keys to a successful research project is good organisation and a most successful means of achieving this is to keep a research diary.

Keeping a diary of your research process may be regarded as a task that places more stress on an already overworked student. This is not the case; a diary used well reduces stress levels because it keeps you on task and helps to keep ideas and actions in one place! It is one of the most useful tools for someone new to formal research. The diary is:

- ⊃ a means of helping you to organise your ideas and thoughts
- ⊃ a place to record your actions and to note your data
- ⊃ a place to record the process
- ⊃ a place to consider aspects of analysis.

As part of your employment, or within prior study, you will have developed skills in observing, recording and analysing children's development through writing case studies and making focused observations. Some of you will use recording methods in your workplace or placement as part of everyday practice. There is a requirement in many courses to keep a record of your perceptions of the taught modules and your workplace experience in a personal and professional log. The sequential focus of such activities prepares you for diary writing. You will find that keeping a research diary is easy to organise and it is an effective means of recording the detail required for effective reflection and analysis. The diary may also be used as an approach to research – a research method if the quality of the entries is carefully controlled and organised. The diary method fits well within a framework of qualitative research methods. Figure 10.7 illustrates the many uses of a diary.

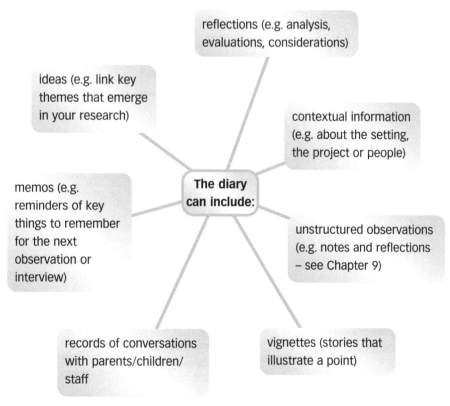

reflections (e.g. analysis, evaluations, considerations)

ideas (e.g. link key themes that emerge in your research)

contextual information (e.g. about the setting, the project or people)

memos (e.g. reminders of key things to remember for the next observation or interview)

The diary can include:

unstructured observations (e.g. notes and reflections – see Chapter 9)

records of conversations with parents/children/ staff

vignettes (stories that illustrate a point)

Figure 10.7
Keeping a diary

The diary is a record of your research and can be used to provide a wide range of qualitative data to support your research study as shown in Figure 10.8.

Qualitative data to support your research study may include:	
A detailed record of your research process	Both factual and reflective
A record of your personal development	Noting your ideas, your responses to your research and your reactions to incidents
Relevant data	Records of conversations and informal interviews Transcripts of taped conversations Observational records
A record of your responses	To your reading. Note bibliographical references
An analysis of your reflections	The process of reflection over time
A construction of your own theories and comparisons with others	Using your readings from the academic literature, websites, journals and the media

Figure 10.8
Qualitative data you may include in your diary

Because you will be using the diary weekly, perhaps even daily, throughout your research project, opportunities will arise for you to recognise emergent patterns within your data. This may be, for example, in the ways children interact with adults, how adults question children or how children respond to particular contexts or stimuli within outdoor play.

Time spent on ensuring the quality of the diary will be rewarded. In some ways, a good research diary will be more valuable than other types of research methods in that it can present a series of sequential snapshots, it can reflect personal development and it can show investigative strands in ways that are not possible through the use of questionnaire or interview.

In terms of personal development, the research diary is particularly important as it documents your perceptions and insights through the different stages of your research project. It should be noted here that the approach to writing the diary should be honest. It should note apparent failures as well as the successes. Reflection is concerned with analysing events and issues in a ways that are not simply superficial or descriptive.

Recording the sequence of events is important so that events can be revisited and reflected upon in more detail and an overall picture may emerge.

What should the diary look like?

Writing a diary is a very personal matter and every writer develops his or her own style. The diary will include details that you may not want to share with others, as well as extracts which will be useful for essays and your research study. You will find that with practice you will develop your own ways of recording information. There may be sections where you use a form of note taking, using bullet points or your own type of shorthand that may be rewritten at a later date. You may use a particular form of layout or develop new ones. We have our own idiosyncrasies, but as long as you can understand and retrieve your thoughts and data from the diary this does not matter. You will rewrite the data recorded in your diary to meet the needs of different readers, in this case your research study tutor.

There is a temptation to use a ring binder because you can compile a compendium of different types of data; for example, annotated photographs and children's work, questionnaires and other data. The research diary could take this format or you could use a bound book. The advantage in using a bound book is that there will not then be the temptation to add or take away things from the sequential record. (You have the problem then of where to put all the extra materials. The additional materials you collect may be gathered in a file; this will form your archive.) There are no hard and fast rules so find a format that you can use with confidence. Whatever form the diary takes you should leave spaces or margins to make additional comments, analysis and reflections. These later entries could be made distinct by using a different colour of ink. You will find that strands begin to develop within your research; these could be noted by using 'highlighters' of different colour.

Use your time effectively

Write diary entries regularly – and at a regular time. If you establish a habit it will be easier to maintain. You should quickly establish a pattern of writing your personal log at regular times. You should identify points to note within lectures, in your reading that relate to your study which you can reflect upon at home. Keep field notes in your practice setting. These could be made on sticky notes, on a clip board or in any other format used within the setting for noting children's development. Transfer these notes to your diary at the end of the day and reflect upon them.

At the end of the first term or semester, if you have not kept up to date with your diary entries, or if you have not done them at all, you may find it difficult to get started. Don't despair; start in a small way, and as soon as possible. Build up your confidence by setting small achievable targets and increase the frequency and detail of the diary entries over the next few weeks.

Making entries

As this research method is in diary format each entry should be organised in a systematic way. It is easier to follow and to track trends if you order your work. You will, of course, include the date and time of your observation or interaction. You should include contextual information; for example, where the research is taking place, what is happening, who is involved, the focus of the observation and anything else that seems important.

Although this is a personal document, it is useful to be disciplined in how you write your entries. You may wish to use headings. The system of numbering sections and paragraphs is particularly useful as this makes referencing sections of your work easier.

> **Activity 6**) **Your skills**

1 Consider the skills that you are developing. These skills might include:
   ⊃ a range of interpersonal skills gained by talking to children, parents/carers and to other professionals
   ⊃ skills in systematically recording observations and conversations.
2 Discuss your findings with your critical friend.
3 Write a short analysis of your personal development in research skills.

Ethical considerations

Children form a vulnerable group, and their rights need to be protected. Recent events have brought into question photographing and video filming of children. Some settings will not allow this; others will require parental permission. You will need to check carefully on the regulations in your setting. Your college or university may have specific guidelines for ethics in research, which you must follow. In the absence of these, the following details should be followed.

Guidelines for ethical conduct in research

There are issues of consent in relation to children and you should indicate in the introduction to your study that you have observed ethical procedures. Your study should contain a statement indicating how you have ensured that the study is conducted in an ethical manner, an ethical protocol. Your statement should answer the questions shown in Figure 10.9.

You should be clear, honest and open about what you are hoping to achieve in your research. This should be conveyed to parents and carers in language that is clear and unambiguous. They should be able to give consent based on a clear understanding of the purpose of the research. You must be sensitive to the children. Their needs take priority over the research.

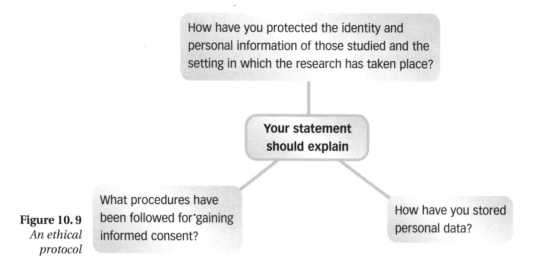

Figure 10. 9
An ethical protocol

How have you protected the identity and personal information of those studied and the setting in which the research has taken place?

Your statement should explain

What procedures have been followed for gaining informed consent?

How have you stored personal data?

Further reading in the area of ethics may be required at some point in your research. Coady (2001) presents a clear focused discussion of a range of issues related to informed consent, deception in research, confidentiality and privacy and cultural issues.

Case Study 7

Organising your time

Claire has two children under five years of age. She works in a pre-school two days a week, Thursday and Friday, and attends university one day and one evening during term time. For her research, Claire has chosen a curriculum-related topic and she uses her weekly experience in the pre-school to undertake her research. She puts information on sticky notes during the sessions and writes up her findings as notes during lunch. She has to prepare for the Friday morning session at the end of Thursday afternoon and does not have time to record the afternoon findings until later in the evening, when her children are in bed. Saturday is a family day, so no university work is done until Sunday evening. Claire finds that working at this time is slow as she is very tired. She now sets aside some time during lunchtime on the day she is in university to write up her notes. Claire finds that after she has been to the evening session at university her mind is buzzing and she uses this time to write up her diary.

Approaches to small-scale enquiry

In this section the range of research methods will be explained in more depth.

Experimental designs

In an experimental design, the experimenter introduces some sort of change and the effects of this are monitored. The aim is to find out whether this treatment (the change) has an effect on some outcome (the effects of the change). At the same time, the researcher tries to control other factors that might affect the outcome, to avoid the possibility that effects due to other factors are confused with effects caused by the treatment.

Observational designs

In an observational design, there is no change introduced by the researchers; they simply study 'things as they are'. It is still an issue, in an observational design, as to whether some degree of control is needed, for the same reasons as in experimental designs. It is important also to realise that observational designs are not the same as observation methods. Observation methods, that is, watching and recording behaviour, are widely used in early years' research. They can be used in both experimental and observational studies, which is a bit confusing! The key point is that observational studies do not involve the researcher changing something to see what happens; if that is done, the study is by definition an experimental one.

Questionnaires

Questionnaires are a popular method of gathering data. Questionnaires ask questions. They look easy and quick to construct; but they are not. To write a questionnaire that will provide valid data, that is worthwhile research and that is not biased, takes time and effort.

Before writing a questionnaire it would be useful to examine why you wish to use this method for your research (see Figure 10.10).

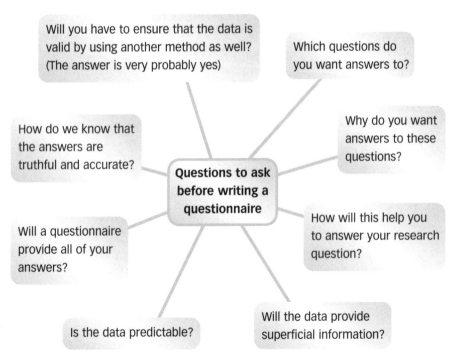

Will you have to ensure that the data is valid by using another method as well? (The answer is very probably yes)

Which questions do you want answers to?

How do we know that the answers are truthful and accurate?

Questions to ask before writing a questionnaire

Why do you want answers to these questions?

Will a questionnaire provide all of your answers?

How will this help you to answer your research question?

Is the data predictable?

Will the data provide superficial information?

Figure 10.10
Writing a questionnaire: initial considerations

To check on accuracy and ensure validity of your findings you should test the results by using another method, such as interview. If the results match, you know they are likely to be more accurate than if you had relied on one method. We have all experienced being a recipient of a questionnaire; we therefore know the frustrations of having to select from a limited range of answers. It sometimes appears that the person who has devised the questionnaire already knows the answers and wants you to confirm them by ticking a box. It is easy to analyse data provided in a small range of boxes. The accuracy and value of the findings from such research depend on how the questions have been written. The interviewee may respond in a way that acknowledges you, changing the accuracy of the data in order to provide the answers the interviewee believes you wish to hear.

Gillham (2000) in *Developing a Questionnaire* provides a useful extended and detailed examination of the use of questionnaires within research.

Observation

Observation is used extensively as a method of obtaining information within early years settings (see Chapter 9). The familiarity of the use of observation to record, assess and monitor children's development provides security for practitioners. Using observation as a research tool is somewhat different in focus. Rather than observations being used to help your understanding of an individual child's progress and needs, you will observe, analyse and reflect upon wider issues.

The presence of outsiders as observers may be intimidating. The possibility of the presence of an observer intentionally or unintentionally influencing the action is very real. Evidence obtained through observation is subject to personal interpretation.

It is not an easy technique to use effectively, as it is difficult in terms of concentration, in focusing on making decisions about what to record and in sustaining the level of quality if they are undertaken, as they should be, over a prolonged period of time.

Observation as a research method is most effective when used in combination with other methods. You can confirm what others tell you in interview through your own observation. Data from questionnaires may relate to context-based activities, which could be confirmed through observation.

Nason and Golding (1998), in a discussion of the comparative advantages and disadvantages of using observation methods, highlight time, expense and opportunity as key issues. You may wish to consider the questions highlighted in Figure 10.11.

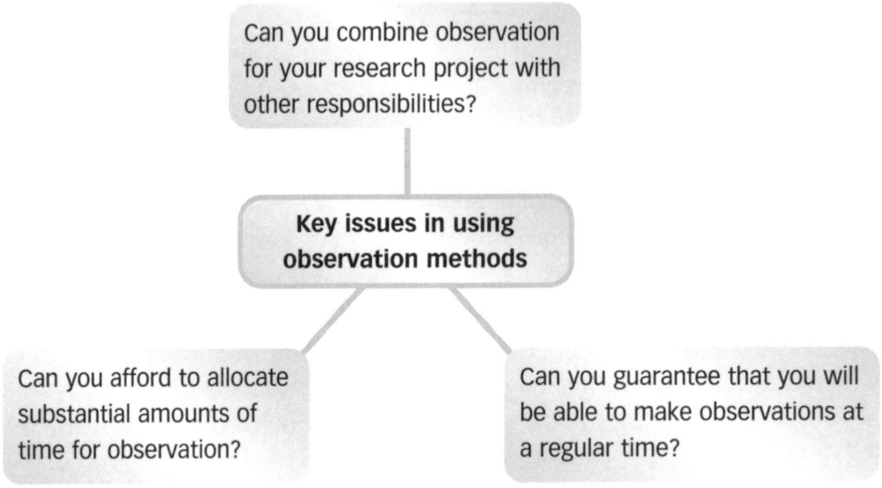

Can you combine observation for your research project with other responsibilities?

Key issues in using observation methods

Figure 10.11
Using observation methods

Can you afford to allocate substantial amounts of time for observation?

Can you guarantee that you will be able to make observations at a regular time?

> **Activity 7** **Self-assessment exercise**
>
> Reflect on your first-hand observation of children. How has your prior experience, for example, participation in professional activities such as assessment of children, helped you to make measured judgements of children's capabilities and progress? Are these judgements entirely free from bias?

Interviews

Interviews may be a means of eliciting information from groups of people or individuals who would be reluctant to respond to questionnaires. They are useful when combined with other methods to confirm validity of your data and your findings. They are easy to undertake and you can be sure of the response – unless something drastic happens to your tape recorder or pen.

There are two approaches to conducting interviews but between the two extremes there are many variations. Interviews may be unstructured or structured.

Unstructured interview

In an unstructured interview you may engage someone in conversation and focus on a number of key areas of questioning. You should record as much of the conversation as possible on paper (or laptop). When you have written up your interview you can check with the interviewee for their thoughts on the accuracy of your report. In some situations, particularly in semi-structured interviews, where there is an indication of the range of question topics, the interviewee may not object to your tape recording the conversation. This is valuable as a source of data, as the tape-recorded conversation can be transcribed and analysed.

In the interview schedule (your list of questions) ensure that the questions are not over directive, that they are free from bias and that they allow the

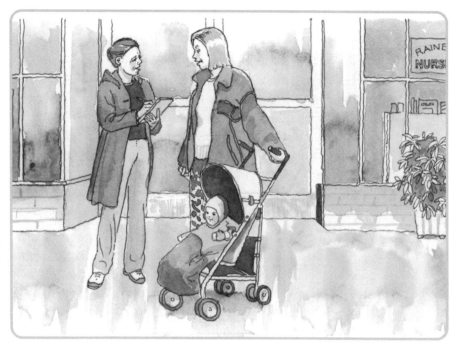

Whether structured or unstructured, interviews can be a valuable way to gather information

interviewees to speak 'with their own voice' and not to be influenced by you. Be conscious of time if you use 'open' questions, which allow the interviewee free range to answer. If you use 'closed' questions with a narrow range of answers, take care to be unbiased. Interviews and questionnaires may cause people to become self-conscious. Are the answers that people give really what they think or what they believe?

Do answers to questions change depending upon the audience? Would someone say something to you, which they would not say within earshot of a manager? In informal interview, the way in which a question is answered may be very different from the response provided in a written evaluation, which the manager may see. Some people prefer to write, others to talk.

Case Study 8

A survey of special needs

Dawn was undertaking a survey of special needs provision in a large national network of pre-school providers, which followed a specific philosophical approach to early childhood. The brochures provided by the organisation indicated that a special need was integrated into all teaching. Practice observed by Dawn indicated that this was the case and yet in questionnaires and interviews conducted with staff, responses indicated that there was no specific provision for children with special needs. There was clearly conflict between understanding of practice and practice within the workplace, communication of ideology and practice, and self-awareness of practice.

Case study approach

Many courses of early childhood studies use case study as a means of illustrating theory in practice, legislation and policy in action within a setting or context. Often such cases illustrate and examine relationships between members of a group, a family or interactions between agencies and families. A case study approach will look in detail at a particular group. For example, the study may focus on relationships within a group, interactions between members of the group. It may relate to responses or reactions by members of the group to outside agencies or the influence of such agencies on group members. As such interactions and relationships are complex, focusing on the group through a case study approach will enable you to gather rich and detailed data.

If your research question lends itself to a case study approach you will probably use a number of different methods to gather data. It therefore has the potential to give a more complete picture of a situation than most other research designs. Corroboration of the validity of data, the opportunity to test reliability of data is one of the advantages to this approach. Several sources of data allow for cross-checking. Data from informal or semi-structured interviews can be compared with formal interview/questionnaire, observation and diary entries.

A case study can be a short project or a long-term, longitudinal study. Often case studies undertaken at stage two of a degree course result in findings that provide an exploratory platform for further study and can be extended into research for a longer and more tightly focused dissertation. The case could be used as a means of understanding a complex relationship or as a descriptive illustration of events, which are then tested in another setting or context. Case study research is very well covered in some detail by Stake (1994).

Case Study 9

Revisions to the Code of Practice 2001

Bev is a special needs nursery nurse and works with a KS1 class. Her study focused on the revisions to the Code of Practice (2001), which required closer collaboration with parents than was previously expected. A case study approach offered opportunities for Bev to examine the documentation in detail, to compare this with practice in other countries (she has contacts in Australia) and to track the implementation of the Code of Practice with one child and her parents.

Practitioners in early years settings relate well to cases as a means of professional development. Familiarity with issues raised in specific cases can be used to draw other colleagues into your research. They may be able to offer support and comment in a number of ways that will enhance your research. Comments may develop into conversations and then into informal interviews. A secondary development of using this approach may be to encourage practitioners in your workplace to review their own practice. If your project does develop into a more collaborative research project, it may well be that you could look at action research as a possible extension.

Action research

As an approach to small-scale research, action research appears well suited to the needs of a researcher conducting research in educare settings. It is a very applied approach, one that links the research process closely to the early years context and has a practical purpose clearly visible to participants. It has often been used by groups of staff to review current practice and to introduce and implement new practices or procedures, a curriculum and professional development strategy. Action research is essentially a form of self-reflective enquiry, undertaken in order to improve practices. If you do wish to work with colleagues in this way you will find that your study will be reflective. It will address praxis, your own understanding of theory and practice, your own practice, and the relationships between context and practice.

Action research projects lead to change and have a focus on enabling participants to improve aspects of their own and their colleagues' practices. It is an experimental means of testing ideas and hunches, going through repeated cycles and changing each time.

It is essentially a collaborative activity, although often led by an individual. It is possible to undertake a small-scale research project as an action research project where you set up an experiment, implement it, analyse and refine it and implement it once more to measure any change.

There are similarities between the High/Scope approach and the action research cycle: Plan–Do–Review.

For further reading in this area two key texts are recommended, one by Elliott (1991), who is a key figure in the use of action research as an educational research tool, and the other by McNaughton (2001), who presents a clear and detailed discussion of the research method.

Analysis of data

You will now have researched the literature, selected and implemented your research project and have amassed a large amount of data. Sift carefully through your data. Mark with a specific colour those sections that are relevant. Put aside all those other interesting but not entirely relevant data!

Activity 8) Interpreting your findings

1 Check that you are taking care to look at your findings in an objective manner and that you can support your interpretations with evidence.

2 Check that you are taking care not to jump to conclusions and seeing things within the research that cannot be subjected to close scrutiny.

3 Check that you are not influencing the sample you are researching

Look at ways in which to present your material that conveys your findings clearly and unambiguously. Will this be as a series of charts, graphs or tables? If you have questionnaires, go through and identify similarities and differences of response. There may be no other alternative than to address each issue raised as a distinct entity in a separate paragraph. The key to a good presentation of data and analysis is to make it concise and clear.

Activity 9) Checking for clarity

1 Is there any evidence of bias in my observations, in my reflections or in my analysis? If so, what can I do to counteract my bias?

2 How subjective am I in my observations and reflections?

3 Have I left out any evidence that would not support my argument?

4 Have I checked my findings through triangulation?

5 Do my analysis and conclusions match the evidence provided by the data?

6 How useful is this research for others?

7 Are the findings generalisable or do they present understanding of issues?

Reflection and ideas for further research

It is often permissible and sometimes a requirement to conclude your study with a section that includes a reflection on your own development and ideas for further development of your area of research. Your research diary will provide you with ample material upon which to reflect. The following pointers may be helpful in constructing your conclusion.

Activity 10) Reflect on your development

1 What aspects of research have you particularly enjoyed?

2 What have you found difficult or demanding?

3 What new learning has taken place?

4 How could you improve your research skills?

5 How would you extend this research?

Conclusion

The purpose of this chapter has been to encourage you to engage in research and to feel confident in tackling some of the issues related to linking theory with practice. Coverage of the issues has been very brief. I hope that your enthusiasm for research has been fired!

References and further reading

Aubrey, C., David, T., Godfrey, R. and Thompson, L. (2000), *Researching Early Childhood Education: Debates and Issues in Methodology and Ethics*. London: RoutledgeFalmer
This book provides an introduction to a range of issues relating to research in the early years.

Bell, J. (1999), *Doing Your Research Project* (3rd edition). Maidenhead: Open University Press
A sound basis for organising and undertaking a research project.

Blaxter, L., Hughes, C. and Tight, M.(1996), *How To Research*. Maidenhead: Open University Press.
A clearly written text which has proved popular with students.

Coady, M. (2001), '*Ethics in early childhood research*' in MacNaughton, S., Rolfe, G., and Siraj-Blatchford, I., *Doing Early Childhood Research*. Maidenhead: Open University Press. pp 64–72

Delamont, S. (1992), *Fieldwork in Educational Settings: Methods, Pitfalls and Perspectives*. London: RoutledgeFalmer
A sound analysis of issues. Although the book is now rather dated, it remains a classic text.

Denscombe, M. (1998), *The Good Research Guide: For Small-scale Social Research Projects*. Maidenhead: Open University Press
A clear and accessible text. It defines and clearly illustrates many research terms.

Edwards, A. and Talbot, R. (1999), *The Hard-Pressed Researcher: A Research Handbook for the Caring Professions*, (2nd edition). London: Longman
A clear review of qualitative methods.

Elliott, J. (1991), *Action Research for Educational Change*. Maidenhead: Open University Press

Gillham, B. (2000), *Developing a Questionnaire*. London: Continuum International Publishing Group
A useful source for further reading about quantitative research.

Gomm, R. and Woods, P. (1993), *Educational Research in Action*. London: Paul Chapman
Useful examples of qualitative and quantitative approaches to educational research.

Harrison, L. (2001), 'Quantitative designs and statistical analysis', in MacNaughton, S., Rolfe, G., and Siraj-Blatchford, I., *Doing Early Childhood Research*. Maidenhead: Open University Press. pp 93-116

McNaughton, G. (2001), 'Action Research' in MacNaughton, S., Rolfe, G., and Siraj-Blatchford, I., *Doing Early Childhood Research*. Maidenhead: Open University Press.

MacNaughton, S., Rolfe, G., and Siraj-Blatchford, I. (2001), *Doing Early Childhood Research*. Maidenhead: Open University Press
This book has an emphasis on research that relates directly to early childhood. A very full range of issues are addressed in detail including research methods and anlaysis and the process of research.

Sinclair, R., Cronin, K., Lanyon, C., Stone.V. and Hulusi, A. (2002), *Aim High Stay Real*. National Children's Bureau/British Market Research Bureau: Qualitative and Children and Young People's Unit. London: Children and Young People's Unit.
Available from mailbox@cypu.gsi.gov.uk or Children and Young People's Unit. 4E Caxton House, 6–12 Tothill Street, London SW1H 9NA. Ref No CYPUAHSR. A good example of a research report relating to early childhood.

Stake, R. (1994), 'Case Studies' in Denzin, N. and Lincoln, Y. (eds), *Handbook of Qualitative Research*. London: Sage Publications Ltd.

Useful websites

British Educational Research Association (BERA) Ethical Guidelines
www.bera.ac.uk/guidelines

British Psychological Society (BPS) Code of Conduct and Ethical Guidelines
www.bps.org.uk

International Bibliography of the Social Sciences (IBSS)
www.bids.ac.uk
A useful starting point

Policy, practice and current legislation in the early years

11

Janet Kay and Iain MacLeod-Brudenell

In this chapter, a range of legislation affecting the early years will be analysed in terms of how it influences and shapes services to children and families, and how legislative change impacts on content and delivery of early years care and education. The legislative framework comprises laws influencing education and care, and relevant policies, guidelines and regulations.

The ways in which the legislative framework not only shapes, but is also shaped by, practice and by theoretical and empirical developments will be explored as will the role of the practitioner within this developmental process. Key considerations for practitioners working within the legislative framework will be discussed, in terms of strategies for achieving and maintaining high standards of care and education for young children. The ways in which legislation changes and develops over time will be touched on in this chapter, and explored in more detail in Chapter 12 (Critical Issues).

In the educational aims for the Sector-Endorsed Foundation Degree (DfES, 2001:16) there is an expectation that students have an appropriate understanding of the regulatory and legislative framework for early years and that they should be prepared to work within this framework.

This chapter addresses the following areas:

- ⊃ The Children Act 1989
- ⊃ Legislation for education
- ⊃ The Special Educational Needs Code of Practice
- ⊃ 'Birth to Three Matters'

At the end of this chapter the student will

1 understand that legislation shapes practice and that practice influences legislation
2 consider, within the legislative framework, factors which ensure quality of care and education of children
3 demonstrate understanding of the Children Act and its implications for practice
4 understand the relationship between the range of legislation for early years education
5 be able to identify those aspects of the regulatory and legislative framework which apply to your chosen educare setting.

Introduction

Legislation affecting early childhood is, in the simplest terms, the product of government activity and is designed to control and shape expectations and behaviour within early years service development and delivery. But legislation is influenced by changes in beliefs and understandings about the best approaches to early years care and education. These understandings may be part of wider social policy developments affecting a broader range of the population. For example, social policy developments around social inclusion currently driving government activity have not only impacted significantly on early years care and education, but have also introduced benefits to support parents returning to work or study and a raft of retraining and upskilling measures to improve an individual's employment chances.

Legislation is also shaped by the work of practitioners and their understandings of that work, research findings in the field, and events that have highlighted flaws in existing legislative structures.

Factors contributing to developments in policy and legislation are given in Figure 11.1.

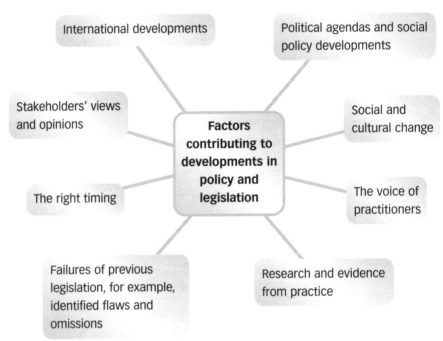

Figure 11.1
Developments in policy and legislation

Legislation can be seen as a social construct, in that it is a product of a particular set of social and cultural conditions and, therefore, will differ between diverse social and cultural settings, and will change over time as societies develop. The key importance for practitioners in recognising legislation and policy as social constructs lies in their understanding of legislation, not as an immutable force developed outside the early years context, but as changeable, subject to many forces, and developing in line with a particular set of beliefs and opinions within the field. This means that we can disagree with the principles and theories underpinning legislation and we can believe that a different approach may be better.

As practitioners, possibly as researchers, we may have the opportunity to contribute to changes in beliefs about principles and practices, enshrined in policy and legislation, as do other stakeholders. This means we may work sometimes within legislative frameworks that do not necessarily entirely support our own views on 'best practice'. It is important for practitioners to recognise that they can contribute to the debate on legislative change and that legislation is a product of human activity and therefore may be flawed. For example, the debate about whether policy to encourage 4- to 5-year-olds into Reception classes is appropriate for children of this age continues.

Discussion Point 1

Role of legislation in developing quality services in early years

There is a number of issues that need to be considered when discussing the role of legislation in developing quality services in the early years. These include:

- ⊃ reflection on the value and effectiveness of legislation and policy in shaping and supporting quality services in the early years
- ⊃ recognition that legislation is not 'set in concrete' but subject to change and development
- ⊃ understanding of the processes by which legislative change is driven
- ⊃ the social, cultural and political basis of legislation.

The Children Act 1989

The Children Act 1989 was one of the most significant pieces of legislation influencing the protection of children and the promotion of their welfare for many years. Many different influences shaped the legislation, both in terms of timing and content. These are given in Figure 11.2.

One of the key issues in child welfare legislation is the balance between the role of the state and the role of the family in supporting children's growth and development. The extent to which different states intervene in the role of the family in nurturing and raising their children varies, but 'The Children Act Now: Messages from Research' (DoH, 2001) an evidence-based review of the Children Act 1989 points out three common factors.

The first of these relates to the role of a state in nurturing children and promoting their best interests.

> The principles of the 1989 UN Convention on the Rights of the Child, for example, support the view that concerted attention should be given by families and the State to various aspects of children's lives, including education, care, recreation, culture and health, and children's social behaviour. (DoH, 2001:3)

Some influences on the development of the Children Act 1989 include:	
'Children in Care' report, 1984	Recommending a review of the law which was 'at best, complex and confused, and, at worst, contradictory' (DoH, 2001:5)
White Paper 'The Law on Child Care and Family Services', 1987	Outlining the principles on which new legislation should be based
Law Commission reviews of private law affecting children	
Failures in practice	Including the conclusions of the child death inquiries during the 1980s in respect of: ⊃ Tyra Henry ⊃ Jasmine Beckford ⊃ Kimberley Carlile
The inquiry into the Cleveland child sexual abuse crisis, 1987, during which more than 100 children were removed into care within the space of a few months	Practitioners' concerns included: ⊃ gaps in provision, for example, no order to enforce assessment of children ⊃ a 'back door' into care, through which children who had been in voluntary care for 6 months could be made subject of a Care Order without a court hearing ⊃ the increasing and inappropriate use of Wardship by Local Authorities ⊃ inadequate emergency protection provisions for children
The United Nations Convention on the Rights of the Child also came into force in 1989	This strongly influenced the underlying principles of the Children Act 1989, in terms of children's rights issues.

Figure 11.2 *Development of the Children Act 1989*

The second theme relates to children's rights as citizens embodying their rights to be party to decision-making about them and to have their wishes and feelings taken into account.

The third theme relates to protecting children from harm. The role of the state within this process is determined by where the boundaries are placed between the responsibilities of the family and the duty of the state to intervene. This boundary is variable between different cultures and countries, and where this boundary is placed will influence the type of services delivered to children and families and the ways in which they are delivered. The Children Act 1989 is the main piece of legislation providing for child welfare in England and Wales, and therefore embodying these themes. In this section, the ways in which the Act has developed these themes within the particular cultural setting and the type of 'balance' between children's and adults' rights and the role of the state versus the privacy of the family is explored.

The Children Act 1989, implemented in 1991, embodies both public and private aspects of legal proceedings related to children. It brought together a range of already existing legislation under one Act, and introduced some new measures. The Children Act 1989 provides:

- ⊃ for the protection of children from abuse
- ⊃ for the welfare of 'children in need'
- ⊃ measures to ensure the welfare of children in private proceedings such as divorce.

It is based on a set of underlying principles that changed the ways in which children and their families were viewed within legal proceedings, some of which were drawn from concepts of children's rights. In addition, it is important to consider some of the criticisms of previous legislation in more detail to understand the ways in which the Children Act 1989 came to be constructed. Some of the problems identified in practice prior to the implementation of the Children Act included:

- ⊃ poor information sharing between agencies, which often contributed to faulty judgements being made about the welfare of children
- ⊃ children being removed from parents on inadequate evidence of abuse
- ⊃ focus on working with parents, rather than children, contrasted with lack of genuine partnership with parents in decision-making processes
- ⊃ lack of effective permanency planning for children in care, resulting in children drifting in and out of care or lacking a stable permanent home.

In the following discussion, the impact of the Children Act 1989 on practice issues and the shape of services to children and families will be discussed, with reference to quality and other key issues for early years practitioners. It would be helpful to read or refer to Chapter 15 (Child Protection and Children's Rights) in which the provisions within the Children Act 1989, relating to protection of children from abuse and children in need, are described in more detail.

Underlying principles

The Act introduced a range of new principles on which the spirit of the law rests. The underpinning ethos behind these principles is the belief that the concerns of children and their families should be located much more firmly at the heart of legal procedures affecting them. The paternalistic approach, which had dominated proceedings until that point, had resulted in many families being 'acted upon' rather than 'worked with'. Research findings, particularly about the outcomes for children subject to welfare legislative proceedings, had led to a widely held belief that improvements in the quality of welfare services for children could only be achieved through a different emphasis on their rights within procedures.

Organisations such as the Family Welfare Association had spent several years lobbying for parent's and children's rights to be more central to proceedings, and they had highlighted flaws in practice where children and families did not have a say in the decision-making processes about them. For example, many children who came into the care system did not have continuing contact with their families and other significant individuals. There was a lack of consistency in practice around ensuring contact between children and families, and the onus was often on families to ensure that contact took place, despite a range of practical and psychological barriers.

Case Study 1

Effects of lack of contact

Jane's baby went into foster care at 9 months of age after Jane had allowed an abusive boyfriend back into her home, despite repeated warnings from social workers that he was a risk to her child. Jane's two previous children had been taken into care and then placed for adoption after she had failed to protect them from a series of abusive boyfriends. Eight years later when she was asked to agree to her son's adoption by his foster carers, she told this story:

'I wanted to have him back then, but it was hard to visit because they lived a long way away and when I turned up once without phoning the social workers were angry. They (the foster carers) were nice enough, but they thought I was a rubbish mother for letting him down and he seemed so happy there. He didn't recognise me and I never felt comfortable there, so I stopped going. I knew they would say I wasn't bothered about him, but I knew I wouldn't get him back because of the other two, so why bother? Then when I went and took him after school, they went mad and I couldn't go anymore.'

Failure to ensure contact was maintained often opened the door to permanent separation of children from their families. The impact on children growing up in care with no knowledge of, or contact with, birth families was often very negative. A sense of dislocation and lack of sense of self, low self-esteem and poor levels of confidence were common among children who had lost contact with their birth families and/or had little or no knowledge about their own origins and early lives or the processes that had brought them into the care system.

Research in the field and practitioners' own experiences created a belief that many children's life chances could be greatly enhanced if they had a better understanding of their experiences in the care system and links to their families. The more widespread use of 'life story' work to help children in care to understand their past developed in the 1980s, alongside a better understanding of the problems children faced when events in their past remained unclear. However, the belief that children in care were best served by a 'clean break' from birth families had also by then been challenged by research findings.

Case Study 2

Restoring contact with family members

Chris was 12 when the small children's home he lived in suggested that he might benefit from fostering. Chris had lived in a variety of settings after coming into care when he was 5 years old, including the homes of several family members and a number of different children's homes. He had never been placed for fostering because of some behavioural difficulties and his own resistance to being placed with a family. Chris had begun to want to live with a new family, but felt that he needed to know more about his past before he could be fostered. With the assistance of one of his workers, Chris went back through events in his early life using photos to record significant events, and to provide a permanent record on which many discussions about his early life were based. Chris came to understand much more about why he had ended up in care and to recognise that his separation from his family was not his own fault. After some time, contact with some family members was successfully restored and Chris went to live with an uncle and aunt who were willing and able to care for him.

Influenced by the United Nations Convention on the Rights of the Child, the Children Act 1989 sought to improve and balance the rights of both the child and family within child welfare law by introducing the following underpinning principles.

Children are better off with their families

This principle underpins the whole of the Children Act 1989 and influences the ways in which the Act was constructed and implemented. It clarified the goals of welfare work with children and families and changed practice to some extent, in that the central goal of work with children and families became to support and maintain family functioning wherever this is possible. The exception to this is in cases where the child cannot be safeguarded effectively within the family. This principle militated against poor practice where children were removed into care for trivial reasons because of concerns about their general welfare, often resulting in long-term or permanent separation from families of origin. Resources had to be focused on maintaining families where unmet needs made this difficult without service provision.

Avoiding delay

Delay in the progress of court proceedings had come to be seen as harmful to the child's welfare. For some children, childhood meant long periods of uncertainty about the future and a sense of impermanence in their living situation. Were they going home, or being adopted, or returning to live with their families of origin? For some children, there were long delays in determining these issues, while their childhood passed by. The Children Act 1989 introduced the 'no delay' principle to ensure that children's futures were settled much more quickly than previously. For example, Emergency Protection Orders by which children can be removed from parental care where there is considered to be risk of 'acute physical harm', last only 8 days with a possible 7-day extension. This Order replaced the Place of Safety Order, which lasted 28 days, a period of time during which there may have been no contact between children and parents.

In some proceedings (Section 8 and care proceedings) the court is required to draw up a timetable to ensure delay is avoided.

The non-interventionist principle

This principle was based on the belief that a court should only make decisions in respect of a child if this step is best for the child. Legal intervention came to be viewed as a last resort in efforts to resolve public or private disputes about a child's welfare. In terms of both the child and family's best interests, legal action should be minimised and only used if all other avenues have been explored unsuccessfully. In addition, if a court is presented with a request for legal action in respect of a child, it has to determine whether making an Order is in the best interests of the child. Otherwise the court should do nothing.

The non-interventionist principle means that those responsible for children's welfare must make every effort to resolve welfare issues in respect of a child without recourse to the law. The intervention of the courts is considered to be heavy-handed and inflexible compared to a voluntary arrangement between those involved with a child, which can be reached amicably. This also applies to children in private proceedings, such as divorce, where Orders are now only made in respect of contact between non-resident parents and children if no agreement can be reached.

This principle facilitated some important changes in practice. For example, when a child is considered to be in 'acute physical danger' and therefore immediately 'at risk', it is the responsibility of social workers to secure the child's safety as soon as possible. However, within a non-interventionist approach, this no longer means an immediate recourse to legal action. Before considering legal steps, the Children Act 1989 demands that social workers must explore alternative methods of ensuring the child's safety. These could include methods shown in Figure 11.3.

Legal intervention, in the shape of an Emergency Protection Order to remove the child into the care of the local authority, should only be used if all other options to safeguard the child fail. However, where there is to be a transfer of care of the child to the local authority, through the making of a Care Order,

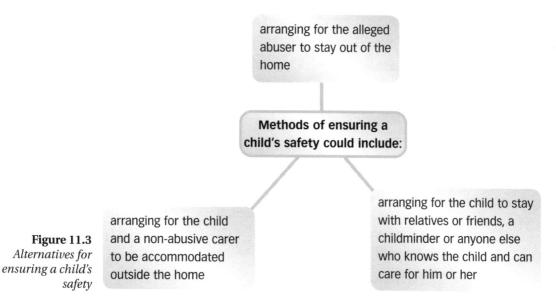

Figure 11.3
Alternatives for ensuring a child's safety

arranging for the alleged abuser to stay out of the home

Methods of ensuring a child's safety could include:

arranging for the child and a non-abusive carer to be accommodated outside the home

arranging for the child to stay with relatives or friends, a childminder or anyone else who knows the child and can care for him or her

the Children Act 1989 deemed that this could only be done thorough a full court hearing where 'significant harm' to the child has been identified or the child is beyond parental control. This approach ensures that children could no longer go in to care through other routes, which did not involve a full hearing at which parents could be legally represented. Effectively, this principle supports the rights of families to privacy from State intervention, except where it is imperative in order to protect the child from harm.

The feelings and wishes of the child

The Act introduced an explicit requirement that the wishes and feelings of the child should be elicited and taken into consideration in proceedings related to him. Although good practice had, for many years previously, demanded that the child should be consulted before decisions were made about his future, the lack of emphasis on this requirement and variations in practice meant that this did not always happen effectively. In order to elicit the child's wishes and feelings and ensure the child is properly represented in proceedings, the court can appoint those officials identified in Figure 11.4.

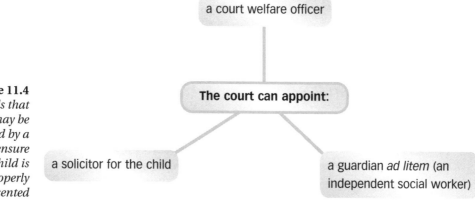

Figure 11.4
Officials that may be appointed by a court to ensure that a child is properly represented

a court welfare officer

The court can appoint:

a solicitor for the child

a guardian *ad litem* (an independent social worker)

Underpinning this principle is the recognition that the child's best interests may not be represented by either the local authority or by his parents.

The extent to which a child's wishes and feelings are considered depends on the child's age and level of understanding. These are critical factors in determining the weight that is placed on the child's view and feelings. Younger children may have very limited influence on outcomes affecting them because they are not considered to have sufficiently developed understanding about the issues under consideration. Similarly, the court cannot allow children to act against their own best interests. If the child's wishes and feelings contradict his or her best interests, the child's best interests remain paramount. For example, a child may want to live with a particular parent, but if that parent is unable to care safely for the child, then the child's wishes will be denied.

This principle reflects the increased emphasis on the rights of children within legal proceedings.

Parental responsibility

The concept of parental responsibility replaced the notion of parental rights within the Children Act 1989. The concept of parental rights was seen as outmoded, representing a view of children as the property of their parents that was out of step with the children's rights ethos shaping the principles underpinning the Children Act 1989. The notion of parental responsibility was intended to emphasise the view that parents should have responsibilities to their children rather than rights over them. Similarly, the extent to which parents can legally lose their parental responsibility for a child was curtailed. Under previous legislation, parental rights ceased when a Care Order was made in respect of the child. Under the Children Act 1989, parental responsibility is retained by the parent through all childcare procedures unless the child is adopted. If a child is subject to a care order, parental responsibility is shared between the parent(s) and the local authority. Sharing of parental responsibility between individuals and between individuals and the local authority was introduced to ensure that children retained contacts with all significant others, whether they were in the care of the local authority or not.

However, parental responsibility is not automatically conferred on all parents (see Figure 11.5).

It was thought by some that the Children Act 1989 had not gone far enough in establishing and securing parental responsibility for unmarried fathers. However, the automatic retention of parental responsibility by both parties after divorce is seen as a positive move in efforts to retain links between children and their fathers after family breakdown. Similarly, retention of parental responsibility when children are subject to a care order was seen as a positive step in encouraging parents to maintain contact and possibly to eventually resume the care of their children. This principle attempts to

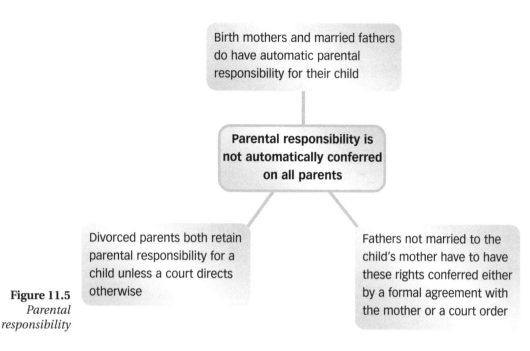

Figure 11.5
Parental responsibility

Birth mothers and married fathers do have automatic parental responsibility for their child

Parental responsibility is not automatically conferred on all parents

Divorced parents both retain parental responsibility for a child unless a court directs otherwise

Fathers not married to the child's mother have to have these rights conferred either by a formal agreement with the mother or a court order

support both increased rights for children in relation to their parents, and the maintenance of parental responsibility as a link between parent and child as a goal for legal proceedings where at all possible.

Partnership with parents

The Children Act 1989 was built on the premise that parents and children needed to have their rights much more clearly recognised within the legislative process. As such, local authorities have a general duty to ensure that parents are party to legal processes involving their children. This duty raises a number of difficult questions about how practitioners can remain in partnership with parents when involved in actions that may be seen as adversarial by those parents. The obligation to discuss options with parents and to ensure that they have all relevant information about the social services' views and actions may be difficult to fulfil when serious child abuse has taken place. The principle was introduced partly to reduce this adversarial element to the relationship between social services and parents, but the involuntary removal of children from the care of their parents very often raises extremely strong feelings, making dialogue with parents difficult and sometimes even risky. Despite this, practitioners involved with children and families retain this duty and the onus is on service providers to ensure that it is fulfilled.

In terms of services to children in need and their families, there is an emphasis on partnership with parents to provide appropriate services to support the family where unmet need threatens family functioning or stability. Initially, the concept of a 'child in need' was interpreted solely at local authority level, producing a wide range of different service levels depending on location. To remedy this disparity, the *Framework for*

Assessment of Children in Need and their Families (DoH, 2000) was introduced as a national tool for assessing need. It ensures that:

- ⊃ families receive equitable access to services with clearer boundaries for when service provision should be triggered
- ⊃ all the child and family's needs are identified and responded to through a comprehensive assessment process
- ⊃ family strengths should be identified and worked with
- ⊃ services provided should be acceptable and seen as helpful by children and parents
- ⊃ resources should be used wisely by ensuring services are appropriate, effective and targeted on identified need.

The underlying principles of the Act reflect concerns with child welfare, children's rights and the protection of children from harm. The principles support a particular approach based on partnership between agencies and between agencies, children and families. The rights of both children and parents have been enhanced within the Act through the application of the principles discussed above. However, in some areas there are continuing problems in applying these principles effectively. Failures or limitation on the effectiveness of inter-agency partnerships continue to be at the root of many criticisms of child welfare in the UK. Legislation also shapes the ways in which services are developed and delivered. In the next section, this will be discussed with reference to child protection services.

Responsibility for child protection within the Act

The Act places a duty on local authority social services departments to investigate and take steps to prevent child abuse taking place. The NSPCC and the police are given more limited duties to protect children. Although health, education and other professionals have a responsibility to provide information and support social services in protecting children, the legal responsibility for investigating and responding to abuse lies firmly with social services departments within local authorities.

Shaping services through legislation

This allocation of legal duty has shaped the ways in which child protection services have developed. Although there is a strong emphasis on joint agency and multidisciplinary responses to child abuse both at strategic planning and individual case level, the fact that ultimately legal responsibility lies with social services has meant that they continue to dominate the child protection process, with ramifications for the perceived roles of other agencies and professionals. Although social services may have regular contact with families in need and families where abuse has already been identified, other agencies are much more likely to have contact with children where abuse may be ongoing but not yet identified. In addition, as family support services have developed in a range of

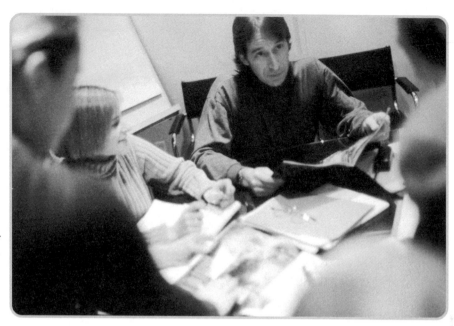

Members of multidisciplinary teams bring a range of expertise to child protection cases

agencies including health, education and charitable and voluntary sector organisations, there has been a split in the delivery of services to children that has left child protection services isolated from other provision.

Health visitors, early years practitioners and teachers have a key role in initial identification and response to child abuse and monitoring of children where abuse has taken place. Yet expertise in these areas continues to be located largely within social services, ensuring that child protection work takes place outside the provision of mainstream services to children. Although health and education are specified as having a duty to being involved in child protection within the legislation, their role is minor compared to social services and professionals in these agencies are much less likely to have had relevant training and staff development. This is significant in terms of the balance of roles within multidisciplinary child protection teams. For example, social workers take the lead in child protection case conferences, which are normally organised and chaired by social services. There is evidence that, despite the emphasis on 'working together', in fact other agencies drop out of the multidisciplinary core groups designed to implement child protection plans soon after the initial investigation.

Guidelines to promote an integrated multidisciplinary approach

Efforts to ensure that services are effectively integrated and that a multi-disciplinary approach is maintained have been promoted through the DoH guidelines *Working Together to Safeguard Children* (DoH, 1999), which outline the roles of all practitioners working with children in the child protection process. The requirements of these guidelines, which all establishments and workers with children should comply with, are given in Figure 11.6.

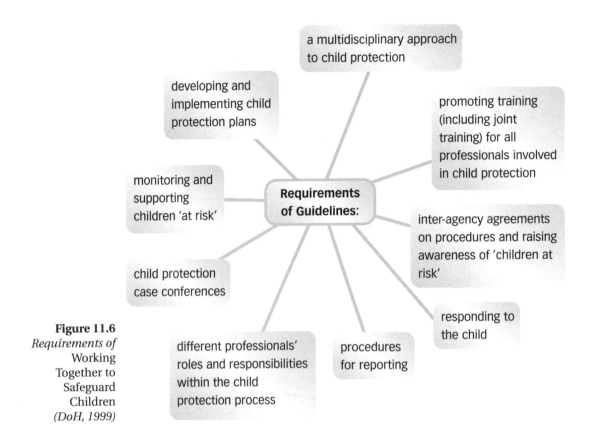

Figure 11.6
Requirements of
Working
Together to
Safeguard
Children
(DoH, 1999)

The diagram shows "Requirements of Guidelines:" with connections to:
- a multidisciplinary approach to child protection
- developing and implementing child protection plans
- promoting training (including joint training) for all professionals involved in child protection
- monitoring and supporting children 'at risk'
- inter-agency agreements on procedures and raising awareness of 'children at risk'
- child protection case conferences
- responding to the child
- different professionals' roles and responsibilities within the child protection process
- procedures for reporting

Despite this, there have been considerable failures to establish effective partnerships between all relevant agencies, as exemplified by the Laming Report into the death of Victoria Climbie (DoH, 2003; see Chapter 12, Critical Issues).

'Every Child Matters'

The Green Paper, 'Every Child Matters' (DfES, 2003) has been influenced by:

⊃ the political agenda around social inclusion for all children

⊃ the tragic death of Victoria Climbie

⊃ perceptions of flaws in existing arrangements to ensure inter-agency cooperation and communication (see Chapter 2).

Attempts to involve all relevant agencies and professionals in the child protection process have recently been stepped up, particularly in response to the death of Victoria Climbie, which exemplified failures in communication and information sharing between agencies, amongst other things. 'Every Child Matters' (DfES, 2003) indicates that to some extent attempts to develop partnership between agencies have been superseded by proposals to merge education and children's social services under a single directorate. Key stakeholders in the child protection process have greeted these proposals with cautious enthusiasm. The NSPCC commented that to achieve success by integrating services consideration must be given to the following:

these measures will only work if local authorities are given both a legal duty and the resources to integrate key services and to ensure that key professionals within them work together more effectively to safeguard children. (www.nspcc.org.uk)

They go on to argue that in order to achieve effective protection of children, legal steps should be taken to ensure that children have equal rights to protection from assault as adults and that parents should be given a 'positive duty of care' through the law in England and Wales, as is already established in Scotland.

> **Activity 1** **Taking legal steps**

Read Case study 3, below, and, with reference to the provisions of the Children Act 1989, discuss the legal steps that could be taken to protect Shaun, and the circumstances in which they would be relevant. Then, with reference to the discussion above:

1 Describe the parent's rights within this situation.
2 Describe the child's rights.

Case Study 3

Child abuse

Shaun is 4 years old. He lives with his single mother and her parents. Shaun and his mother went to live with the grandparents after being evicted for non-payment of rent. Shaun attends a nursery school and is about to enter Reception class. The nursery has been concerned for some time about Shaun, who is an aggressive little boy with a number of developmental delays, especially in his communication and social skills. Shaun's mother rarely collects him and, therefore, there have been limited opportunities to discuss concerns with her. Shaun's grandmother normally collects him, but she is a quiet, self-effacing woman who has little to say. Other parents have said that Shaun's mother goes out a lot and leaves Shaun in the care of his grandparents, and that she and the grandfather have an acrimonious relationship. Attempts by nursery staff to discuss concerns with the grandmother have been fruitless. Today, Shaun appeared at nursery with a bruise on his face, across the cheekbone. Unusually, the mother dropped him off and made a point of telling staff that Shaun had fallen over in the yard. At break Shaun is sent in from play for fighting. A nursery nurse sits with him and ask him what the matter is. She asks him if his face hurts from the bruise. Shaun tells her that his grandad hit him when he didn't want to play a game and that he hates living with his grandad, who often hurts him. He tells the nursery nurse that he has tried to tell his mother, but she won't listen. The nursery nurse asks what the game was that Shaun's grandad wanted to play and Shaun replied, indistinctly, '... hurting willies'.

The proposals within 'Every Child Matters' are aimed at placing child protection within the context of other services to children and families, rather than as an additional (and sometimes unwelcome) duty for the majority of early years practitioners. The integration of education and children's social services within local authorities and the grouping of a wider range of children's services within Children's Trusts is intended to achieve a much higher level of cooperation between services than currently exists. The identification of education as the key agency in this process has significant implications for the roles of many early years professionals in the child protection process, and for the type and range of training and qualifications early years practitioners may anticipate in the future.

In terms of the three common themes of children's legislation discussed above, the implementation of the Green Paper proposals would place the emphasis firmly on nurturing children through services designed to support their development and prevent them coming to harm, with the balance between adult and children's rights shifting towards the latter. In order to achieve this there will need to be legislative changes to support a higher level of state intervention in the privacy of the family, particularly in the area of information sharing between agencies on a much wider scale.

Legislation for education

Practitioners often deal with education legislation on a 'need-to-know' basis, rather than considering how and why these requirements are made. As a practitioner you may be familiar with the requirements of the curriculum in theory and in practice, and yet you may not have considered how legislation influences what you do with children in the classroom. The term 'practitioner' is used to refer to anyone working in a paid or unpaid capacity with babies and young children. The term does have formal recognition and there are specific responsibilities that accompany this role. The term 'practitioner' is specifically used within early years education and care, as it can be used in a wide range of contexts and be used to describe people with varied training and areas of professional responsibility. It may in different circumstances include, for example, qualified nursery nurses, voluntary workers and teachers. The term practitioner relating to legislation for the Foundation Stage means any person who teaches the Foundation Stage in a Foundation Stage setting.

New legislation in education often reflects political response to change in social and cultural conditions. Factors that contribute to such developments in education policy and legislation include those given in Figure 11.7.

Legislation relates very closely to social and cultural settings. Education law reflects social context, its cultural needs and aspirations and will differ between countries. An example of such difference has been demonstrated by recent reports of the introduction of legislation in France forbidding the wearing of 'overt' religious symbols in schools; preventing the wearing of

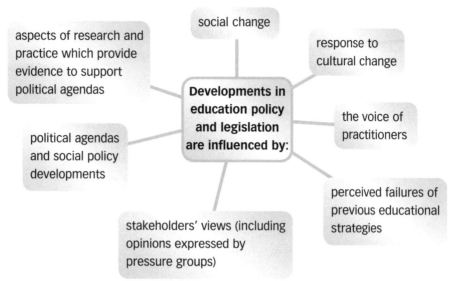

Figure 11.7
Developments in education policy and legislation

the *hijab*, the head covering worn by some Muslim girls and the *kippah* or *yarmulkah*, the 'skull cap' by Jewish boys. A similar proposal would not be tolerated in England, as this would contravene legislation in relation to racial and religious discrimination. Educational processes and systems reflect the values of the society in which they are located. In practical terms these values are embedded in legislation. As a culturally diverse society, the United Kingdom recognises the rights of children and adults to comply with religious and cultural requirements within the school context.

Legislation for education broadly relates to three key aspects:

- ⊃ the curriculum, i.e. what is taught
- ⊃ the regulation of where the curriculum is located and taught
- ⊃ the regulation of those who work with and teach children.

The curriculum

The Statement of Requirement indicates that senior practitioners should have an informed understanding of legislation relating to the curriculum and to its implementation. The difficulty for some practitioners in education, particularly those working in Key Stage 1 classrooms and nursery classes, is that the curriculum has been subjected to frequent change. Reflective practitioners will be aware of change in legislation not simply by response to directives but through questioning for meaning and purpose, reading media reports and critically analysing government documentation.

Making comparisons

Foundation degree students, particularly those working in early years settings that receive government funding, will be familiar with the curriculum requirements of the country in which they work. As students of early childhood it is useful to compare and contrast the curriculum, which they support in their workplace, with those of our nearest neighbours.

There is much to be learnt from such comparison. Differences in approaches to learning and teaching methods, which at first appear sharp in contrast, may diminish after studied comparison.

The structure of the education system in the United Kingdom has changed considerably over recent years. The introduction of national assemblies has provided greater autonomy in many areas of policy making, including education. Educational policy is determined by the departments of education for each of the four countries which comprise the United Kingdom and there are four distinct national systems of education. The policies that determine the curriculum and funding for education in Scotland, England, Wales and Northern Ireland reflect the philosophical approaches to education of the different nations. The curriculum for Wales was, for example, until the establishment of the Welsh Assembly similar in content to that of England. Recent developments in Welsh educational circles have encouraged greater response to local need and indeed to the philosophy of education. Divergence of approaches to testing of young children between Wales and England is emerging as a fundamental difference in philosophy between the two countries. Philosophical differences have been present between the Scottish and English approaches to curriculum from the outset. Scotland, unlike England, does not have a legally prescribed national curriculum but provides guidelines for teachers.

Using government websites

There is an expectation of students on a degree course of study that they will consult web-based resources. Much of the legislative material we describe within this chapter is accessible through government websites, although much of this is in more formal language than that which we have used. In order to help you to extend your understanding of curriculum provision in the United Kingdom and to develop your skills in ICT, it is suggested that you access and compare the curriculum approaches demonstrated on government websites given at the end of this chapter.

An interesting quotation from the British Council website indicates, for international reference, that changes in the structure of education systems within the United Kingdom are:

> ...*reflecting successive governments' aims to improve quality, increase diversity and make institutions more accountable to students, parents, employers and taxpayers.*

Accountability for policy is controlled by the voting public; however, it would be highly unlikely that early years education policy, or indeed any social policy would be the cause of not re-electing either an individual or a parliamentary party.

The National Curriculum

The Education Act (1988) proposed an approach to education which would bring about a greater consistency in the quality of educational experience of children who are of statutory school age, that is those who enter formal school settings in the term following their fifth birthday. The National Curriculum for England and Wales (1988) was introduced into schools in England and Wales, in order to provide a broad, balanced and coherent system. Prior to the introduction of the National Curriculum, curricula were devised at local level, by means of a common curriculum framework with clear guidance on what subjects must be taught and how they would be tested. The curriculum set out what pupils should study and how standards would be monitored.

The first National Curriculum in England and Wales is divided into four age-related Key Stages (KS), three core subjects (English, mathematics and science) and nine non-core foundation subjects. Throughout the first years of implementation there was regular change to documentation, and of expectations of children and teachers. Documents were 'slimmed down' to help teachers to manage apparent overloads of paperwork and testing was reduced to core subject areas. Changes to curriculum content were often the result of pressure from particular lobby groups. This was particularly noticeable in relation to the curriculum for English.

Political intervention

The substantial and frequent change that has taken place in the National Curriculum in the last 15 years is not discussed here, but it is sufficient to say that change is neither always negative, nor is it always positive. Mistakes have been made and acknowledged and no doubt there will be further development and change to curriculum content to reflect government policy. Political intervention is the driver of curriculum change in England. Educational development strategy is not considered in isolation, it is closely connected to ideas and initiatives in other aspects of social policy. This is clearly seen in the links between the introduction of literacy and numeracy strategies in schools and adult and family literacy and numeracy initiatives.

As a practitioner, you will already be conversant with a form of curriculum, either the Foundation Stage Curriculum or the National Curriculum. You may well have followed the practice of many others by focusing solely on the teaching content when reading the documentation for the curriculum; this is a mistake. It is important to read the introductory sections of key documents as it provides the reader with a rationale for the delivery of the curriculum.

The National Curriculum is provided as a means by which all children in maintained schools may be taught a prescribed range of subjects through a broad and balanced curriculum. The literacy and numeracy strategies may be regarded as factors in breaching the last requirement as their introduction has resulted in a reduction of the time available for the effective experience of other curriculum areas. Nonetheless the requirement is that schools should still provide a broad and balanced curriculum.

Reflecting the needs and values of society

The curriculum should reflect the needs of society and legislation relating to equality and non-discriminatory practice applies to all school settings. Careful and considered planning for the delivery of the National Curriculum is essential in order to achieve equity of experience for all children. Breadth applies to the relevance of the curriculum for children regardless of culture, gender, religion or physical difference. All children are entitled to have equal access to the curriculum.

The curriculum reflects the values of society expressed through legislation and these values are present within National Curriculum documentation. Party political views and values on education issues are indicated in manifesto commitments. The values of the present government are clearly demonstrated in legislation. Higher priority is given to some aspects of education rather than to others.

These values are visible in the high proportion of space allocated in the current National Curriculum documents to philosophical and promotional messages; two pages for each curriculum area compared with a similar or slightly larger allocation of space for the curriculum detail.

The promotional messages contained within the documents provide justification for the importance of each curriculum area by drawing on a wide range of 'experts' from all walks of life: popular entertainers, media personalities and academics. For example, the National Curriculum for English (DEE 1999:14–15) incorporates short statements by the author Anne Fine; the poet, writer, actor and broadcaster Benjamin Zephaniah; Professor Lisa Jardine and the writer Ian McEwan.

> ## Activity 2) The National Curriculum
>
> Select a National Curriculum foundation subject: Physical Education, Geography, History, Design & Technology, Music, or Art.
>
> Read the introductory section in the National Curriculum for this area (for England, details may be obtained from the DfES Department for Education and Skills website). The rationale for each curriculum area is clearly articulated in formal statements and aims and also through quotations from selected personalities and experts in the curriculum.

1 Provide your own rationale for children studying this curriculum area.

2 Why study it?

3 What does it mean to young children?

4 Why is it a life skill?

Consideration of the purposes of the curriculum will not only provide you with a sense of real purpose in teaching this area but also help you to understand the purpose for the inclusion of the subject in the legislative curriculum framework.

Subject areas within a curriculum will vary between countries

It is important to remember that the subject areas selected for inclusion within a curriculum will vary from one country to another. The English National Curriculum contains subjects that are not present in exactly the same form in the curricula of other countries.

National Curriculum Key Stage 1 documents provide statutory curriculum detail for the teaching of 5-, 6- and 7-year-old children. The content of the curriculum builds on the traditions of existing early childhood curricula, which were current in England at the time of writing the first statutory orders in 1988. Nowhere was this more clearly seen than in the curriculum for Design and Technology in the first Statutory Orders (DfES, 1988). The link between planning, identifying a need for making something, making and evaluating an object was present in best practice in many early years classrooms. This approach to best practice was promoted by support with curriculum guidance materials; an idea now promoted in Foundation Stage documentation (DfEE/QCA, 2000). The Design and Technology example is particularly apt, as it is an area that does not appear as a distinct curriculum area in many other national curricula. Britain is a world leader in technological innovation and it may be judged appropriate that this subject appears in the curriculum from its earliest stage. The design technology curriculum has changed many times over the last 15 years, but in essence it still helps teachers to provide children with opportunities to develop their thinking skills as well as their abilities to control and manipulate materials. There are strong links between subjects studied within the National Curriculum by children in Key Stage 1 (for children in Year 1 and above) and children following the Foundation Stage curriculum (those who have not yet transferred to Key Stage 1) in the term following their fifth birthday.

The Curriculum for the Foundation Stage

The Education (National Curriculum) (Foundation Stage Early Learning Goals) (England) Order 2003 (Statutory Instrument 2003 No.391) provides for curriculum provision and assessment of the education of children within the Foundation Stage.

Children in England begin formal education at a much earlier age than in most other European countries. There is no compulsion for children to attend pre-school in England; the statutory school starting age remains the term following the child's fifth birthday, but social and political factors have significantly extended part-time education to the under-fives.

The Foundation Stage was introduced as a distinct phase of education for children aged 3- to 5-years-of-age in September 2000; however, within two years this phase was incorporated within the National Curriculum (Education Act, 2002). In effect, this formalised a curriculum structure for children of 3 and 4 years of age. The legal definition of 'foundation stage setting' means a maintained school, a maintained nursery school or establishment where nursery education is provided under the arrangements mentioned in section 77(2)(b) of the Act at which the Foundation Stage is taught.

Guidance for the Foundation Stage is the key document to be used by all practitioners who work with children in the Foundation Stage to plan their teaching and thus the learning experiences offered to children. The range of life experience, ability and understanding is probably more diverse with this age group of children than with any other in the educational system. This guidance is intended to help practitioners to plan to meet these diverse needs.

> **Activity 3** **Curriculum Guidance for the Foundation Stage**

Think about the *Curriculum Guidance for the Foundation Stage* and make notes on the following. You may need to read around this issue and talk to colleagues or your mentor to clarify your ideas:

1 What are the underlying principles of the Guidance?
2 How are these different to principles underpinning practice prior to the Guidance coming into force?
3 Where did these principles come from and who or what influenced their development?

Interpreting the Guidance document

In order to ensure clarity in interpretation of the Guidance, special emphasis is placed on the rationale for the government's aims for the Foundation Stage, their interpretation of principles for early years education and the approved approach to learning and teaching within documentation for the Foundation Stage.

The use of the term 'guidance' is interesting, as it would appear to imply that there is an element of choice in its use. There is ambivalence in the intent and to some degree the purposes of this terminology. Children of 3-

to 5-years old **may** attend educational settings for the purpose of educational experience if their parents or carers so wish. The range of educational experiences on offer is broad and ranges from private early years settings, which receive no government funding and, therefore, devise and regulate their own curriculum to other settings, which are required to follow a nationally prescribed curriculum that is inspected and tested in order to receive government funding. Funded providers include:

- ⊃ childminders
- ⊃ pre-schools in the voluntary , the private and the independent sector
- ⊃ maintained (state) or voluntary-aided (often church sponsored) nursery schools
- ⊃ nursery classes attached to primary, first or infant schools.

Nursery or kindergarten provision may also be funded by the government for early years settings affiliated to international educational bodies such as Montessori or Waldorf/Steiner (see Chapter 1), although some may maintain their independence through self-funded provision.

It is clear that the type of early years setting will present challenges for the provision of all of these areas. The differences in Ofsted inspection reflects this variety: one-day inspections of voluntary and private provision and more lengthy inspections of nursery schools in the maintained sector. There are concerns of equity in terms of comparability of quality of provision and the initial and ongoing training of practitioners.

Managers of private and voluntary settings as well as head teachers are required to ensure that curriculum guidance is used within their settings. It is clear that the government aims to ensure that all managers take responsibility for effective delivery. The practice of total delegation by managers to those having 'front line' delivery responsibility for implementation of the Guidance is no longer regarded as acceptable. This may be seen as a policy strategy that aims to ensure that managers have an active interest and involvement in the delivery of the curriculum.

Practitioners who receive government funding for provision of educational experience for 3- to 5-year-olds are required to plan and provide a curriculum that is based on the six areas of learning in the Foundation Stage Curriculum.

Six areas of learning

The six areas of learning are seen as a bridge between informal learning in the home and the more formal structure of the curriculum in Key Stage 1.

The expectation that most children will achieve and some, where appropriate, will go beyond the early learning goals by the end of the Foundation Stage indicates that the writers of the curriculum believe that the levels are appropriately pitched. Emphasis on achievement of basic skills is clearly presented within planning guidance.

The six areas of learning, which now have the status of being statutory, are closely related to the areas of the National Curriculum for Key Stage 1. The *Early Learning Goals,* which provide summative assessment for these areas of learning, provide expectations of testable attainment for children at the end of the Foundation Stage. Each area of learning has a set of related early learning goals; however, it is in the 'Stepping stones', exemplar materials and vignettes, that the practitioner is supported in his or her understanding of the means through which the knowledge, skills, understanding and attitudes that children need may be achieved. Curriculum guidance for the Foundation Stage is intended to help practitioners plan to meet the diverse needs of all children so that most will achieve and some, where appropriate, will go beyond the early learning goals by the end of the Foundation Stage. The guidance gives 'examples of what children do', which help practitioners to identify significant developments and plan the next steps in children's learning. It also gives examples of what the practitioner needs to do to support and consolidate learning and help children make progress towards the early learning goals.

See Figure 11.8 for an illustration of the links between National Curriculum subjects and areas of learning (the sixth area being personal, social and emotional development).

National Curriculum Subjects	Areas of Learning
Mathematics	Mathematical development
English	Communication, language and literacy
Art	Creative development
Physical Education	Physical development
Information Technology	Knowledge and understanding of the world
Science	Knowledge and understanding of the world
Design and Technology	Knowledge and understanding of the world
Geography	Knowledge and understanding of the world
Music	Creative development
History	Knowledge and understanding of the world

Figure 11.8
Links between National Curriculum subjects and areas of learning

The Qualification and Curriculum Authority

The Qualification and Curriculum Authority (QCA) was established under section 21 of the Education Act 1977. This body has produced much of the documentation that has supported the development of the National Curriculum. More recently, the QCA has extended its range of involvement in early years education and has produced the two key curriculum guidance documents for the Foundation Stage: Curriculum Guidance for the Foundation Stage (2000) and Planning for Learning in the Foundation Stage (2001).

The QCA has a tradition of consultation with practitioners and has drawn on the expertise of professionals in the development of curriculum content and materials. The involvement of representatives of relevant groups of practitioner stakeholders and professionals in early years education has been largely in the design of the curriculum and in materials used for its delivery. This attempt to develop partnership between curriculum designers and professionals in the field has had some success. It may be argued that full representation of the range of views relating to a curriculum area or educational issue is not possible when organising a writing group. This pragmatic view does lend itself to focused and rapid production of materials. It does not, however, guarantee clarity and precision in the content and organisation of areas of learning. The numerous revisions of the National Curriculum lend weight to this statement. Development in the legislative arena of education must be recognised as an essential aspect of the search for quality. Political intervention is largely focused on the achievement of quality.

The usefulness of the curriculum guidance materials, which supported the National Curriculum in its earlier versions, has been recognised and the model has been incorporated in the design of the Foundation Stage Handbook. The link between familiar early childhood theory, which has formed a part of teacher training for many years, and a loosely structured curriculum syllabus approaches has been received with cautious optimism by many practitioners in early years settings.

Planning for Learning in the Foundation Stage

It is intended that *Planning for Learning in the Foundation Stage* (PLFS) (DfES/QCA, 2001) should be read alongside *Curriculum Guidance for the Foundation Stage* (DFEE/QCA, 2000). It has been developed to provide a framework for planning, which will meet the legislative requirements. Some Foundation Stage practitioners, for example those in the maintained sector in the Pre-School Learning Alliance and in Montessori nurseries, have had a great deal of experience in planning in their training as well as in practice. For others, this may be a new and challenging aspect of their work. Some early years settings will follow a particular philosophical tradition such as Montessori or Steiner or an approach to learning such as High Scope. PLFS acknowledges that different early years settings may require a different focus in the way that learning experiences are planned.

In order to provide ready evidence for the Ofsted inspection process it is highly likely that established forms of planning used by practitioners may be modified to conform to the format outlined in the PLFS.

Differences such as number and age of the children and the number of staff are also recognised as influential in determining forms of planning.

There is an attempt in the PLFS to provide guidance on long-term and short-term planning which will encourage development of current practice in a range of settings.

Support in planning is given to voluntary and private sector pre-school settings by peripatetic qualified teachers. This goes some way towards helping those who are less experienced at formal planning. For those with more experience, it will help when reviewing their plans. The implementation of the Foundation Stage curriculum has gone a long way in changing expectations and practice in the non-maintained sector and nowhere more so than in approaches to planning. Planning which acknowledges the length of time spent by a child in a setting is particularly important for private and voluntary sector pre-schools and this has been recognised within the document.

> **Activity 4** **Planning**

Make notes on the following issues. You may need to consult colleagues or your mentor to clarify your ideas:

1 What is the underlying purpose of *Planning for Learning in the Foundation Stage*?
2 Where did the need for a definitive approach to planning come from and what influenced its format?
3 Talk to colleagues or your mentor to identify how the introduction of *Planning for Learning in the Foundation Stage* has enhanced or changed practice in your setting.

The education of children of 3 and 4 years of age in formal settings remains a contentious issue; nevertheless, for these children a National Curriculum provides a uniform range of curriculum content and a cohesive approach to early learning.

Promotional materials provided by the British Council indicate that in the United Kingdom:

> *pre-school education is available (often on a fee-paying basis) for children aged two to four/five through playgroups and nursery schools. The emphasis is on group work, creative activity and guided play. Compulsory education begins at five in England, Wales and Scotland and four in Northern Ireland. There is little or no specialist subject teaching and great emphasis on literacy and numeracy in early years.*

This statement belies the complexity of provision and the efforts of central government to encourage a consistent and uniform approach to planning educational experiences for pre-school children.

In the past the experience of some children of nursery age in Reception classes has not been appropriately pitched to their needs and their age. This was due to a number of factors, including a shortage of trained early years teachers and pressure exerted within schools for children to prepare for progression to the National Curriculum. The inclusion of the Reception year within the Foundation Stage has clear implications for the training of teachers and other practitioners working in early years settings.

Training is seen by the government as a vital element for success in the delivery of the Foundation Stage. Note is made that those who support and train practitioners have a crucial role to play in the success of this new curriculum for early years. On initial training courses for teachers and other early years professionals, and in-service courses for practitioners, clear guidance must be provided.

Foundation Stage Assessment

The Education (National Curriculum) (Foundation Stage Profile Assessment Arrangements) (England) Order 2003 (Statutory Instrument 2003 No.1327) provides a national assessment scheme for the Foundation Stage. Introduced into schools and settings in 2002–3 to provide a single national assessment system for the Foundation Stage, the Foundation Stage Profile replaced a variety of baseline assessment schemes, which were being used throughout England.

This Order applies to maintained schools, maintained nursery schools and early years settings and people providing funded nursery education under the arrangements mentioned in section 77(2)(b) of the Education Act 2002. The Foundation Stage Profile Handbook describes in great detail how assessment will be conducted.

The Profile has 13 summary scales covering the six areas of learning. These must be completed for each child receiving government-funded education by the end of his or her time in the Foundation Stage.

This formal assessment of children is completed for children in the final term of the Foundation Stage, the Reception Year and not later than 4th July falling in that term if earlier. If it cannot be completed within this period, the legal requirement is that it shall be completed as soon as is practicable following completion of the Foundation Stage.

Purpose of the assessment

The purpose of the assessment is to determine the level of attainment achieved by the child in each of the areas of learning and the early learning goals. It also functions as a means of recording this attainment through the use of attainment scales and the completion of a Foundation Stage Profile of the child.

The Explanatory Notes in the Foundation Stage Profile indicate the following:	
The age of the children who will be tested	Children who are in the final year of the Foundation Stage
The settings in which children will be tested	Maintained schools, maintained nursery schools and non-maintained nursery education settings, funded by a local education authority
The areas which will be tested	Each of the areas of study for which early learning goals have been specified (pursuant to an Order made under section 87(2)(a) of the Education Act 2002)
When the assessment will be used	Both throughout the final year and when the profile will be completed in the final term of the Foundation Stage
The form the assessment will take	A record of attainment based on progress against the prescribed assessment scales that relate to each of the early learning goals
Who will undertake the assessment	'Practitioners and others' who are responsible for conducting Foundation Stage profiles…*
The criteria for assessment	Confirmation that the Foundation Stage Profile Handbook will be used
External verification	The role of the LEA (local education authorities) in monitoring the way in which the assessments and Foundation Stage Profiles are being conducted by teachers to ensure consistency and proper implementation of the statutory provisions. (It should be noted that there is some inconsistency in who assesses the children – practitioners and others/teachers (see * above)
The Order also requires details of the results of the foundation stage profile assessments and related information set out in the Schedule to the Order to be provided	To: ⊃ Parents ⊃ the local education authority and by the local education authority to the Secretary of State at the end of each school year

Figure 11.9
Explanatory Notes in the Foundation Stage Profile

The Foundation Stage Profile assesses children in each of the six areas of learning in the Foundation Stage curriculum. It encourages teachers to use focused observation as a means of recording children's achievements throughout the year. These observations lead to a summative record of children's achievements at the end of the Reception year. The requirement is to conduct the assessment at the end of the Foundation Stage with an added rider that this is usually the end of the Reception year.

Implementation of testing in educational contexts, in the SATs (now STAs) and in teacher assessment has shown that interpretation of levels may vary between teachers. Processes for ensuring consistency will include agreement trialling meetings of those assessing chidren's work to view work and agree on judgements and moderation. These methods have been shown to be useful in ensuring consistency in the assessment of children's work at Key Stage 1.

Orders often include Explanatory Notes, which, although they are not part of the regulations, provide further detail, for example in the expectations for implementation. It is often this form of guidance that influences and forms practice.

Figure 11.9 clearly indicates the cycle of assessment and the lines of reporting that are required by law.

Foundation Stage Profile training

Allocation of additional funding to a project is always a key indicator of the relative importance of a legislative strategy. The importance attached to training for practitioners in the use of this assessment method is indicated by the funding allocated to support both training and supply cover. All funding allocated for baseline assessment has now been transferred to Foundation Stage Profile training In addition, arranged LEA training can be supplemented by the Foundation Stage Fund and the Early years Training Grant if agreed as part of a Local Authority/Early years Development Childcare Partnership implementation plan.

The 'e'-Profile

Emphasis on the use of ICT within schools and educational settings has been further strengthened by the introduction of the 'e-Profile'. This electronic version of the Foundation Stage Profile is available to schools that wish to link it to any existing electronic system they use for assessment records – or it may be used as a means of introducing electronic record keeping. The message is clear; it is expected that electronic recording will be introduced. A uniform system of recording will facilitate the provision of data for LEAs, which, in turn, are required to provide this information for wider publication.

It is intended that all children who attend a Foundation Stage Setting should have access to the Foundation Stage Profile, in order to ensure equity of access for children with special educational needs.

1 Consider how a child with special needs will access the Foundation Stage Profile.

2 How are Foundation Stage Profile Scales cross-referenced to the P-scales?

It would be useful to consult the summary of the findings of the second pre-test for the Foundation Stage Profile (produced by the National Foundation for Educational Research and Birmingham City Education Service, September 2002), which is accessible through the DfES website, details of which are given at the end of the chapter.

Implications of collaboration

There are major issues for collaboration between private and voluntary sector settings and the maintained sector, which have not yet been fully addressed. In Section 4 of the Foundation Stage Profile acknowledgement is given to the part played by previous practitioners. There may be substantial variation and difference in available material depending upon the experience a child has before entry to the Reception year. For some children, the Foundation Stage Profile may rest entirely on judgements made by staff within the maintained school setting; for others, it will be enriched by comment from nursery school, pre-school or comments from parents who have been active in their child's education, where no pre-school experience was available for their child.

The purpose of the Foundation Stage Profile may thus be questioned. Is this a record of the development of a child during the whole Foundation Stage or a record of achievement and attainment during the final year of the Foundation Stage?

Moderation of work undertaken by children during the Reception year goes some way towards standardising assessment practice. This is built on extensive work over the years in Key Stage 1 assessment procedures within schools and between schools through LEA support.

The 'responsible person'

Staff in early years settings work as teams, but within the team individuals have responsibility for different and distinct tasks. (This is considered in more detail in Chapter 2, The Reflective Practitioner.)

Legislation for the Foundation Stage Profile distinguishes one 'responsible person' within the early years setting who, as the title suggests, will be responsible for a number of key implementation and reporting tasks. The responsible person will usually be the head teacher in a maintained school or maintained nursery school. The responsible person within a funded setting will usually be the person who has managerial responsibility for the provision (section 77(2)(b) of the Act).

Duties

Within the early years setting the 'the responsible person' will:

- ⊃ make arrangements for each child to be assessed throughout the year by a practitioner in relation to each of the areas of learning and early learning goals
- ⊃ enable a Foundation Stage Profile and a record of attainment to be completed in the final term of the Foundation Stage
- ⊃ be responsible for ensuring that conduct for the assessment of children is completed in relation to the Foundation Stage Profile. The document is very clear on procedures for assessment and these should be followed
- ⊃ be responsible for providing information to the parent of a child
- ⊃ arrange for provision of information to the LEA
- ⊃ provide information to a child's new school if the child moves to a new school during the final year of the Foundation Stage.

The directions contained within legislation for 'responsible people' are clear. They are instructions for managers, which will ensure that staff are available for formative, ongoing assessment, summative assessment in the final term of the Foundation Stage and that assessment procedures will follow those stated in the Foundation Stage Profile. They are also required to ensure good lines of communication with the LEA, with parents and with schools to which children transfer during the final year of the Foundation Stage.

Those practitioners who are responsible for the completion of assessment for and completion of Foundation Stage profiles are also required to follow the directions applied to the profile in terms of their conduct.

The legal requirements for practitioners and governing bodies are translated into practical terms within the Foundation Stage Profile (DfES/QCA 2003:123–124). The governing body of a maintained school or maintained nursery school has responsibility for ensuring that the Foundation Stage Profile is completed for each child.

Monitoring of assessment arrangements

Within the Act there is clear indication of the responsibilities of the Local Education Authority (LEA) relating to moderation and for reporting. They are required to make provision for monitoring of the assessment process in all Foundation Stage settings maintained or funded by the LEA at which, in any school year, Foundation Stage Profile assessments are administered to children. Settings must liaise with the LEA to support the implementation of assessment in a number of ways:

- ➲ allow entry to the relevant Foundation Stage setting at all reasonable times in order to observe the implementation of the arrangements for the completion of Foundation Stage Profiles
- ➲ permit the LEA (monitoring authority) to inspect and take copies of documents and other articles relating to those Foundation Stage Profiles and assessments
- ➲ provide to the LEA (the monitoring authority) such information relating to such Foundation Stage Profile and assessment as they may reasonably request.

Provision of information

The Act implies the necessity for good communication at many levels (see Figure 11.10).

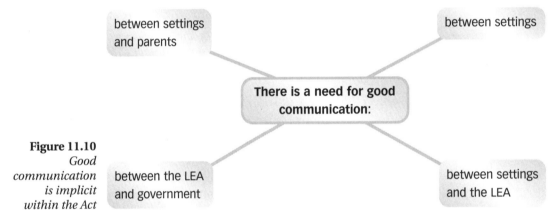

between settings and parents

between settings

There is a need for good communication:

between the LEA and government

between settings and the LEA

Figure 11.10
Good communication is implicit within the Act

> ## Activity 6) Communication

Liaison between settings and the Reception class staff is crucial but may not be easily achieved.

1 What do you see as the key difficulties?
   (Cost; supply cover for private and voluntary providers; differing priorities?)
2 What measures could be taken to improve communication?

Regulation

Ofsted (Office for Standards in Education) has a duty to enforce and monitor legislation; it is the key regulatory body for early years provision in care and education in England. Ofsted's function in relation to education is widely known. Its role in relation to the regulation of care may be less familiar.

The five main regulatory functions in relation to childcare, which Ofsted provides, are shown in Figure 11.11.

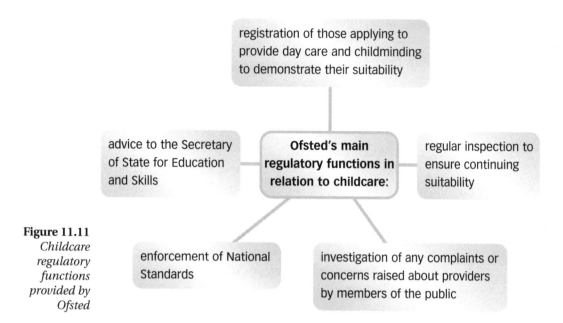

Figure 11.11
Childcare regulatory functions provided by Ofsted

registration of those applying to provide day care and childminding to demonstrate their suitability

advice to the Secretary of State for Education and Skills

Ofsted's main regulatory functions in relation to childcare:

regular inspection to ensure continuing suitability

enforcement of National Standards

investigation of any complaints or concerns raised about providers by members of the public

Ofsted's aims are to ensure that all children are safe and well cared for, and that they take part in activities that will help them to learn and develop.

Great strides have been made in the last 10 years to provide access to high quality educational experience for all 3- and 4-year-olds. An integral strategy used by successive governments has been to use inspection as a means of ensuring consistency of quality between different types of provision and thus greater equity of experience for children in pre-five settings. Variety in the expectations of the delivery of the curriculum by different providers is a key issue for equity of experience for children and one that cannot be easily resolved. Questions of equity and comparability of provision, which may be posed by parents and other stakeholders and for which the government are seeking answers, may relate to issues as diverse as how a childminder can provide a rich and 'suitable' curriculum for 4 year olds, which compares with the curriculum offered in a maintained nursery school? How, for example, can a pre-school, organised by the Pre-School Learning Alliance, provide the breadth of experience for children that is offered in a Montessori nursery?

Such real and live issues as these are of great importance in an education system that has such diversity of provision. One answer is that that comparison should not be made between early years settings, as they offer very different experiences.

The richness of experience may relate to a number of factors. Examples include:

⊃ adult-child ratio within a setting
⊃ the training and commitment of the practitioners to a particular philosophical approach to working with children
⊃ flexibility of approach
⊃ structured and supported learning.

Inspection of early years settings will provide evidence of the ways in which response is made to particular conditions which contextualise learning.

Reading and critically reviewing Ofsted inspection reports on its website reveals the differences in provision for children's education throughout the country and the responses made by inspectors to these differences.

Consideration must be given to the experience and training of those making judgements, the Ofsted inspectors. Selection and training of inspectors is an area that continues to require scrutiny.

Ofsted also draws on the expertise of those with specific experience and knowledge. The inspection of care provision requires distinct and different skills, qualifications and experience from that of education. The dual role, inspecting care and education, places Ofsted in a vulnerable position for a number of reasons:

- ⊃ matching the initial training qualifications of inspectors to inspection responsibilities
- ⊃ ensuring relevance of the professional work place experience of its inspectors to the settings they inspect
- ⊃ maintaining current understanding of working practice with children.

Activity 7) Diversity issues

Using the Ofsted website, access two reports of early years provision. It is useful to compare reports of different types of setting.

1 Scrutinise and evaluate the comments made on particular areas of learning.
2 Look at comments and responses to provision for cultural diversity in settings with few and many children from minority ethnic backgrounds. Reflect upon your findings.
3 Compare full school inspections with those one-day inspections undertaken in some Foundation Stage settings. Consider any comment about children with special educational needs.

An awareness of the context in which an issue occurs may help a practitioner to make informed comment in response to questions raised during Ofsted inspection. Often practitioners are aware of the response made by their own early years setting and not that of the wider issue. Reading Ofsted reports provides a broader contextualisation of an issue.

Regulation for educare provision is complex

Educare provision for children under 8 years of age is complex and there is wide variety in the types of setting that provide for care and education.

There are at least eight different pieces of legislation, which currently relate to such settings; these include:

- ⊃ the Children Act (1989)
- ⊃ the School Standards and Framework Act (1998)
- ⊃ the Tax Credits Act (2002).

The difficulties that arise from such complexity of regulation and bodies to which they are reported has been indicated in relation to the case of Victoria Climbie. Fisher (2002:27) draws our attention to the variety of children's educare experiences through description of a 3 year old going from home in the morning to a childminder, from the childminder to half-day nursery provision, then to playgroup, back to the childminder and then to home. This disjointed experience is not unusual for many children and it is easy to see how lack of coordination, or an absence of shared information, may lead to a poor quality of experience for children as well as the obvious inherent dangers for vulnerable children.

Care and education services do not fit easily into existing frameworks or categories and a range of issues arises from this complexity of regulation. Ofsted have addressed this by developing models for combined inspections under different Acts. In practice this is difficult. Progress on these attempts may be viewed on the Ofsted website as shown in *Early Years- the first national picture* (Ofsted, 2003).

Special Educational Needs Code of Practice

The SEN Code of Practice aims to support schools and Local Education Authorities in interpreting those aspects of the1996 Education Act, the 2001 Special Educational Needs and Disability Act and Regulations arising from these Acts, which relate to the support of children with special educational needs.

The Code of Practice was introduced in 1994. Guidance on implementation was provided at its introduction and this has been further strengthened with training for practitioners and by web-based resources. Revisions were made to this document in 2001, which came into force in January 2002. These revisions have been informed by a number of research projects and papers undertaken by Ofsted: OFSTED (1996), 'The Implementation of the Code of Practice for Pupils with Special Educational Needs', OFSTED (1997), 'The SEN Code of Practice: two years on' and OFSTED (1999), 'The SEN Code of Practice: three years on'. In these surveys the voice of practitioners is evident and this is reflected in the revisions introduced in 2001.

The Special Educational Needs Code of Practice 2001 provides guidance for educational settings, schools and local educational authorities (LEAs). The Code does not have the force of law, but it is a requirement that 'notice' must be taken. Figure 11.12 illustrates what the SEN Code of Practice covers.

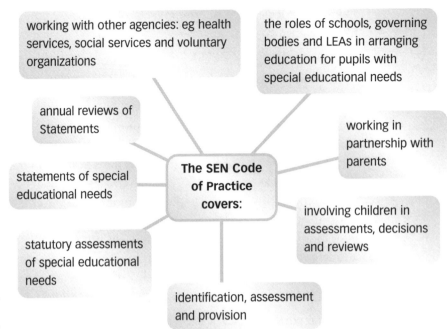

Figure 11.12
The SEN Code of Practice: an outline

working with other agencies: eg health services, social services and voluntary organizations

the roles of schools, governing bodies and LEAs in arranging education for pupils with special educational needs

annual reviews of Statements

working in partnership with parents

statements of special educational needs

The SEN Code of Practice covers:

involving children in assessments, decisions and reviews

statutory assessments of special educational needs

identification, assessment and provision

The underpinning principles of the SEN Code of Practice are given in Figure 11.13.

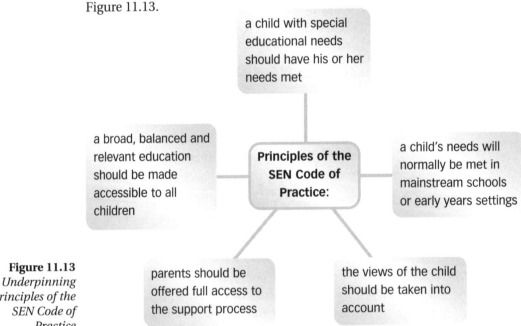

Figure 11.13
Underpinning principles of the SEN Code of Practice

a child with special educational needs should have his or her needs met

a broad, balanced and relevant education should be made accessible to all children

Principles of the SEN Code of Practice:

a child's needs will normally be met in mainstream schools or early years settings

parents should be offered full access to the support process

the views of the child should be taken into account

Activity 8) Parent partnership service

Local education authorities now have to provide information and advice to all parents of children with special educational needs. This information and advice is available through the Parent Partnership Service. Contact your local PPS to find what types of support are offered.

The Schools Admissions Code of Practice (2002) and the Code of Practice (Schools), which covers the disability discrimination aspects of the new Special Educational Needs and Disability Act are available on the Department for Education and Skills website.

Birth to Three Matters

The rapid expansion in childcare within the last few years has provided many challenges for providers of out-of-home care for young children. The introduction of formal, accountable education for children of 3 years of age through the introduction of a 'Foundation Stage', a nationally prescribed curriculum, opened the door for a more rigorous approach to childcare and education for very young children. It may, therefore, be seen as a logical progression to introduce a framework for all those who work with and care for children from birth to age 3 years. The Framework is set within the context of the *National Standards for Under Eights Day Care and Childminding* (DfES, 2001) and provides a link to the *Curriculum Guidance for the Foundation Stage* (DfES/QCA, 2000).

The Framework *Birth to Three Matters* is intended for use with all children, including those with a special educational need or disability. It is, therefore, an 'entitlement curriculum', a range of educational experience to which special needs children have as much right as other children. The justification and rationale for the introduction of this Framework appears to be located in a desire to acknowledge the importance of children's earliest experiences in relation to their subsequent development. The intention of the Framework is that it should be used flexibly. It is hard to see how it could be used otherwise if it is intended to respond to children's needs. There is a strong emphasis on readiness to learn, preparedness for school and avoidance of underachievement. Providing what to all intent and purpose is a national curriculum for children from birth to age 3 years in out-of-home settings may be regarded as contentious and, in its defence, the government stresses that the document was developed with experienced practitioners. There is no doubt that the document is well intentioned and the aim to improve, refine and enhance children's opportunities for developmentally appropriate provision is laudable.

The main users will be practitioners working with babies and children from birth to age 3 years in out-of-home settings individually and in groups, and their priority will be the well being of children in their care.

A milestone in government intervention in child care

A Framework to support practitioners working with children from birth to age 3 years is a milestone in government intervention in the area of child care. The Framework aims to provide support for the wide range of practitioners who have responsibility for the care and education of babies and children from birth to age 3 years. Recognising and valuing the role of practitioners in this area of educare is closely linked to an acknowledgement of the abilities of babies and children from birth to age 3 years. There are two strands that run through the document: the aim to raise the professional esteem of practitioners in this area, closely linked to encouraging the recognition of the developmental needs of the individual child.

The Framework recognises the importance of professional practice and in order to extend and enhance practice the document provides examples of appropriate practice. Case studies are used to illustrate the sixteen Components in practice. Ideas to support organisation and planning and resourcing are provided. Professional practice is also encouraged in special needs, equal opportunities and in strengthening relationships with parents.

Reflection on practice is encouraged throughout the Framework, as is the realisation that this may present a challenge for some practitioners. It is acknowledged that working with children of this age presents a challenge and often there may be no ready answers. A section within the Framework poses questions and presents some answers to a range of problems that practitioners may encounter. The principles that permeate the Framework are shown in Figure 11.14.

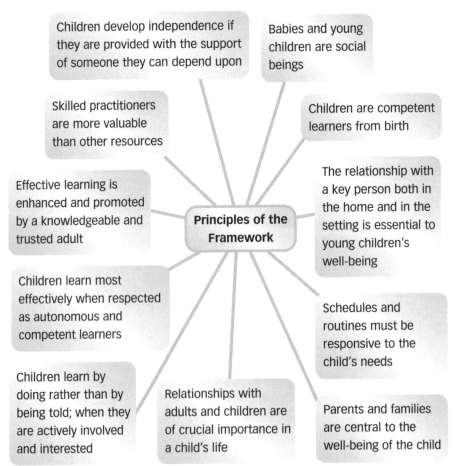

Children develop independence if they are provided with the support of someone they can depend upon

Babies and young children are social beings

Skilled practitioners are more valuable than other resources

Children are competent learners from birth

Effective learning is enhanced and promoted by a knowledgeable and trusted adult

Principles of the Framework

The relationship with a key person both in the home and in the setting is essential to young children's well-being

Children learn most effectively when respected as autonomous and competent learners

Schedules and routines must be responsive to the child's needs

Children learn by doing rather than by being told; when they are actively involved and interested

Relationships with adults and children are of crucial importance in a child's life

Parents and families are central to the well-being of the child

Figure 11.14
The Framework for supporting practitioners

Practitioners are encouraged to recognise the central role that they play in the place of a child's development, that learning is encouraged through interaction with people and supported exploration of the world around them. Recognition of the 'holistic' nature of development and learning and an awareness of their individuality and capabilities is central to the purpose of *Birth to Three Matters*.

For some children, development may be delayed or inhibited in particular areas. These areas are shown in Figure 11.15.

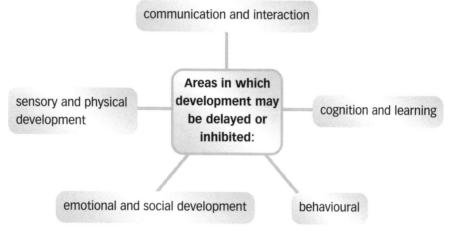

Figure 11.15 *Childhood development: areas that may be delayed or inhibited*

The Four 'Aspects' and their Components

The learning experiences are presented as separate Aspects and Components. The four Aspects are:

- ⊃ a strong child
- ⊃ a skilful communicator
- ⊃ a competent learner
- ⊃ a healthy child

Each Aspect is divided into four Components, as shown in Figure 11.16. Practitioners are required to recognise that learning experiences will cross over these areas and that there will be a need to consider all aspects in order to plan effectively.

Conclusion

The role of policy and legislation is significant in determining the type and range of services available for children and their families at any particular time, within the cultural context. Practitioners need to be aware not only of the provisions within current legislation shaping their roles and responsibilities, but also of the principles that underpin that legislation and give it a meaningful context. These principles are not static but subject to development through complex processes influenced by a wide range of

A Strong Child	
Me, myself and I	⊃ encouragement of self awareness, and awareness of capabilities ⊃ emotional safety, trust and a positive self image
Being acknowledged and affirmed	⊃ response to positive affirmation ⊃ promoting confidence
Self-assurance	⊃ developing self confidence within the context of supportive relationships
A sense of belonging	⊃ promotion of security in order to support learning
A Skilful Communicator	
Being together	⊃ development of social relations ⊃ friendship ⊃ empathy ⊃ sharing emotions and experiences ⊃ becoming a competent language user
Finding a voice	⊃ promoting confidence ⊃ extend their range and increase their skills ⊃ making sense of sounds around is understanding 'conversation'
Listening and responding	⊃ encouraging appropriate listening and response ⊃ understanding the importance of paying attention to sounds and language ⊃ interpreting non-verbal signals ⊃ imitating, repeating and mirroring others
Making meaning	⊃ developing an awareness of the conventions of communication
A Competent Learner	
Making connections	⊃ discriminating and making connections between different objects and experiences
Being Imaginative	⊃ sensory stimulation ⊃ role play ⊃ imaginative play ⊃ pretend play
Being creative	⊃ encouraging imagination ⊃ exploration ⊃ discovery ⊃ experimentation ⊃ using sound, media and movement

Representing	⊃ giving time and encouragement to share their thoughts, feelings, understandings ⊃ encouraging the use of drawings and words to 'represent' ⊃ using movement, music and dance ⊃ imaginative play
A Healthy Child	
Emotional well-being	⊃ developing relationships ⊃ expressing feelings ⊃ developing strategies to cope with new, challenging or stressful situations
Growing and developing	⊃ emphasis on the importance of health and its relationship to the ability to respond to learning ⊃ confidence in asking for help when needed
Keeping safe	⊃ being protected ⊃ becoming confident and skilful in a range of movement ⊃ large and fine motor control

Figure 11.16
The Four 'Aspects' of the learning experience and their Components

factors including political objectives, lessons from practice and research, and the dominant cultural norms. Stakeholders within the early years are part of these influences and play a role in shaping policy and practice. Practitioners in early years settings need to be aware of developments that may lead to changes in policy and legislation and the ways in which policy and legislation shape services and determine their objectives.

Legislation, therefore, needs to be considered within the cultural and policy context and not as an isolated phenomenon. It is not unusual, for example, for problems to be identified in legislation when it is put into operation. Often issues and difficulties that may not have been foreseen emerge in the light of practice. This has occurred in education legislation as well as in child protection. Practitioners in early years settings are required to work within the current policy and legislative framework, but this requirement should be fulfilled alongside a critical appraisal of that framework and an understanding of the processes by which it may be changed.

References and further reading

The Children Act 1989

DfEE (1994), 'Code of Practice. On the Identification and Assessment of Special Educational Needs'. London: HMSO

DEE (1999), 'National Curriculum for English'. London: HMSO

DfEE/QCA (2000), 'Curriculum Guidance for the Foundation Stage'. London: HMSO

DfES/QCA (2001), 'Planning for Learning in the Foundation Stage'. London: HMSO

DfES/QCA (2003), 'Foundation Stage Profile'. London: HMSO

DHSS (1984), 'Children in Care'. London: HMSO

DHSS (1987), 'The Law on Child Care and Family Services'. London: HMSO

DoH (1999), 'Working Together to Safeguard Children'. London: HMSO

DoH (2000), 'Framework for Assessment of Children in Need and their Families'. London: HMSO

DoH (2001), 'The Children Act Now: Messages from Research'. London: HMSO

DoH (2003), 'Every Child Matters'. London: HMSO

DoH (2003), 'The Victoria Climbie Inquiry: Report on an Inquiry by Lord Laming'. London: HMSO

'Early Years – the first national picture' (Ofsted 2003).

Education (National Curriculum) (Foundation Stage Profile Assessment Arrangements) (England) Order 2003 (Statutory Instrument 2003 No.1327).

Education (National Curriculum) (Foundation Stage Early Learning Goals) (England) Order 2003 (Statutory Instrument 2003 No.391)

Education Act (1988)

Feldman, L. and Mitchels, B. (1990), *The Children Act – A Practical Guide.* London: Longman

Herbert, M (1993), *Working with Children and the Children Act.* Leicester: BPS Books

Mallinson, I. (1992), *The Children Act – A Social Care Guide.* London: Whiting and Birch Ltd

National Curriculum for England and Wales (1988)

OFSTED (1995), *Handbook for Inspecting Primary and Nursery Schools.* London: HMSO

School Standards and Framework Act (1998)

Tax Credits Act (2002)

Websites

www.britishcouncil.org.uk/education/system/se/sestruc.htm
British Council

www.dfes.gov.uk
DfES Department for Education and Skills website

www.doh.gov.uk
DoH Department of Health

www.ofsted.gov.uk
Ofsted

www.learning.wales.gov.uk
Wales: National Assembly Training and Education Department (NATED)

www.nc.uk.net
National Curriculum in England

www.accac.org.uk
National Curriculum in Wales

www.nspcc.org.uk/html/home/newsandcampaigns/responsetogreenpape
rfull.htm
NSPCC 'The Green Paper; Every Child Matters – the NSPCC's Initial
Response'

The Scottish Executive Education Department
www.ltscotland.com/curriculum

Curriculum Guidance Scotland
www.scotland.gov.uk

Scottish Executive Education Department (SEED)
issues guidance which provides broad detail for the curriculum areas.
www.ltscotland.com/curriculum

Northern Ireland Council for Curriculum, Examinations and Assessment.
www.ccea.org.uk
As with all national curricula the Northern Ireland Curriculum has also
been subject to change and as can be seen from their website aims to
provide an approach to teaching and learning which builds on local
traditions, needs and aspirations.

www.deni.gov.uk
The curriculum in Northern Ireland is the responsibility of the Northern
Ireland Council for Curriculum, Examinations and Assessment. Northern
Ireland within the Department of Education in Northern Ireland (DENI)

Critical issues in early years care and education

12

Janet Kay and Iain MacLeod-Brudenell

The aim of this chapter is to encourage your awareness of topical and critical issues that affect practice in early years care and education. As a practitioner working with young children, you will have responsibility for their well-being, their care and their education. Your understanding of the requirements of this role and the legal framework in which early years services operate does not exist within a vacuum. All aspects of childcare and early years education are influenced by the particular social and cultural context in which they take place. Early years care and education will also reflect changes within the social and cultural context, which occur as part of natural evolvement. The expectations placed on early years practitioners are not immovable – they are not 'set in stone'. They change with time and respond to events in the wider world and, more particularly, in the immediate social setting.

The term 'critical issues' is used to indicate areas of discussion that are topical and contested, are subject to debate, within the area of early childhood.

Critical issues are:

➲ live and contentious, and have an impact upon the quality of educational and care experience for young children and their families

➲ become the subject of debate because they are the source of tension between the values and expectations of different groups.

Occasionally a particular critical issue arises in response to an incident or event, which demonstrates a failing in the system to provide adequate and appropriate care or education for children. Other critical issues arise from ongoing debates about the principles and values underpinning approaches to care and education.

Recognising the existence of critical issues and determining what creates contentious debates in the early years field is crucial to your personal and professional development. Understanding the ways in which particular issues become topical and contested is part of your development towards becoming a reflective practitioner.

Critical issues are often contentious and there is often more than one viewpoint. In order to develop your understanding as a practitioner, you need to discuss these issues with colleagues, both in learning situations and in the workplace, to gain a range of viewpoints. Awareness of a number of views will enable you begin to consider the validity of the evidence you have to support your own opinions. Most references to literature within this chapter are not, as you may expect, to books and journals but to web-based resources and the media. This is because the relevant issues are critical and although you may wish to research the historical context of an issue, the key aspects of a critical issue are related to the current time.

This chapter is divided into two main sections, addressing:

1 The role of critical issues in the early years

2 Current critical issues in the early years

At the end of this chapter you should have knowledge and understanding of:

⊃ defining 'critical issues'

⊃ quality issues

⊃ stakeholders in critical issues

⊃ the role of government

⊃ reflective approaches

⊃ individual practice

⊃ practice in settings

⊃ values and perceptions

⊃ personal values

⊃ values in practice

⊃ provision and the regulation of settings

⊃ assessment

⊃ working with parents as partners

⊃ equity and equality

⊃ the role of teaching assistants

⊃ smacking

⊃ the Victoria Climbie case

⊃ The role of critical issues in early years practice

This section introduces you to the concept of critical issues and the importance for a reflective practitioner to engage with such debates.

Defining 'critical issues'

If this chapter had been written 10 years ago, the range of critical issues would have been different. The contents may have included such issues as the introduction of a standard curriculum for the under-fives; base line assessment; subject emphasis within the National Curriculum; funding of pre-school places for 4 year-olds; and the emerging emphasis upon skills in numeracy and literacy. These issues were very contentious at that time and in most cases they still have relevance today. They may be less topical because events have changed policy and practice in the area of early childhood education and care.

A change in emphasis

Some areas remain topical, but the emphasis has changed. Perhaps, for example, the value of a standardised curriculum for 3-and 4 year olds may still be debated, but now this would be from the standpoint of experience of delivery and inspection of this provision. Assessment of very young children may now be more acceptable than it was previously, but the critical question is whether the Foundation Stage Profile will be workable and effective in the measurement of achievement of children at the end of the Reception Year. The use of literacy and numeracy strategies remains an issue in the debate about breadth and balance within the National Curriculum. It may be argued that the time allocated to these strategies within the school day restricts opportunity for children's physical, emotional and creative development. There is less time for teaching other curriculum areas. On the other hand, the value of dedicated time for literacy and numeracy development has strong support from many quarters.

New areas of concern

It is clear then, that 'critical issues' change in emphasis over time, but often remain 'live', with new areas of concern, questions and debates to be considered in respect of any particular issue. Another example relates to the care of young children 'looked after' by local authorities. One of the key issues in the past was about permanence and the extent to which efforts should be made to rehabilitate children to their birth families before making decisions about a child's long-term care. This issue is still of great importance, but a more critical key issue in this field is the educational, health and welfare outcomes for children 'looked after' and the impact of failures to ensure these outcomes are positive on the child's long-term life chances. 'Critical issues' are those that impact on children, families and professionals within the field at a particular point in time.

The nature of critical issues is that they will change in both the priority given to them at different times and in different places and also in the emphasis placed upon them for political and economic purposes. For example, in recent years emphasis has been placed on reduction of class size for very young children in England. This may be viewed simply as an attempt to provide a better experience for children, but there are also political reasons for this action and associated financial costs.

Quality issues

At the heart of any discussions of critical issues is the debate about quality. Quality of experience and outcomes for children is the overriding issue and is central to all of the themes discussed in this chapter. However, notions of quality in early years care and education change over time, with developments in our understanding of children's needs and how best to meet them. In order to take part in debates about critical issues, practitioners need to have a concept of quality and how it can be achieved. One of the reasons why topics become 'issues' is because changes in views on quality in early years care and education alter our perceptions of existing services and practices. For example, the growing dissatisfaction with separate care and education services in the UK developed from perceptions that quality in early years services was very variable; there was lack of equity in provision for different children depending on family income and location, and the child's cultural background; ability and social class. In addition there was a confusion of different provision, which was fragmented and often failed to meet the real needs of children and their families.

Debate about integrating care and education

Therefore, the debate about how to better integrate care and education services began and culminated recently in proposals in the Green Paper *Every Child Matters* (DfES, 2003) to integrate social care and education services and draw all children's services together within Children's Trusts. Another debate that has recently resulted in a raft of policy developments and changes in practice is the outcomes for children in public care as described above. The Utting Report (1997) identified disastrous outcomes for children, who had been 'looked after', in terms of their education, qualifications, employment chances, criminality, drug and alcohol abuse and homelessness. New policies in the shape of 'Quality Protects' were introduced to improve the quality of health and education monitoring and services for children 'looked after' in response to Utting's recommendations.

Some of the key beliefs that currently dominate views of quality in early years services and practice are shown in Figure 12.1.

> **Activity 1** **Change in quality issues over time**

Beliefs about quality are not static and will develop over time. Look at the beliefs about quality issues identified in Figure 12.1 below and, with reference to your own childhood, try and make notes about two or three areas in which ideas about quality have changed. For example, relationships between early years practitioners and parents have changed dramatically in the authors' lifetime. 'Partnership with parents' has become a key element of good practice in care and education, whereas 20 or 30 years ago it was not recognised as significant in the same way.

Think about practices in your workplace and write down two or three areas in which you think that quality is not as evident as it should be. Why do you think this?

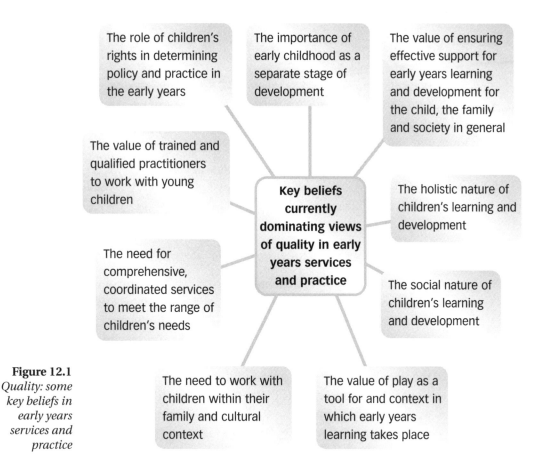

The role of children's rights in determining policy and practice in the early years

The importance of early childhood as a separate stage of development

The value of ensuring effective support for early years learning and development for the child, the family and society in general

The value of trained and qualified practitioners to work with young children

Key beliefs currently dominating views of quality in early years services and practice

The holistic nature of children's learning and development

The need for comprehensive, coordinated services to meet the range of children's needs

The social nature of children's learning and development

The need to work with children within their family and cultural context

The value of play as a tool for and context in which early years learning takes place

Figure 12.1
Quality: some key beliefs in early years services and practice

The concept of raising quality in early years care and education is inextricably bound up with beliefs about what quality entails. Developing an understanding of debates about what constitutes quality in early childhood is a crucial part of self-development towards becoming a reflective practitioner. Examination of critical issues encourages reflection on your own personal experiences and values. The quality of experience offered to children is often a direct result of the practitioner's awareness of these issues.

Stakeholders in critical issues

What do you understand by the term 'stakeholder'? It may be a term that is unfamiliar to you, but we are all in a sense stakeholders in the care and education of children; some, however, are more active and vociferous in our need to influence provision and delivery of these services. Stakeholders appear in all walks of life, for example, shareholders in the financial world and users of the health services. The role of the community as stakeholders in the local provision of education and care is self-evident. Faith and community groups may be the most obvious groups of people with a strong interest in shaping the educational experiences of children in a community. Businesses, emergency services and social services may be less obvious but are of equal importance.

> **Activity 2** **Stakeholders in the care and education of young children**

The structure of the education system in the UK has changed considerably over the recent years, reflecting successive governments' aims to improve quality, increase diversity and make institutions more accountable to students, parents, employers and taxpayers.

List all those people, agencies and organisations you consider to be stakeholders in the care and education of young children. Discuss your list with a colleague or mentor and ask if they have other ideas.

The influence of the media as stakeholders

In this chapter, you are encouraged to consider some of underlying factors that may influence your perceptions of a particular issue. For example, awareness of a critical issue may emerge within the workplace, but the way in which the issue is presented in the media may be at odds with your personal experience. The approach taken by different sections of the media may be expressing a standpoint, which some may consider biased. Contradictory viewpoints may be expressed within and through the media. The media are some of the stakeholders in education and care and, as such, may represent viewpoints of individual commentators, editors and different shades of political and public opinion. 'Stakeholder' is a term used to identify those who have an interest in the quality and effectiveness of the provision, but also may wish to actively influence decision-making. Stakeholders may be passive, in that they have a role to play but may not exercise their right to be involved, or they may be active. Some stakeholders may have the public ear or eye, such as the media, politicians and professional bodies but some less prominent individuals and groups may be influential at other levels. Stakeholders such as school governing bodies, Local Education Authorities and Ofsted effect change through application and interpretation of legislation. Parents and carers may make their views known in other less obvious ways.

Pressure groups

Pressure groups exert influence and they may have power that is disproportionate to their numbers, as exemplified in the discussion about smacking on page 396. The National Curriculum has had numerous revisions and the influence of pressure groups may be seen in the way in which subject content has changed from one revision to the next. Comparison of the content of the curriculum for England with that of Scotland clearly indicates a different set of values and interest in equity.

Comparison of approaches to the curriculum within the United Kingdom is facilitated by ready access to curriculum documentation on the Internet. See the websites listed at the end of this chapter.

The role of government in shaping provision is central; however, the influence of pressure groups should not be underestimated. The place of those who influence decisions is often given little consideration by practitioners and yet the ways in which influence is exerted is worthy of reflection.

Stakeholders have varying levels of influence

Different stakeholders have different levels of influence on the development of specific critical issues, depending on the issue itself and the various roles of those involved. Some stakeholders have consistently more or less influence than others. For example, parents and carers are primary end-users of educare as much as children. However, the familiar theme of 'parents as partners' does not always encompass the concept of children as partners in their own care and education. As such, children may be seen to have only a limited influence on their own care and education; they have much to contribute to the relevant debates.

> ## Activity 3) Using the media to analyse issues

Consideration of your personal experience and the values that underpin your opinions may help you to identify factors that influence parental involvement in educare. You may be aided in this venture by making a point of using the media to support your analysis of issues. In consideration of a particular critical issue currently under debate, read newspapers and watch television reports, consult local and national press and relevant websites. Most importantly be aware of bias. This will raise your awareness of critical issues currently appearing in the media and identify some of the underlying factors that may influence your personal stance on the issue.

The role of government

It is useful to reflect upon how national policy influencing early childhood education and care is decided and by whom. Who are the national stakeholders in care and education in the early years? Political agendas can be determined from a variety of sources. For example, examination of relevant documentation will indicate how the expectations of political opinion are represented in the curriculum guidelines, in terms of both the content and delivery of the curriculum. Other sources are government papers, local authority guidelines, legislation and discussions on legislation. Many early childhood organisations monitor government policy closely and publish commentaries on developments (see websites listed at the end of the chapter).

Policies affecting early childhood care and education may well be part of wider agendas. For example, many policies currently affecting early childhood are part of the government's wider agenda on social exclusion and raising skills and educational standards within the workforce. The focus of government policy can be found in both the type of critical issue prominent at the time and the type of developments made within a particular critical issue. Government does not operate in a vacuum; it is influenced by wider public opinion, research, and developments in similar areas of interest and concern in other countries.

Reflective approaches

The concept of reflective practice is now firmly rooted in our understanding of the development of quality in early years services and the need for practitioners to continue personal and professional development post-qualification. Reflective practice is the process through which practitioners come to understand their role more fully, and through which improvements in service content and delivery are made. Reflective practice should lead to better quality for children by improving their access to services and to experiences that contribute to their holistic development. The role of the reflective practitioner is discussed in detail in Chapter 2.

Kolb (1984) describes reflective practice as a cycle of activity, as shown in Figure 12.2.

Reflective practice is the process by which change is driven within early years services. It is rooted in the belief that quality is both subjective and based on cultural assumptions and, therefore, to determine what quality is and to achieve quality will require different processes at different times. If we look back to approaches to childcare and education in the past, it is clear that they are based on many different principles and practices to those that are currently considered 'best practice'. Changes include, amongst many other things, the ways in which we support children's learning, the content and style of child-adult relationships, methods of control and our understanding of children's needs and the interrelationship

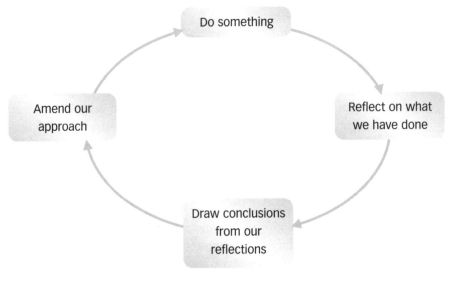

Figure 12.2
Reflective practice is a cycle of activity (after Kolb, 1984)

between them. Reflection is the key to recognising and responding to critical issues at practice level. Practitioners need to make the links between their knowledge and understanding of critical issues and their own practice. For example, one of the key findings from the Laming Report (2003) into Victoria Climbie's death (discussed on page 401) related to lack of effective training in child protection for relevant professionals. But, what does this mean in practice? How should this finding be translated into action by individual practitioners and settings? Reflection can help to determine flaws and gaps in policy and practice that need addressing in order to improve quality and raise standards. Reflection is the process by which practice is considered and judged against expectations and standards, drawing on a range of information sources to make this comparison.

Woods (1998) describes several aspects of reflective practice, which are shown in Figure 12.3.

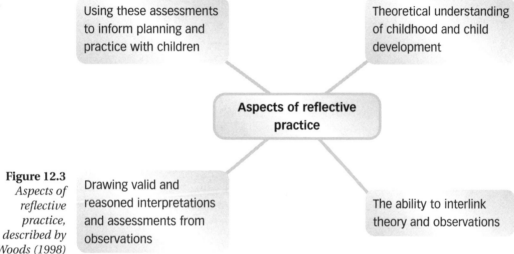

Using these assessments to inform planning and practice with children

Theoretical understanding of childhood and child development

Aspects of reflective practice

Figure 12.3
Aspects of reflective practice, described by Woods (1998)

Drawing valid and reasoned interpretations and assessments from observations

The ability to interlink theory and observations

These aspects highlight the links between developing the knowledge-base; reflection on real practice; applying theory to real practice in the light of knowledge and experience; and changing or modifying practice in response to new understandings.

Individual practice

Practitioners need to reflect on their own experiences and ask 'What works/does not work?' and 'What evidence do we have to confirm our views?' Judging the effectiveness of one's own practice involves considering the factors that shape that practice and the underpinning processes that resulted in a particular set of factors having influence at any particular point in time. For example, key theories currently influencing approaches to the curriculum emphasise the social nature of children's learning development and the need for expert support by more experienced others in the learning process. However, research by Elfer (1996) has shown that

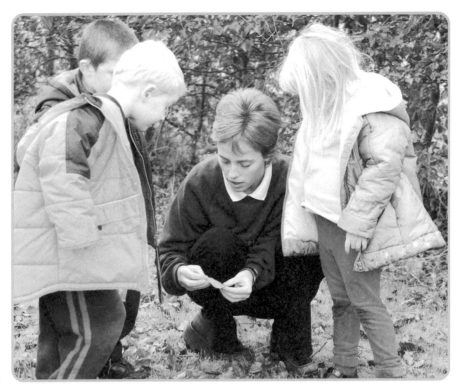

Practitioners need to spend time building up relationships with children in their care

there is a lack of warmth in relationships between adults and children in nursery settings, and other research shows that direct involvement of adults in play activities is often very limited. In this example, individual practitioners may need to consider why practice does not meet the expected requirements of the field. They may draw their information from observations of other's practice and reflections on their own research findings that support a view within this issue; policies and guidelines that determine expectations (national, local and within the setting); and other sources of information. An individual practitioner who reflects on this issue may conclude that more time needs to be devoted to building relationships with children and playing with them in order to provide a high quality learning environment in which the child's emotional and social needs are effectively addressed.

Practice in settings

Practice in settings is usually determined by policies designed to regulate the care and education of young children, many aspects of which are determined by external legislation and guidelines. However, many areas of practice are open to interpretation in their implementation. For example, recent research has emphasised the need for young children to have access to drinking water at all times in school or nursery. Studies have shown that children's learning can be adversely affected by dehydration and that many children become dehydrated during the school day. In one example of a setting, flasks of water were provided for each child and then withdrawn because of spills on tables and the carpet. The comment was that 'it was too much trouble to provide water for the children'. Reflection on this issue could have helped to remind the setting manager that the problem was not that the children needed drinking water, but the method chosen to ensure they had it. Reflection may have reminded the staff that the reason for having the water was sound, and that there is more than one way of making water accessible to the children. At this level, reflection takes place more at team level, and should be part of teamwork processes to raise standards and improve practice.

Values and perceptions

Values underpin all aspects of our work with children and families; personal values and beliefs; the values generally agreed upon within the communities in which we work; and the values that are promoted by our elected representatives in parliament.

Personal values

The term 'values' is open to wide interpretation, so it is important to consider and clarify our understanding of the term. When we consider the range of values that may affect our own approaches to life we begin to realise how influential they may be; these may include social, cultural, moral, ethical, religious and political values, but you may well think of others. How do these affect teaching and learning?

> **Activity 4** **Effects of religious beliefs**

Write down notes on the following questions:

1 In what way may a strongly held religious or atheist belief affect the ways in which an educator works with children?
2 Can religious and moral values enhance practice?

This remains a critical issue for many practitioners. For those practitioners who hold atheist or humanist beliefs, this may influence their participation in quasi-religious practice such as 'broadly Christian' school assemblies. Observant practitioners of a faith who wish to demonstrate their belief through their work may find similar conflict of interest.

Values affect our perception of critical issues. They are at the root of agreement or disagreement about fundamental issues in our professional role. Values are different from opinion or preference and in this respect we must be vigilant to separate our personal from our professional views. This is illustrated in the discussion on smacking as a critical issue in this chapter, which highlights the possible distinction between personal views of smacking as a disciplinary tool in both private and public arenas. Values underpinning the various roles within care and education of young children are broadly outlined within relevant policy and legislation and on most issues relating to these roles there will be agreement.

Personal values may conflict

There will be occasions when dissension may arise because personal values and their impact on professional understanding will result in conflict and thus make the issue a critical one. Examples of this are provided in this chapter in the discussion of the relationship between professionals in the workplace prompted by the changing demands placed on classroom teaching assistants. The value placed on the professional role of teaching assistant and advanced practitioners by local and national government through salary and promotional structure is clearly a critical issue. It relates to a perception of the status of practitioners and to what some see as exploitation of personal commitment by offering inappropriately matched financial reward. Conversely, some would argue that reliance on the personal values of voluntary as well as paid practitioners to undertake their essential roles in childcare and early education is justified. Satisfaction of undertaking such a worthwhile job could be argued to be sufficient reward. This critical issue raises issues of value such as equity, exploitation, expectation and reward.

Values in practice

Practitioners need to consider their own values and principles as well as those influencing their role externally. External values will be those indicated in curriculum documentation and the views expressed by the local community.

Values play an important part in the implementation of legislation and particularly in the delivery of the curriculum. In general, the implementation of policy and legislation is based on broadly held principles that practitioners and parents will support. A critical issue may arise when legislation conflicts with the religious or moral beliefs of parents or practitioners. The use of ICT within schools has presented a critical issue for those practitioners who work with children from families who for religious reasons reject the use of computers. Interpretation of modesty in dress within a school setting, in physical activity (particularly in swimming) has had an impact in the recent past for practitioners in fulfilling their role as required in delivering the curriculum, or so it appeared to them at the time. This critical issue was largely resolved by accommodating values so as not to exacerbate conflict. The delivery of the Foundation Stage remains a critical issue for many practitioners; for example, there are wide variations in how the concept of learning through play is interpreted. A clear and well-documented expectation that the Foundation Stage curriculum will be largely delivered through play activities is still open to wide interpretation because there is no definitive definition of play that is accepted by all. There is no complete agreement on this matter because the purposes and form of play is so closely linked to personal values and beliefs. The perceived value of play as a tool and context for learning and other aspects of development differ widely in and between individuals as well as between and within the professions working in this sector. Another dimension is added to critical issues relating to the early years curriculum in that it is presented in so many different frameworks for children who are not required by law to be in a formal educational setting.

Values are visible in the curriculum offered to children and the quality of experience provided by staff delivering that curriculum. Many practitioners do not fully appreciate the role that political value judgement plays in shaping the early years curriculum.

A comparison of the curriculum offered in England with Scotland or another European country quickly reveals differences as well as similarities in values through the selection of curriculum areas, the curriculum content and the means of teaching. The differences between the curriculum offered in different countries are also an expression of the differences of values between as well as within societies. The values underpinning the various roles within care and education of young children in England are broadly outlined within relevant policy and legislation. For example, there is a clear and well-documented expectation that the Foundation Stage curriculum will be largely delivered through play activities, based on the perceived value of play as a tool and context for learning and other aspects of development. However, there is also scope for the implementation of policy and legislation to be based on individual or setting-wide values, as well as being in line with the broader sweep of underpinning principles. So, within the delivery of the Foundation Stage there are wide variations in how the concept of learning through play is interpreted.

Activity 5) Values

Values are evident in a wide range of critical issues relating to perceptions of what children should be taught and in what manner and when this should take place. There is debate in England between the merits of particular approaches such as HighScope, Montessori, Steiner and that demonstrated in the Foundation Stage. Philosophical approaches are value driven; they are often the subject of passionate belief and truly reflect deeply held beliefs. The critical nature of this dissension or contention is further demonstrated if the debate extends to the European Community.

In the context of provision of education and care within the European Community make notes on the following issues. Comparison of provision and approach to delivery will indicate why these issues are critical.

School starting age

Comparison of starting ages across Europe indicates differences in values relating to the place of care and educational experience in early childhood.

A useful starting point would be the study 'School Starting Age' by Caroline Sharp, available at www.nfer.ac.uk.

Curriculum content

Comparison of the curriculum offered to 3 to 5-year-old children and 6 to 8-year-old children indicates considerable difference between European countries.

Training of early years staff

The training of staff to work in early years settings varies between European countries.

1 Which of these issues do you consider being critical or simply a matter of passing interest?
2 Research in this area may be undertaken by reading professional journals such as *Nursery World* and through the use of the Internet. This will provide answers to some of the questions that may arise from consideration of these critical issues.

Values are at the heart of our work with young children. If the concept of the reflective practitioner is fully recognised it follows that the professional role will be subjected to analysis and evaluation. Reflective evaluation and analysis of practice will often lead to comparison of practice in order to improve and develop professional competence. It is in the comparison of the experience of children and the role of the supportive educator and carer in their setting, the wider community and between systems operated in different countries that the critical nature of the equity of experiences will arise.

Current critical issues in the early years

In this section, a range of contemporary critical issues will be examined to highlight the ways in which particular topics become crucial to debates about quality and services in the early years. The key arguments that determine that an issue is critical at a particular time will be considered in the examples given, and the ways in which such issues can influence changes in policy and practice will also be considered. The relevance of each debate to the study of early childhood for early years practitioners is discussed, in addition to the significance for early years practitioners.

Provision and regulation of settings: key points

In 1988 the National Curriculum was introduced into schools in England and Wales, making for a broader, more balanced and coherent schooling system. The curriculum sets out what pupils should study, what they should be taught and the standards that they should achieve. The National Curriculum in England and Wales is divided into four Key Stages (KS), three core subjects (English, Mathematics and Science) and

*nine non-core foundation subjects. In Scotland there is no legally
prescribed national curriculum but the Scottish Executive Education
Department sets out guidelines for teachers. (www.britcoun.org)*

This statement by the British Council presents, for international
consumption, a view of critical provision of education in England and
Scotland. It may be argued that parts of this statement present a not
entirely accurate or representative picture. Are children in England and
Wales provided with a broad, balanced and coherent system of schooling?
How much time is allocated to the non-core foundation subjects? It may
be argued that the issue is contentious. Some would argue that the
guidelines provided for Scottish schools may be regarded as a model for
the early years curriculum in that the curriculum is presented for teachers
to interpret and to teach rather than to 'deliver'.

Relevance to the study of early childhood

The situation in early years provision is no less contentious and this
chapter addresses issues relating to curriculum practice and provision in
relation to pre-school children.

There is an on-going debate about the age at which children should enter
formal education and central to this debate is the role of practitioner.

The role of the practitioner in a private or voluntary setting is changing
rapidly, no more so than because the curriculum demands this change.
Changes resulting from the imposition of a national curriculum in England
for children of 3- and 4 years of age are contentious and critical. The
delivery of the curriculum for pre-school children is a critical issue that is
ongoing, as it affects all providers and users of early years educational
provision in England.

Equity in delivery?

Identification of the range of settings in England now regarded as places in
which young children have access to education reveals a very disorganised
and diverse picture. This is a critical issue in terms of equity. The
educational experiences offered to 3- and 4-year-old children vary
markedly between settings using the Early Learning Goals as a framework
for planning. Different experiences will be offered by childminders,
voluntary pre-school settings, maintained nursery schools, private pre-
schools and nursery provision following Montessori or Steiner principles.
These differences may result from the range of resources, the levels and
type of training which staff have experienced. Staff pay structure in
different types of setting varies markedly. This presents settings delivering
the same curriculum with inequitable problems for delivery. These
differences are critical. One may argue that diversity presents opportunity
for selection of an appropriate setting to meet the needs of the individual
child. This can only be true where there is genuine choice.

It may be argued that the division between the maintained and voluntary sectors of pre-school education is breaking down as pre-schools in the voluntary and private sector follow the prescribed Foundation Stage curriculum.

1   Make notes on the key differences between the ways in which the curriculum is offered in maintained, voluntary and private settings.

2   What are the differences between the approach to care offered in these settings?

Starting points for discussion:

⊃ how the curriculum is taught and offered

⊃ the range of experience offered to children in settings

⊃ expectations of parents/carers

⊃ the training of early years practitioners

⊃ the range of qualifications of those working in early childhood settings as educators.

Delivery of the Foundation Stage differs from the National Curriculum as it occurs in so many different types of setting. These differences are substantial. It is acknowledged that there is not an entirely cohesive range of provision and that a very mixed experience for children moving from one region of the country to another is unavoidable. A review of schools provision for delivering the National Curriculum will also identify other critical issues. A critical issue in many rural schools is the teaching of mixed age groups, of Reception-age children in the Foundation Stage working alongside older children working through the National Curriculum. In small schools, there may not be opportunity to experience a full and rich curriculum in areas where resources are limited. In settings providing National Curriculum experience children may be attending an Infant, Primary or First school with differing facilities. There will, however, be no allowance made for this in the range or depth of responsibilities of the early years educators within the various settings.

Inspection process is variable

In this context of variable experience a means of attempting to regulate and ensure comparability of experience for children is undertaken by the Office for Standards in Education (Ofsted) through inspection. It is clear that this process is also inequitable as different processes are applied to the maintained sector compared with non-maintained settings. The penalties applied for non-compliance are also different. In short, different types of inspector with different levels of training and experience are inspecting these two ranges of educational setting for the same curriculum.

All practitioners who work with children are subject to complying with sets of rules and regulations. Many practitioners will regard these requirements as little more than part of routine other than when an Ofsted inspection is impending. Reflective practitioners will be concerned with the process as well as the implications of legislation. An awareness of the regulatory frameworks is an aspect of professional life that enhances understanding and the quality of provision and thus provides for some practitioners a heightened awareness of the critical nature of Ofsted inspection.

> **Activity 7** **Out-of-home educational opportunity**

What is the range of out of home educational opportunity for 3 and 4-year-old children in your location?

1 Look at Ofsted reports for the private, voluntary and maintained (state sector) settings in your location; these are available on the Ofsted website (www.ofsted.gov.uk).

2 Note and comment on the range of experiences offered to children in these settings.

There are many issues that are raised by practitioners before, during and after Ofsted inspection. The fact that many of these issues are common indicates that they are of critical concern. Stress, paperwork, uncertainty, lack of trust – the range of issues is broad but consistent. Comparison of experience of Ofsted between groups of practitioners often reveals inconsistency, or perceived inconsistency in the standards applied to inspection. The critical nature of inspection as a tool for improving standards is clear. At the heart of this debate lies the need for clarity in determining the purpose of assessment and whether this can be achieved through inspection. Assessment of Ofsted appears to be a critical issue in terms of accountability to all of the stakeholders in the education and care of young children, parents, practitioners and ultimately to the children who are the primary end users of the system.

Assessment: key points

The assessment of children takes many forms and is used for many purposes. The debate relating to formal testing of children by means of Standardised Assessment Tasks in England has been a critical issue of concern for parents and carers as well as teachers for over ten years. Testing as a means of providing data for a range of political purposes is well established. You may conclude from analysis of school roll numbers and test results that there are clear links between national target setting, the league tables of test results and the popularity of particular schools. This may be demonstrable in some locations, but strength of parental support and community involvement in schools and settings under threat of closure would appear to indicate that test results and outcomes of formal inspection procedures reflect a partial picture of the relationship between assessment and parental opinion.

Relevance to the study of early childhood

Assessment of very young children would at first appear to be a contentious issue. Should 3- and 4-year-old children be formally assessed? A critical aspect of this discussion must be in arriving at a definition of what constitutes a formal assessment procedure or process compared with an informal one. The introduction of the Foundation Stage Profile (QCA, 2003) has formalised assessment procedures for recording children's development. Although emphasis is placed on assessment as part of the learning and teaching process (QCA, 2003:1) the document provides little acknowledgement of the formative use of the document for children who do not achieve the Early Learning Goals by the end of the Reception Year. There is marked variation in the age at which children will join Year 1 infant classes in England; this will range from 5.0 for an August-born child to 5.11 for a September-born child. If one takes in to account the differences of rate in development of children, as well as their age, the need for assessment that is child centred becomes clear.

Significance for early years practitioners

Critical debate around the need for formalised assessment is buoyant and illustrates the divergence between political opinion and that of professionals in the field of education. Correlation between SATs results and teachers' assessment grading is close and would appear to indicate the redundancy of formal testing. The critical nature of the issue lies in the wide differences that appear between those who legislate and those who deliver – early years teachers. Tests record achievements that are measurable against narrow criteria and are, therefore, easily quantifiable. It may be argued that this process is less subject to bias than assessment located in one person's judgement.

Financing of educational provision

Critical and contentious issues relating to the financing of educational provision are closely linked to assessment. These issues are illustrated in Figure 12.4.

There are many other issues that have a bearing on this debate. Spending on education and care has been a major priority in England and is set to develop even further. It is clear that such spending requires accountability of purpose and clarification of achievement. Testing and assessment provides data to justify further spending as well as vindicating existing and past policy. The extent to which stakeholders are involved in the micro as well as the macro political decisions appears to be the cause of some tension in some limited areas. Increased development of early childhood services through substantial funding is welcomed; however, the

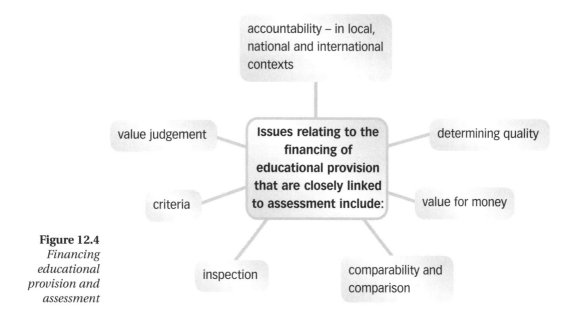

accountability – in local, national and international contexts

value judgement

Issues relating to the financing of educational provision that are closely linked to assessment include:

determining quality

criteria

value for money

inspection

comparability and comparison

Figure 12.4
Financing educational provision and assessment

restrictions that apply to the forms of education and care stipulated by the government do not receive unqualified support. Changes to pre-school practice have been most noticeable in the area of voluntary provision. Playgroups have generally become pre-schools. Perhaps the terms do not change forms of practice; play may still be a central theoretical basis for learning but with a new emphasis on more tightly focused approaches to learning indicate a compromise.

> **Activity 8** **Taking an objective approach**

Within a discussion of critical issues there may be those who have opposing but equally valid views on a subject. There may be advantages and disadvantages within an issue, which becomes blurred because of the adversarial nature of some discussions. A reflective practitioner will have an objective approach to critical issues and consider and carefully evaluate evidence before making decisions.

1 Consider two opposing viewpoints for an issue. Note advantages and disadvantages for both sides of the discussion and provide a balanced conclusion.

Working with parents as partners: key points

Most early years practitioners will be familiar with the term 'parents as partners' and also with the concept of parents as the first educators. The expectations of parents are clearly outlined in some documents, for example in Curriculum Guidance for the Foundation Stage and in the Foundation Stage Profile, but in others the message is more covert.

The way in which the curriculum is presented in the growing number of leaflets for parents presents a particular approach to partnership. It could be argued that the leaflets present a covert, hidden agenda as they present a single approach to learning and one that may be targeted at a particular socio-economic group. Conversely, supporters may argue that provision of guidance for parents is provided for those who wish to have access to it.

Significance for early years practitioners

In the light of this discussion it is useful to consider bias in one's own approach to this issue. Have you thought about the way in which your views are influenced? Are you informed or influenced by the ways in which issues are presented on television, radio, and in newspapers? Do you consider the views of colleagues, parents of children in your workplace or with parents with whom you have contact at a social level when forming your own opinions?

Now note and consider the validity of the evidence parents use to support their opinions.

> **Activity 9** **The expectations of parents and carers**

What do you consider to be the key issues for parents of young children? Is it the curriculum? Are there other issues that are of greater importance for parents? Are these issues critical for you because they challenge school or nursery policy?

Some parental concerns may challenge as well as support government policy and legislation.

Look at the government's expectations of parents and carers set out in the Curriculum Guidance for the Foundation Stage and answer the following questions.

1 Do you consider these expectations to be realistic and appropriate or have you formed other opinions?
2 Do these expectations acknowledge that some parents may have difficulty in supporting their children due to their own lack of competence?
3 Note any evidence to support your responses.

Equity and equality: key points

This area is a contentious issue. How we perceive 'equality' as a concept may relate to our own personal experiences and values. To address this issue it is necessary to attempt to identify the underlying factors. Interpretation of terminology differs according to context and personal values; what is seen as a gender-related issue in one context might be viewed as racism in another. A high priority may be ascribed to an area of 'equality' by one person; for example, the needs relating to a physical disability may figure prominently in the personal concerns of one individual and yet the same area may be judged to be of peripheral concern by another. This may be the case even when those two individuals have the same disability. Racism may be perceived as a social control mechanism, a political act, verbal or physical abuse or simply an act of unkindness. How one views the term depends very much on personal experience.

Significance for early years practitioners

There is much emphasis in Ofsted inspection of realised and missed opportunities for enhancing and developing children's learning experiences.

As a practitioner it is necessary to consider what factors may have a bearing on equal opportunities offered to children. List these factors and try to tease out why you have selected them. This may involve you in testing your own value judgements. Before examining what equality of opportunity means in practice we should consider the following:

➲ What is our understanding of opportunity in early years educational settings?

➲ What are opportunities?

➲ What opportunities are expected to be equal?

➲ Do these opportunities relate to the children we work within our placements or settings?

In order to help you to begin your reflections on this issue it may be useful to consider the role of human interaction – how people relate to one another. Do you make a conscious attempt to treat everyone with equal respect: children and staff? What effect do you think that this has on role modelling? Role models at home provide children with varying experience, which may be at variance with that which they experience in the nursery or school. Therein lies a critical issue, which as with most critical issues is not easily and readily resolved.

> ### Activity 10) Equity within the workplace

As a student working towards a qualification as a senior practitioner it would be appropriate for you to look at an issue of equity within the workplace.

Make notes on two of the following issues, one that is very relevant, is 'live' within your workplace and another that is less familiar.

1 What issues relating to gender affect children, their families and staff in early years settings?

2 What issues relating to race affect children, their families and staff in early years settings?

3 What are the issues relating to difference, in terms of special or specific need, that affect children, their families and staff in early years settings?

4 What are the issues relating to physical difference that affect children, their families and staff in early years settings?

The role of teaching assistants: key points

The role of teaching assistants is an example of an issue that has developed over a period of time before becoming 'critical'. The growth of a the range of non-QTS staff in schools, supporting teaching and learning, caring for children and providing school-wide support services has been apparent for some years. The range of qualifications, roles and titles for such practitioners has grown rapidly and confusingly, although many have similar roles and responsibilities despite diverse pay and qualifications.

The DfES allocates all classroom support staff the collective title of 'teaching assistant' to cover this diversity, and this term will be used in this discussion. However, 'teaching assistants' come in many forms, have many pay scales and responsibilities. They are often involved directly in the care and education of groups and of individual children with special needs, in planning and delivering the curriculum, in preparing materials and activities, recording, assessment and reviews. They have detailed knowledge of the curriculum, often across the National Curriculum and Foundation Stage, of child development and strategies to support children with special needs and a range of other issues specific to their own role, school and community in which they work. Many are skilled in talking to parents, communicating with children, planning school-wide events and contributing to school development at all levels. Some are unqualified, some have childcare qualifications and others have specific qualifications in supporting particular key stages or types of children; for example, the CACHE Specialist Teaching Assistant Award (STA) for teaching assistants supporting learning in Key Stage 1. However, despite the growth in both the range and complexity of the teaching assistant's role, most are low paid and two-thirds remain unqualified, and there is no central control over pay.

In nursery classes and primary schools, the role of teaching assistants has developed in line with the increased demands of and complexity of the early years curriculum. Numbers of teaching assistants across all sectors have grown to 216,000 full-time equivalents, an increase of 80,000 since 1997 (Ward, 23/10/02). Many teaching assistants have also gained higher levels of responsibility partly in response to the increasingly varied and complex roles of teachers. Yet many teaching assistants are unqualified or do not have qualifications or training relevant to all their roles.

Plans to extend the role of teaching assistants

In 2002, plans were revealed to extend the role of teaching assistants to contribute more fully to teaching and learning in classrooms up to and including whole class teaching. Proposals included establishing Higher Level teaching assistants who would receive training to take classes, among other duties, under the supervision of qualified teachers. Supervision would not necessarily mean having a qualified teacher in the classroom. The rationale was that teachers would then be freed to devote more time to planning and assessment within school hours. It was proposed that 10 per cent of teacher time should be given to these tasks. The role of teaching assistants became a critical issue overnight in response to these proposals. The NUT responded by refusing to agree to the new workload arrangements for teachers arguing that:

> *key government plans to give more responsibility to teaching assistants in a bid to lighten workload undermine the teaching profession. (Curtis, 3/7/03)*

Eighty per cent of NUT members were quoted as being opposed to teaching assistants covering for teachers:

> *one teacher described teaching by classroom assistants as being similar to receiving an operation from a hospital porter (Curtis, 17/12/02)*

The response from many sides was extremely critical of the proposals. Accusations were launched at the government, of 'dumbing down' and undermining standards within the teaching profession. The role of teaching assistants came under media and professional scrutiny, with many and varied responses to their value. On the one hand, teaching assistants were praised as the vital component of school cohesion, providing a wide range of essential services and skills to support children outside and within the classroom. The sheer range of their roles and responsibilities, skills and talents, knowledge and ability drew praise and confirmation of the essential nature of their professional role. On the other hand, teaching assistants became the object of abusive comments and denigration of their role and skills, as exemplified by the quote above. The concept of teaching assistants taking whole classes was strongly criticised on the grounds that they did not have the skills and ability, they lacked appropriate training, experience and qualifications, and in short, they are not teachers.

Relevance to the study of early childhood

The traditional structure of the workforce in early years has long been subject to divisions in pay and conditions between those involved in 'care' and those involved in 'education'. The blurring of the distinction between care and education services, which has been central to recent policy developments, and attempts to integrate care and education in the early years through the development of new types of services, have had to work around this traditional hierarchy to date.

Significance for early years practitioners

From September 2003, teaching assistants have taken over 24 administrative and clerical tasks from teachers, in order to free teachers for more teaching-related activities as a significant step in changing teachers' roles and responsibilities. Training routes for teaching assistants have expanded rapidly with the introduction of work-based routes into teacher training and Sector-Endorsed Foundation Degrees and other foundation degrees leading to higher level qualifications and the opportunity for some teaching assistants to qualify as teachers. However, not all teaching assistants may have the ability or ambition to become teachers, and many may wish to continue offering the valuable services in schools that are part of their critical role.

> **Activity 11** **The role of teaching assistants**

There are many questions still to consider about the role of teaching assistants. Are teaching assistants destined to become more like teachers and to take on more teaching roles, or are they to continue with a supportive role, taking more time-consuming tasks from teachers to free them to teach? How will a two-tier system of teaching assistants work and will pay reflect their new roles fully? Will teachers be reconciled to these developments and lose their fears of being professionally undermined? How will developments to improve training routes for teaching assistants progress?

Using media reports, the Internet and other sources of information make notes on the progress of this issue at the time you are reading this textbook. Some references can be found at the end of this chapter.

1 What progress has the government made with plans to develop the role of teaching assistants?
2 Have plans changed from those originally made and if so why?
3 Is the role of teaching assistants still critical at the time you are completing this activity?

Smacking: key points

A key issue that has dominated debates in child protection, childcare and the social care of children for some considerable time is the use of smacking as a disciplinary measure or a punishment for young children within British society. Of all the issues in these fields, smacking raises some of the strongest feelings among both those who wish to abolish it and those who fight for the right to continue chastising children in this way.

> *The extent to which parents should be allowed to discipline and punish their children as they think fit produces deeply polarised views over whether the use of physical punishment on children can be justified on practical and ethical grounds, and more generally, over the extent to which the state should interfere with parent's family privacy and autonomy (Fortin, 2003:276)*

The debate around smacking is not simple. It relates to some of the fundamental beliefs we hold about children and their place in both the social and cultural context and within the family. It also relates to beliefs about the roles and rights of parents and concepts of the family as a private institution. Proposals to abolish smacking within the law raise the spectre of a breakdown of the fundamental rights of families to privacy and self-determination. There is also a belief that parents' behaviour in this area is beyond the reach of the law, in that it would be impossible to police (Fortin, 2003).

On the other hand, the anti-smacking lobby, notably the alliance of 250 anti-smacking organisations called 'Children are Unbeatable', root their arguments in the rhetoric of children's rights and child-centred care and education practices. They argue that children as citizens have a right to be protected from physical assault, and the humiliation of corporal punishment.

Confusion still exists about corporal punishment

Proponents of both sides of the argument have made progress. Smacking has been abolished in schools, local authority institutions and other public bodies caring for children for some time. More recently, smacking by childminders was banned in this country. However, despite a strong anti-smacking lobby, there is a high level of confusion within the law about the extent to which children can be subjected to corporal punishment and, as yet, there is no anti-smacking legislation on the statutes in England and Wales. Despite the UN's strongly worded criticism of UK law, the 140-year-old defence of 'reasonable chastisement' still exists for parents who beat their children.

Studies of attitudes towards and behaviour around smacking are also not simple in their findings. A survey by the Newsons in 1969 and studies in the 1990s demonstrated that, while fewer parents now smack their children than 30 or 40 years ago, even fewer parents believe that smacking is an acceptable or positive way of controlling children's behaviour. The implication that some parents who do not support smacking in principle are smacking their children in practice raises a whole raft of issues around why parents smack and what promotes or prevents smacking within the family.

Attempts to outlaw smacking in Scotland in 2002 raised a vociferous response from the pro-smackers. The arguments varied between defending smacking as an effective control on children's behaviour to preserving the right of parents to punish their children as they see fit without state interference. Legislation was passed to prohibit hitting children either with implements or on the head, and also to ban shaking. Proposals to ban any form of physical punishment of under-3s were not successful. In England and Wales, the government gave a response that made it clear that attempts to introduce such legislation were unlikely to be pursued in the near future. Yet such legislation has been passed in a whole range of other European countries, mainly Scandinavian countries such as Sweden where all physical punishment was banned in 1979, but also countries as diverse as Cyprus and Latvia. The Committee on the Rights of the Child (2002) has criticised the UK for not taking steps to ban physical punishment of children and re-educate parents in other forms of discipline.

The anti-smacking lobby

The anti-smacking lobby argue that corporal punishment is out of line with child-centred approaches to childcare, an archaic and outdated punishment that hurts and humiliates children, and provides no effective deterrent to unwanted behaviour. They argue that as a disciplinary measure smacking is ineffective, failing to provide children with guidelines on how they are expected to behave. Whilst smacking may relieve the anger and tension the parent is experiencing, it fails to engage the child in positive approaches to behavioural change. The children's rights lobby argues that children have, or should have, natural rights as adults do, and these should include the right not to be hurt and humiliated by physical punishments. The child protection lobby emphasise the links between physical punishments and physical abuse as an argument against smacking. They point to the possibility of escalation in severity of the punishment and the possibility of a smacked child becoming an abused child. Recently, David Hinchcliffe, Labour chair of the Health Committee, introduced a private member's bill to ban smacking, saying:

> Other countries that have banned smacking have seen a significant reduction in child abuse. In Sweden, not one child has died at the hands of a parent or carer over the last 10 years, compared with at least one a week in this country. (Carvel and Boseley, 10/10/03)

The pro-smacking lobby

The pro-smacking lobby emphasise the rights of parents to choose punishment methods and to raise their children as they please within certain limitations. They refute the argument that there is a significant link between smacking and child abuse. In response to David Hinchcliffe's private member's bill to ban smacking, the Director of Family and Youth Concern said:

> All parents understand the difference between a little smack given as a means of discipline in a loving and supportive relationship and abuse.

The pro-smacking lobby argue that smacking is effectual, that in a loving context it is not harmful to any aspect of the child's development and growth, and that smacking should remain a choice for all parents. Strong arguments are made against the right of the state to pass legislation that interferes so directly in the private domain of the family. This view seems to be upheld by the state. Despite the European Court of Human Rights overturning a ruling by the English courts that it was lawful for a step-father to beat his 9-year-old stepson with a garden cane, a subsequent consultation made it clear that no outright ban would be considered (DoH, 2000).

Relevance to the study of early childhood

Smacking is a critical issue in early childhood studies because it highlights the ways in which concepts of childhood are differentially constructed within cultural contexts and the diverse and opposing views that can develop from these constructions. At the heart of the argument are incompatible views on the nature of childhood and the place of children within the family. Political ideologies influence views on the rights of parents versus the rights of children, and these are reflected in the core arguments coming from each side of the lobby. Yet this critical issue is not global. For countries such as Sweden, where legislation to outlaw smacking has been in place for over 20 years, the issue is much less significant.

Critical issues are not, therefore, developed in abstract, but instead, based in the social, cultural and political events of a particular culture or social grouping. They arise from dilemmas or debates within the dominant belief system, often challenging perceived wisdom or existing practices. Critical issues are dynamic rather than static, related to what is happening within the field at a particular point in time. They arise from social change, new understandings and perceptions of existing situations, cultural expansion or political activity. These factors are not discrete but operate in complex relationships to develop awareness of a critical issue. For example, smacking was an accepted method of punishment throughout the history of childhood, and up until the late-20th century the majority of parents smacked their children without much consideration of the meaning or value of this action. Children were smacked at school, within the community and extended family, and by other authority figures. Questions about the morality and validity of smacking were raised as increasing knowledge and understanding of children's developmental needs steered the way towards child-centred parenting and care. The growth of psychology as a discipline and increased awareness of children's emotional needs through the work of Freud and his followers raised awareness of children's wider needs and how these could be met. In the meanwhile, legislation in other countries put pressure on the state to consider such action here. The result so far has been the abolishment of smacking within the professional field of early years practice (and of course in the care and education of older children). The anti-smacking policies common to early years services are at variance with the continuing use of smacking within the majority of families.

Without the political will for change, smacking will remain a critical issue, although the anti-smacking lobby remains vociferous. The development of children's rights as a principle underpinning legislation and policy in increasing numbers of areas of early years services has been halted within this particular debate. The most influential argument against abolishing smacking is not about smacking at all, but about the rights of parents over their children within the private context of the family. The debate is essentially about different sets of beliefs and values.

This notion of the privacy and autonomy of the family remains a strongly supported concept within the cultural norms of British society, and one that has so far effectively prevented the introduction of anti-smacking legislation in Britain. It is possible that the contrast between private and public behaviour of adults in this matter may be related to this point. While smacking remains a right of parents, it is not considered acceptable in any public care and education setting. This paradox has recently been reinforced – as efforts to ban smacking continue to fail in England and Wales, childminders have been banned from smacking.

Significance to early years practitioners

The debate about corporal punishment of children raises several issues that are significant for early years practitioners. One of the main issues is the difference in approach to discipline between parents and early years practitioners. Whereas the majority of parents continue to use smacking as a disciplinary measure, early years practitioners do not. This disparity can have an impact on partnerships with parents where there are disagreements about best methods of control. Practitioners may have concerns about the extent to which some parents smack their children and there may be child protection issues in a small number of cases. Differences in methods of control between home and the setting may be confusing for some children. Parents and practitioners may see the role of parents differently, in terms of their views on children's rights.

There are no simple answers to these differences because in the UK at present there are different rules about smacking in public and private domains. However, it is important to ensure that practitioners and parents continue to share views on methods of discipline.

> **Activity 12** **Implications of regular smacking by parents as a method of control**

Consider a situation where the parents of a child in your care use smacking as a method of control on a regular basis. Make notes on the following:

1 What sorts of problems could this raise in respect of managing this child's behaviour?

2 How do you respond to this as an early years professional?

3 What sorts of strategies could be used to help parents to consider other approaches to discipline?

4 What are your own views on smacking? With reference to the discussion above and your own reading (see references at the end of the chapter), write down the arguments for and against legislating against smacking and reflect on your own position within the range of arguments.

Smacking has developed as a critical issue over a long period of time, and remained as a critical issue because differences in viewpoints on the morality and functionality of smacking as a disciplinary method have remained polarised. Legislative change may, in the future, move this issue forward from the critical 'deadlock', but in the meanwhile smacking remains controversial and a strong example of the wide range of values and beliefs within early childhood.

In the case of smacking, the critical issue lies in the ongoing debate about the rights of parents and children. However, not all critical issues appear in this particular way. Other critical issues may arise in different ways and may be both more immediate and perhaps more short-lived in their impact. They may be highlighted by single notable events that trigger concerns and bring a particular issue to the forefront of our notice. Media reporting may have a significant role to play in determining which issues are highlighted.

The Victoria Climbie Case: key points

Critical issues in early childhood studies often arise from tensions within the political, social, moral and cultural context in which child rearing and the educare of young children take place. These tensions are often highlighted as a result of specific events that raise awareness of particular issues at a particular time, often influenced by media reporting and possibly fuelled by moral panics about the evils surrounding modern children.

Child abuse

Child abuse has been a critical issue in the field for many decades. Since the 'discovery' of the 'battered baby syndrome' by Henry Kempe and his colleagues in the 1960s (Kempe et al., 1962), the abuse of children and the methods, means and structures by which children are protected from abuse have been a major focus of political, social and media interest and commentary. The abuse, injury and death of children at the hands of those who have the responsibility for their care and safety is a phenomenon that seems to strike at the heart of our cultural beliefs about the social role of the family and the place of children within it. Indeed, child abuse seems to challenge assumptions about our notions of childhood itself:

> *Child abuse presents a direct and unwelcome public challenge to society's most cherished values, beliefs and ideologies about the care of its children, about the tasks and responsibilities of parenthood, and about family life. (Pettican, 1998:175)*

As different types of abuse became better understood throughout the latter part of the 20th century, and research added to our knowledge and understanding of the impact of abuse on children's short- and long-term welfare and their adult life chances, the place of child abuse as a central critical issue in the field has been confirmed. The emergence of evidence in the 1980s that sexual abuse of children is a widespread, rather than rare and isolated, event fuelled fears that children and childhood are under threat in the very place they should be safest (Baker and Duncan, 1985). Child sexual abuse, which challenges some of the most deeply held cultural and social taboos in Western societies, became for some time the central critical issue within this area of concern. The role of the family and behaviour in families came under an intense level of scrutiny, and a range of moral panics followed. Fears of false allegations within and outside families became endemic, with anecdotal reports of fathers afraid to bathe their children or perform intimate care tasks for them, and the development of work practices within early years services that are designed to protect adults rather than children. For example, nurseries where children can only sit on knees with cushions on them; male PGCE students on placement in nursery and infant classes who are told not to touch the children at all; and settings where children can only have nappies changed or be taken to the lavatory by a minimum of two staff.

The emergence of child sexual abuse as an event that can take place in all types of families raised many fears, not just about the myth of families as a safe place in which children are raised in protected environments, but also about concepts of children as 'innocent', and childhood as a period of innocence.

However, the death of individual children at the hands of their carers remains the event that most consistently confirms child abuse as a critical issue, and which has resulted in the sort of political, social, moral and professional responses that lead to legislative and procedural change. The string of child death inquiries in the 1980s (Jasmine Beckford, Tyra Henry, Kimberley Carlile) which highlighted procedural weaknesses, lack of effective training and failures in inter-agency cooperation and communication contributed towards legislative and procedural change in the shape of the Children Act 1989 and its attendant practice guidelines. Long before this, the death of Dennis O'Neill in 1945 at the hands of his foster carers, influenced legislative change to better protect children.

The case of Victoria Climbie, who also died at the hands of her carers, resulted in a massive response in the media and in the field of child protection social work and allied professions. The Laming Report into the circumstances of Victoria's death (January 2003) was described as follows:

> *The public enquiry into the death of Victoria Climbie was the most extensive investigation into the child protection system in British history. (Batty, 26/2/03)*

The report made sweeping recommendations about required changes in the child protection system in response to the revelation of a raft of crucial mistakes made by professionals who had responsibility for Victoria's care. Some of these recommendations have been incorporated in the recently published Green Paper *Every Child Matters* (DoH, September 2003) and its sister report *Keeping Children Safe*, which directly addresses Lord Laming's recommendations. In these reports, Victoria Climbie's case is directly cited as the catalyst for change.

Yet, other children, such as Lauren Wright, died at the hands of their parents and carers during the same period of time without arousing anything like such a significant response. In fact, many children die at the hands of their parents or carers every year. So, why did Victoria's death become central to the critical issue of child protection?

Relevance to the study of early childhood

Victoria's death involved both a shocking level of cruelty and a massive failure of agencies to respond to what seemed to be glaringly obvious indicators of abuse. Lord Laming identified 12 separate occasions on which professionals had the opportunity to take action to protect Victoria from further abuse.

The inquiry was dogged by revelations of mismanagement and failure to comply with basic procedures in the agencies involved. Media interest was intense throughout the inquiry, following the testimony of witnesses and providing information about their personal and professional lives. The apparent reluctance of some professionals to help with the process of the inquiry raised indignation on all sides. Images of the unbearable suffering this young child had suffered haunted the media for weeks at both the time of her death and during the inquiry.

Importance to the field of child protection

Victoria Climbie's case became the specific event that highlighted critical issues in the field of child protection, and also in the fields of private fostering and support for immigrant children. The range of services implicated in the failure to protect Victoria was extensive, highlighting poor communication and failure to share information between agencies, and lack of understanding of the cultural issues involved.

Since implementation in 1991, the Children Act 1989 had provided a more child- and family-centred legal basis for intervention, and much clearer criteria for intervention. The distinctions within the Act between children who had been abused and children in need had helped to clarify the roles of professionals within child protection and family support systems and had channelled resources to both prevention and protection. The practice guidelines *Working Together to Safeguard Children* (DoH, 1999) supported the philosophy of the Children Act 1989, by outlining a multi-agency approach to child protection and emphasising the roles of other agencies, particularly health and education, as well as the responsibilities of child protection social workers. Yet within the child protection process, problems persisted on a number of fronts. The role of non-social services agencies had gained a new prominence, yet many practitioners and professional groups had insufficient training or support to feel confident within this role. For example, teachers reported lack of confidence in detecting the indicators of abuse and in knowing when to pass information to social services. Differences in professional principles, practices and roles meant that 'working together' effectively proved hard to achieve across the boundaries of professional differences (Kay, 2001).

The balance between protection and prevention

By the late 1990s, it was clear that the balance between protection and prevention had not been achieved effectively. In many authorities there was confusion about the threshold for 'children in need' services and separate service provision between child protection and family support services meant that some children and families fell between the two. Concerns focused on the possibilities that some family support services, now provided by a wide range of agencies including health, education, voluntary and community based organisations, were ill-equipped to recognise child abuse, and that their remit to support and promote families meant that they were not necessarily able to perceive indicators of abuse. On the other hand, child protection services focused on the key roles of investigation, legal intervention and monitoring, with concerns about whether sufficient regard was given to finding appropriate support services across the whole range of child and family needs.

> *Many children (and their families) referred, had more general needs which went unmet by welfare workers because of their narrow focus on child protection. (Corby, 2002:145)*

Department of Health commissioned research, published in 2001, into the effectiveness of the Children Act 1989, confirmed these concerns:

> *The critical system of separating child protection enquiries and family support assessment is ineffective and counter-productive to meeting the needs of children and families. The studies suggest that, by separating the two systems, some children have missed the value of early intervention to prevent more intrusive and intensive activity at a later stage. Conversely, some children who need safeguarding because of neglect are slipping through the net of family support services because these services fail to address the importance of safeguarding children's welfare. (DoH, 2001:144)*

The Framework for Assessment of Children in Need and their Families (2000)

This was introduced to provide a comprehensive assessment process to ensure that children received appropriate services whether they were deemed to be in need or abused. The Assessment Framework was designed to try and ensure that child protection concerns are addressed within the context of the child and family's wider needs, and to redress the concerns discussed above.

Despite these developments, and the fact that child protection is one of the most heavily regulated areas of child care, Victoria Climbie died because of the failure of a range of agencies to recognise her many injuries as abuse, and their failure to recognise or meet her most basic needs for protection and care.

In one commentary it was said:

> *Health, police, housing charities and social services failed to work together to effectively protect the girl. (Batty, 26/2/03)*

Significance for early years practitioners

Victoria Climbie's death highlighted the continuing flaws in a child protection system that had become increasingly complex and distant from the everyday work of the majority of health, childcare and education practitioners.

Lord Laming (2003:7) said in his inquiry report into Victoria Climbie's death that:

> *child protection cannot be separated from policies to improve children's lives as a whole.*

The report recommended changes to the service delivery to children to integrate the child protection process more closely with other support for children and families and to ensure that practitioners are effectively trained and aware of their role in protecting children.

Critical issues can develop from single events such as Victoria's death, which reveal, in this case, the extensive flaws that remain in a system. Despite the many procedural and practice developments, fundamental problems continue to exist in inter-agency coordination and inter-professional collaboration within the child protection system. The Green Paper *Every Child Matters* (DoH, 2003) found a number of common threads linking the findings of child death inquiries: these are illustrated in Figure 12.5.

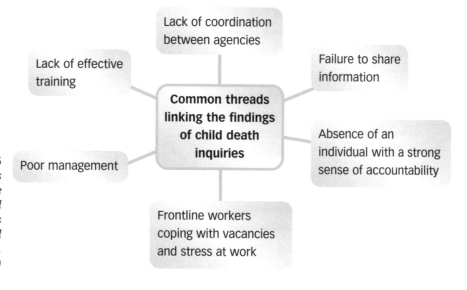

Figure 12.5
Common threads linking the findings of child death inquiries (Every Child Matters, DoH, 2003)

Every Child Matters proposes sweeping changes in structure and approach to protecting children in England, placing child protection services in the context of wider support for children and families. These proposals will have a significant impact on the structure of children's services and the roles of practitioners within those services. The proposals are illustrated in Figure 12.6.

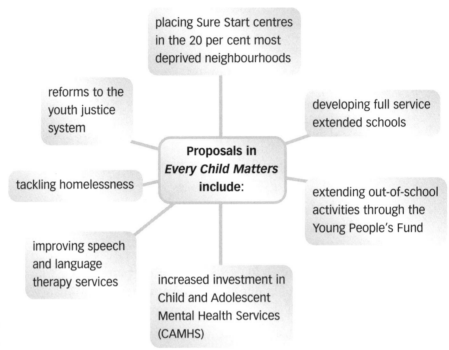

Figure 12.6
Proposals in Every Child Matters

In order to achieve the goals outlined in *Every Child Matters* and to tackle the failures that have led to Victoria Climbie's death and other tragedies, the Green Paper also proposes that to ensure early intervention and effective protection of children changes in service planning and delivery should include:

- ⊃ more effective information sharing between agencies
- ⊃ a common assessment framework for children's services
- ⊃ every case to have a lead professional
- ⊃ on-the-spot service delivery through multi-disciplinary teams based in schools and children's centres.

> **Activity 13** **Assessing the impact of 'Every Child Matters'**

With reference to the discussion above and your own reading (see references at the end of the chapter) write down some ideas about how the proposals within the Green Paper, *Every Child Matters* (DfES, 2003) might impact on the early years service or setting you work in and your own job role. Discuss your ideas with a colleague or mentor.

The Victoria Climbie case became a critical issue because of:

- ➲ the extreme nature of the abuse and the circumstances of her death
- ➲ the number of agencies involved and the range of failures by these agencies to safeguard and support Victoria
- ➲ the cultural and social issues raised by the death of a West African child in England
- ➲ and the recognition by those involved in the aftermath that fatal flaws still remained within the child protection system, despite extensive legislative and procedural developments in recent years.

Other critical issues may arise through different means or the coming together of a range of factors, events or recognitions of flaws or failures in existing systems.

The tensions between policy and practice, legislation and implementation in the workplace may result in a critical issue being addressed and revised legislation emerging to strengthen practice. This is seen in the recent publication of *Every Child Matters* (2003) but also in the revised Code of Practice for Children with Special Educational Needs where the place of parents has been strengthened.

Conclusion

We have tackled a broad range of issues within this chapter. The selection of critical issues in this chapter reflects those issues that are important at the time of writing; however, as change in this area is so rapid you may wish to use our discussion as a model for other critical key issues in the early years. As you reflect on the issues we have identified for you in this chapter you will develop your understanding of issues that underlie practice in early years settings. Some of these issues relate to legislation, others to practice and embedded within your approach to these issues are your values and personal beliefs. To extend your ability and competence in reflection on issues, you may wish to consider an issue that has emerged in the media over the past few weeks. A key aspect of an issue being critical is its relevance to critical debate. Academic books and journals may provide background reading to support your understanding of the issue, but it will be through the media that you will access critical and active debate.

You should now feel more confident in identifying and analysing critical issues. As your studies extend into the second stage of your degree so will the expectations of your skills of critical reflection. Look at the sources of your evidence to see if there is any bias in the approach taken towards an issue. By these means you will be able to present an objective reflection upon a controversial issue and demonstrate competence in reflection and analysis.

References and further reading

Ahmed, K., 'Smacking by Childminders to be Banned', *The Observer* (4/5/03) (www.guardianunlimited.co.uk)

Baker, A. and Duncan, S. (1985), 'Child sexual abuse – a study of prevalence in Great Britain', *Child Abuse and Neglect*, 9: pp457–67

Batty, D., 'Climbie Inquiry: the issue explained', *The Guardian* (26/2/03) (www.guardianunlimited.co.uk)

Carvel, J. and Boseley, S., 'MP Poised to bring in Bill on Smacking Ban', *The Guardian* (10/10/03) (www.guardianunlimited.co.uk)

Christensen, P.H. (1998), 'Difference and similarity: How children's competence is constituted in illness and its treatment', in Hutchby, I. and Moran-Ellis, J. (eds), *Children and Social Competence*. London: Falmer

Curtis, P., 'Let us teach, say teachers', *The Guardian* (17/2/02) (www.guardianunlimited.co.uk)

Curtis, P., 'Miliband calls on teachers to back workload reforms' *The Guardian* (3/7/03) (www.guardianunlimited.co.uk)

Department of Health and Home Office (2003), 'The Victoria Climbie Inquiry: Report on an Inquiry by Lord Laming'. London: HMSO

DfES (2001), Code of Practice. Annesley: DfES

DoH (2003), 'Every Child Matters'. London: HMSO

DoH (2003), 'Keeping Children Safe'. London: HMSO

DoH (2001), 'The Children Act Now: Messages from Research'. London: HMSO

DoH (2000), 'Framework for Assessment of Children in Need and their Families'. London: HMSO

DoH (1999) 'Working together to Safeguard Children' London: HMSO

Eyre, D. (1999), *Able Children in Ordinary Schools*. London: David Fulton

Fortin, J. (2003), *Children's Rights and the Developing Law*. Oxford: LexisNexis

Kay, J. (2000), 'Working Together: the role of schools in child protection', in *ChildRight*, c170, October 2000

Kolb, D.A. (1984), *Experiential learning: experience as the source of learning and development*. Englewood Cliffs, NJ: Prentice Hall.

Kempe, C. H., Silverman, F., Steele, B., Droegemuller, W. and Silver, H. (1962), 'The battered child syndrome', *Journal of the American Medical Association*, 181:17–24.

MacNaughton, G. (2000), *Rethinking Gender in Early Childhood Education*. London: Paul Chapman

Pettican, K. (1998), 'Child Protection, Welfare and the Law', Chapter 10 in Taylor, J. and Woods, M (eds), *Early Childhood Studies: An Holistic Introduction*. London: Hodder Arnold

Roffey, S. (1999), *Special Needs in the Early Years*. London: David Fulton

Sharp, C. (2002) 'School starting age: European policy and recent research' available at www.nfer.ac.uk

Siraj-Blatchford, I. (1996), 'Why understanding cultural differences is not enough', in Pugh, G. (ed), *Contemporary Issues in the Early Years*. 2nd edition. London: Paul Chapman / National Children's Bureau

Wolfendale, S. and Wooster, J. (1996), 'Meeting special needs in the early years , in Pugh, G. (ed), *Contemporary Issues in the Early Years*. 2nd edition. London: Paul Chapman / National Children's Bureau

Woods, M. (1998), 'Early Childhood Studies – first principles' in Taylor, J. and Woods, M. (eds), *Early Childhood Studies: An Holistic Introduction*. London: Hodder Arnold

Useful websites

www.nc.uk.net
The National Curriculum in England website. It provides ready access to all the National Curriculum documents.

www.ltscotland.com/curriculum/
The Curriculum Guidance in Scotland and links to excellent curriculum support materials.

www.accac.org.uk/publications/ncorders.html
The National Curriculum in Wales may be accessed through this site.

www.ccea.org.uk
National Curriculum in Northern Ireland

www.ofsted.gov.uk
This is the key site for all information relating to Ofsted but there are also useful links to other important critical information from other sources.

www.cache.org.uk
Council for Awards in Children's Care and Education

www.dfes.gov.uk
Department for Education and Skills. This site provides a very wide range of information relating to children and families, for example: fostering and adoption, child protection reports and the Children's Green Paper, Every Child Matters.

www.surestart.gov.uk
The Sure Start website:provides government perspectives on all aspects of child care and education included in this initiative.

www.ltscotland.org.uk
Learning and Teaching Scotland provides information on early years approaches in Scotland, which are very useful for comparative analysis with other national curricula.

Working with parents
Janet Kay

13

This chapter explores the principle of 'partnership with parents' across the range of educare provision for young children. The concept of 'partnership with parents' is critically evaluated within early years education and care, and the range of approaches to partnership is examined. Within this, the real value of the concept of 'partnership with parents' to children, parents and practitioners, is considered, as well as the extent to which genuine and effective partnerships can be achieved. In addition, the extent to which the diverse needs of parents can be met through partnership is evaluated. Finally, the chapter addresses some of the issues that prevent or adversely affect the development of effective partnerships between practitioners, agencies and parents and explores some of the strategies that can be used to overcome these issues.

This chapter addresses the following areas:

⊃ the value of partnership to children, parents and practitioners
⊃ the legislative and policy framework for partnership with parents
⊃ types of parents and factors affecting their involvement in partnership
⊃ what partnership means and types of partnerships
⊃ factors supporting the development of effective partnerships
⊃ factors that may inhibit the development of effective partnerships
⊃ what really works to develop partnerships with parents.

At the end of this chapter you should be able to:

1 understand the concept of 'partnership with parents'
2 critically evaluate this concept
3 identify factors contributing to effective partnerships
4 evaluate how to meet diverse needs through partnerships
5 identify factors that can adversely influence the development of partnership.

For the purposes of this chapter, the term 'parent' is used in respect of any individual who has parental responsibility for a child in his or her care.

Introduction

All practitioners in early years settings, at whatever stage of their career, will be familiar with the concept of 'partnership with parents' in the care and education of young children. Every major legislative or policy document currently influencing, or guiding, practice contains reference to 'partnership' and the importance of ensuring that parents are informed about and involved in strategies and approaches to the care and education of their child. The rationale for promoting this approach is based on the belief that children benefit from the cooperation and collaboration of parents and practitioners in their education and care. There is also the underpinning principle of recognising and acknowledging the importance of the parental role. The Curriculum Guidance for the Foundation Stage states:

> *Parents are children's first and most enduring educators. When parents and practitioners work together in early years settings, the results have a positive impact on the child's development and learning. Therefore, each setting should seek to develop an effective partnership with parents.*
> *(QCA, 2000)*

The vast majority of agencies across the spectrum of providers have policies underpinning this approach, which are promoted to parents and others as an indicator of high standards and good quality 'educare'.

In addition, there is a raft of initiatives that promote partnerships between educare providers and parents, including Education Action Zones, Sure Start and the introduction of home-school agreements.

Why partnership with parents?

The value of the concept of 'partnership with parents' is based on the belief that good working relationships, clear and reciprocal communication, and common goals between parents and professionals are crucial to the successful delivery of effective services to children. Wolfendale (2000:2) states that the rationale for parental involvement in children's education lies mainly in raising educational achievement, but also has other aims:

> ⊃ *Boosting children's well-being by having their parents/carers and teachers working to shared goals on their behalf*
> ⊃ *Enhancing teacher satisfaction that parents are supporting their endeavours*
> ⊃ *Increasing parental knowledge of school processes and thus reassuring them that schools are doing their best by their children.*

Common sense and, for many practitioners, real life experience tell us that 'working together' will reduce the incidences of confusion, misunderstanding and hostility between parents and professionals that can adversely influence effective work with the child. Common sense also tells us that effective partnerships between home and school or nursery will mean that all the adults working with a child will have a good understanding of the child's needs and how these can be best met at home and in the early years setting. Yet many questions about both the principle and practice of 'partnership with parents' need to be critically considered in order to ensure that the factors determining effective 'partnership' are genuinely understood.

Wolfendale (2000:3) acknowledges that the value of 'partnership with parents' has been recognised since it was stated in the Plowden Report (1967) that 'by involving the parents, the children may be helped' (Chapter 4), and the fact that many schools now routinely work closely with parents. However:

> *a number of schools have maintained a rather suspicious not to say distanced view of the benefits of closer working relationships and still regard too much parental presence within schools as an intrusion.*

In many areas of educare, there has not been a lengthy tradition of 'partnership with parents' from which to draw on. The development of local authority care and education in separate strands, which dominated early years provision for such a long time, established in some areas the notion of parents as passive recipients of services for their children, taking whatever services they could get in many cases. The more recent rapid development of childcare places through the implementation of the National Childcare Strategy, particularly in the independent sector, and the increased integration of care and education services in recent years, have given some parents more choices; and with increased choice, parents now have more power in determining the types of services their children receive. This development has not been universal for all families. For example, Pugh (2001:15) argues that 'There is still a shortage of quality, affordable childcare, particularly for children under 3 years of age.' Access to childcare still depends largely on income and location, with inner city and rural families still facing a lack of services or extremely limited choices. However, changes have occurred, and while they remain patchy across the range of types of families, and geographic dispersion, some parents have more power to 'vote with their feet' and remove their children from unsatisfactory educare settings than previously.

Achieving partnerships

The current situation reflects the very diverse range of approaches to 'partnership with parents' and the very diverse types of parents with whom educare settings are working. There is neither a simple formula for achieving effective partnerships, nor for ensuring that all parents are involved. However, there are some key points to consider. These are illustrated in Figure 13.1.

One of the first issues to explore is where the common ground between parents and practitioners exists. What sort of areas should be the focus of 'partnership'? Should this include all aspects of the child's care and education, or should it be limited to areas directly related to the services provided by the early years setting? For example, some schools have rules that prevent children from bringing sweets and chocolate bars to school for lunch or snacks. These rules relate directly to an area that may be considered by some to be firmly in the parent's domain – the child's diet and eating habits. Is this an area over which schools should have

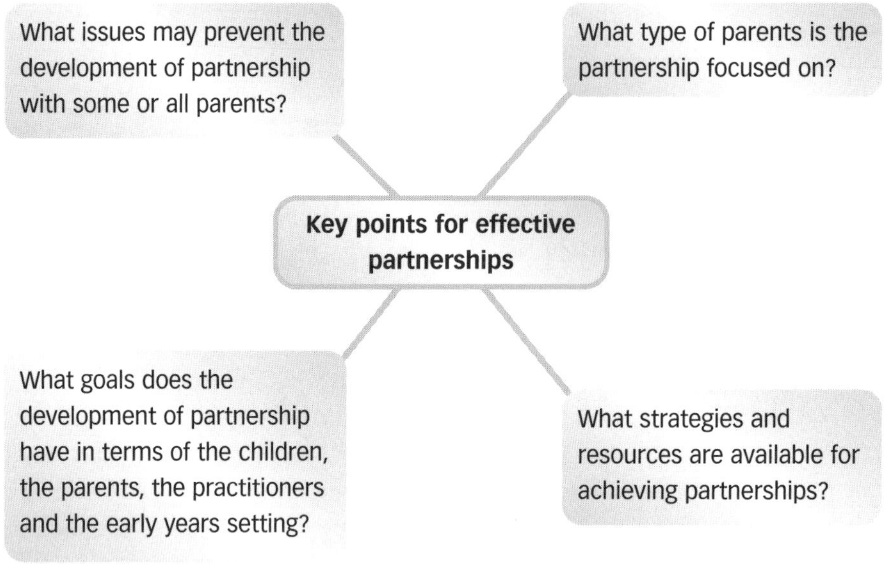

Figure 13.1
Achieving effective partnerships: some key points

What issues may prevent the development of partnership with some or all parents?

What type of parents is the partnership focused on?

Key points for effective partnerships

What goals does the development of partnership have in terms of the children, the parents, the practitioners and the early years setting?

What strategies and resources are available for achieving partnerships?

jurisdiction? Or should they leave this to parents, and concentrate on teaching and learning? Some would argue that parents have a right to feed their children as they like. Others would argue that children's diet affects their overall health and well-being and, as such, has an influence on their ability to learn across the whole curriculum and to access good quality care.

> **Activity 1** **Concerns of parents with young children**

1 Write a list of issues that you think concern the parents of young children. Use your own experience and/or ask others what they think parents are concerned about in respect of their children.

2 Looking through your list, identify which of these issues should be the concern of educarers.

3 Share your ideas with a colleague or mentor and ask for their views.

It is likely that the issues about young children that practitioners will share with parents will be mainly in the areas of:

- learning development
- emotional and social development
- Special Educational Needs (SEN) or disabilities that impact on learning development
- support for parents in the parenting task
- socio-economic disadvantage that impacts on child development.

However, other areas of partnership with parents that may be of concern to some educare settings or services may be:

- parent education and training
- parent input into managing/running/decision-making in the service or early years setting

○ parents developing community-based services to meet their own needs.

○ The value of partnership to children, parents and
○ practitioners

The rationale for developing and sustaining partnerships with parents is based on the belief that, for a variety of reasons, promoting partnerships with parents in the early years will lead to positive outcomes for children, families, practitioners and settings, and communities and society as a whole. In this section, we examine the evidence that supports these beliefs, which underpin the commitment of resources to developing and promoting partnership with parents across a diverse range of approaches, settings and projects.

The value of partnership with parents

It is clear that the ability of parents to engage in activities that support the development of partnership is a strong indicator of success. Families, however, are diverse in their composition, their stability, their effectiveness in parenting their children, and their flexibility in responding to change. The traditional view, that parents from economically successful middle-class homes are likely to be more successful in engaging with partnerships in the early years than families from lower socio-economic groups, needs to be challenged as a stereotype which may hinder the progress of partnership. But how do we measure the contributions of families to the effectiveness of early years education and care? With reference to the role of parents in school, Bastiani (2000:20) argues that the effectiveness of the contributions of the family:

○ *Whose existence as a key player is recognised by many schools and teachers, but underplayed or even ignored by others;*

○ *Whose main influences take place before full-time schooling even begins;*

○ *Which exists independently of much of the everyday life and work of schools;*

○ *Whose responsibilities and influences are both wider and longer term than those of schools'*

is very difficult to assess. Bastiani argues that a family's contribution to school success is largely hidden, and that measuring it is hampered by the fluid nature of family life and wide variations in family types and behaviour.

The problems with measuring the contribution of parent partnership to success are compounded by the diverse ways in which partnership is perceived and implemented. Is a setting successful if compliant parents agree to support their children in ways suggested by the practitioners and sanctioned by the establishment? Or can success be more easily measured

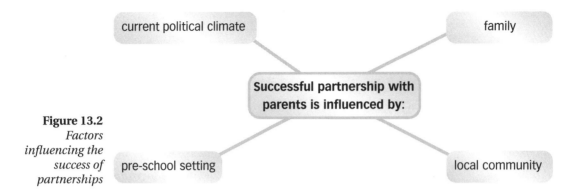

Figure 13.2
Factors influencing the success of partnerships

current political climate

family

Successful partnership with parents is influenced by:

pre-school setting

local community

when parents have a significant influence on the core functions of the setting, such as in some pre-schools that are largely staffed by parent volunteers?

The extent to which 'partnership with parents' is successful depends on a complex range of issues relating to the family, community, establishment, the current climate in early years and many other factors (see Figure 13.2).

Despite the variable nature of partnership and the evidence that many early years settings lack true involvement in and commitment to genuine partnership, Bastiani (2000:21) found a very positive picture in a survey of 11 schools:

> *A majority of the parents and the other main carers in the 11 schools provide regular encouragement and practical support for their children's school learning, are actively engaged as a family in a wide range of 'educational' activities, both in the home and throughout the wider community, and are involved in a range of opportunities that relate to their own learning and development.*

Evaluating benefits

It is probably unnecessary to emphasise to practitioners that developing partnerships with parents requires the commitment of time, resources and energy, and must be based on a firm belief in the benefits of partnership to those involved. Although practitioners are urged to focus their resources on building partnerships with parents, it is not always easy to evaluate the benefits to key individuals. How do we measure, for example, the extent to which partnership helps children's development and learning? Bastiani (2000) suggests a 'What works?' or 'Stakeholder model' for evaluating the contribution of partnership with parents to school effectiveness. This approach is based on a belief that any evaluation must take into account the views of all involved, and draw on evidence from a wide range of sources, charting the perspectives of parents, children and teachers, rather than be based on more limited formal evidence such as OFSTED reports and the extent to which targets have been reached. Evaluation within this model is 'formative and developmental' and 'a continuous task', rather than a periodic snapshot of progress. It is focused on development and using what we know to make further progress and better outcomes.

In order to be effective, this approach to evaluating parent partnership needs to be part of the daily agenda within the early years setting; supported by clearly stated policies and plans for action; and based on an action research type of approach, where evidence is used to plan the next stages of improvement. Although this model is developed with reference to schools, the principles of the approach have meaning for many early years settings. The main benefits of this type of approach are:

- ⊃ ensuring that the effectiveness of partnership is measured from the perspective of all 'stakeholders' – parents, children and practitioners
- ⊃ an ongoing developmental approach within which evidence is translated into action for change
- ⊃ ensuring that there are clear plans and strategies for the development of parent partnership which are embedded in the business of the setting.

How do we know what works and why it works? Evaluating the benefits of different approaches to parent partnership within an early years setting can present a challenge to practitioners. Many approaches that are successful work in a complex range of interrelated ways.

Case Study 1

Parents are invited to school art activities

At one school, parents are invited every year to a week of art activities involving nursery, infants and juniors. The children work on related themes across the classes, and parents are encouraged to work with their children on tasks and projects. At the end of the week, the whole school presents the work in visual images and group performances. The benefits are enormous, involving:

- ⊃ parents gaining a better understanding of what happens in school
- ⊃ parents sharing and developing their own skills
- ⊃ parents having the opportunity to talk to teachers and share ideas and information about their child
- ⊃ children being able to show parents their skills and abilities and share the development of these
- ⊃ children having pride in their own achievements and the achievements of their parents
- ⊃ teachers having the support of other adults to provide a very broad curriculum involving ambitious and complex tasks
- ⊃ teachers having the opportunity to share ideas and information with parents
- ⊃ everybody having fun!

The event is evaluated through many quantitative methods involving feedback from the children as individuals, and through school council; feedback from parents as individuals and through governors and the parents' group; and the teachers' views and perspectives.

Consider one or more of the ways in which partnership with parents is promoted in your workplace. Suggest how the value of the approaches used could be assessed and who would be involved in this.

The value of parent partnership

Parent partnership is of value to all the 'stakeholders' involved. See Figure 13.3.

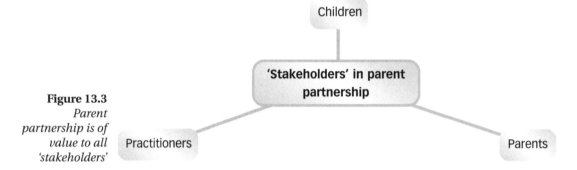

Figure 13.3
Parent partnership is of value to all 'stakeholders'

The value to children

Children benefit from better working relationships between practitioners and the closer involvement of their parents with the early years setting on a number of interrelated fronts. Perhaps the key benefit to young children is continuity, as defined by Draper and Duffy (2001). See Figure 13.4.

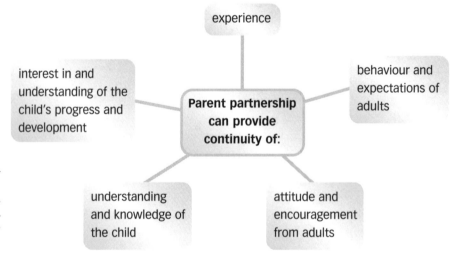

Figure 13.4
Parent partnership can provide continuity (Draper and Duffy, 2001)

Children also learn and develop better in an environment where there are good relationships between the adults around them, based on mutual respect.

Child with a developmental delay

When Davey first went to Cherubs Nursery, he was just 3 years old and developmentally delayed for his age. He received a great deal of support and warmth from one of the nursery staff, who was sensitive to his fears and concerns and who recognised that he became tired and a little anxious towards the end of the afternoon. She would make sure that he had quiet activities when he was tired and during the sing-song, which ended the day, he would often sit next to her for moral and physical support.

Davey's father was relieved to see him gain confidence and start to enjoy the nursery, and he recognised and acknowledged the role of the practitioner in this.

Sharing their ideas and concerns about Davey helped both the father and practitioner to recognise each other's roles and to develop a respect for each other's views and opinions. When Davey's learning difficulties became more apparent and a more structured response was required to meet his needs, the adults in his life had an excellent basis on which to build a closer partnership in order to meet these needs.

An analysis of how the parent partnership in the nursery described in Case study 2 was encouraged is given in Figure 13.5.

Parent partnership in Cherubs Nursery was encouraged by:	
Staff availability at set times	Ensuring that staff were always available at the beginning and end of the day to talk to parents.
Key worker	Having a key worker for each child and ensuring that parents could easily access their child's worker.
Providing a welcome and giving encouragement	Welcoming and encouraging parents to stay for a while in the morning and arrive early to collect so they could see what their children were doing.
Explaining and giving feedback	Explaining the daily activities and giving feedback to parents on what their children had enjoyed and what they had achieved.

Figure 13.5
An analysis of the parent partnership promoted in Case study 2

An analysis of the benefits to children in the Cherubs Nursery is shown in Figure 13.6.

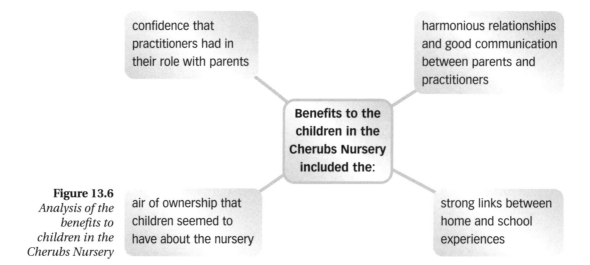

Figure 13.6
Analysis of the benefits to children in the Cherubs Nursery

confidence that practitioners had in their role with parents

harmonious relationships and good communication between parents and practitioners

Benefits to the children in the Cherubs Nursery included the:

air of ownership that children seemed to have about the nursery

strong links between home and school experiences

The value to parents

The role of parenting has changed considerably since the mid-twentieth century. As child-centred approaches to parenting have become increasingly the norm in Western cultures, parenting has become in some ways more complex and in others more uncertain. Parents are subject to a flood of information and advice about their role, some of it conflicting and subject to change (the debate about whether a baby's sleeping position made it more vulnerable to SIDS, and whether babies should sleep on their backs or fronts for safety reasons is a good example of this, as are the many and varied debates about how we should feed our children). Expectations of parents have also changed from those associated with earlier child-rearing styles, which emphasised good quality physical care and access to education. Now parents are expected to be much more concerned about their children's holistic development and, in particular, social and emotional development. The emphasis on early learning in Western societies has raised questions about what sort of stimuli children should and should not be subjected to from pre-birth onwards.

Parenting is a complicated task with multiple demands and a changing context in which parents need to be knowledgeable about a wide range of issues that may affect their child. Yet the majority of parents have little or no preparation for this momentous task. The separation of extended families in many Western cultures has resulted in fewer opportunities for young people to care for and be involved in parenting babies and young children before they become parents themselves.

Roles and attitudes of practitioners

The benefits of parent partnership to parents depend on the roles and attitude of practitioners. A goal of many early years settings is to encourage parents to feel more confident about their role and to understand that role more fully. Parents need to feel welcome and to be acknowledged as the most important people in their children's lives. Practitioners need to share, rather than display their expertise, and to recognise that some parents may be daunted by their professionalism, training and qualifications.

The benefits of partnership to parents include those illustrated in Figure 13.7.

Benefits to parents of partnership	
Support and understanding	Support and understanding for their parenting role from experienced professionals.
Shared ideas and expertise	Someone to share ideas and expertise within the task of supporting children's learning and development.
Reflective and balanced feedback	Reflective and balanced feedback about the child's progress and achievements.
Encouragement and help	Encouragement and help with areas of uncertainty, for example, developing children's play.
Involvement and expertise	A sense of involvement and expertise in the role of child-rearing.
Opportunities for self-development	Opportunities for self-development in the field of childcare and education, possibly professional development.

Figure 13.7
Partnership: benefits to parents

The value to practitioners

The benefits of parent partnership for practitioners are well documented, and focus on improving knowledge in order to better meet the educational and care needs of the children they are involved with. However, not all practitioners feel sure about the benefits of partnership with parents. It may be that their training has helped them to develop skills with children, but less so with adults. Some practitioners may feel uncertain about the prospect of sharing their expertise or lack confidence in explaining the basis and rationale of their approach to childcare and education in the early years. Others may feel that parenting and professional work in the early years are separate issues and should remain so. It may be that some practitioners feel that they are not equipped to work with parents who come from diverse cultural and linguistic backgrounds. However, those who are enthusiastic about and involved in actively developing parent partnerships will be aware of the benefits.

Benefits to practitioners of parent partnership include those factors shown in Figure 13.8.

Benefits to practitioners include learning and sharing knowledge about:	
Specific needs of children	Learning more about the specific needs of the children in their care
Different types of family life	Learning what they need to know about different types of family life, cultures, languages and religions
What parents do with their young children	Learning what parents do with their young children and how this relates, or can be related, to activities in the early years setting
Diversity	Learning about diverse ways of managing children's behaviour, supporting children's learning and helping children to develop across the range of indicators
Range of challenges	Learning about the range of challenges parents face and the support that they can get to face these
Supporting parents in the parenting task	Learning how to support parents in the parenting task and how difficulties may arise within this task
Sharing	Sharing knowledge and understanding, fears and concerns, successes and breakthroughs in the education and care of young children

Figure 13.8
The benefits to practitioners of parent partnership

It is important for practitioners to recognise that many parents are daunted by their professionalism and expertise, and are relieved to discover that practitioners can be warm, friendly and supportive human beings.

The parents who drop off their children as quickly as possible and pick them up in a hurry, without pause for a chat, may not be indifferent to the children's experiences in the early years setting or lacking in concern about how they are behaving, progressing, settling in or achieving. They may simply feel they do not have the experience, the language or the confidence to talk about their children's progress and achievement, activities and developmental stage. Parents may not share a common language with practitioners; they may come from very different socio-cultural backgrounds and have very different views on children's education and care. Practitioners can gain a great deal for themselves, the parents and the children if they take the lead in developing good relationships with all parents.

Practitioners also have a responsibility within the legislative and policy framework supporting the education and care of young children to ensure that the quality of this work is enhanced through effective partnerships with parents.

The legislative and policy framework for partnership with parents

The concept of 'partnership with parents' is rooted in the major legislative and policy documents and guidelines providing a framework for practice across the range of educare provision. This concept is firmly entrenched in political and policy development within the fields of education and early years. Shah (2001), however, argues that within the concept of parents as consumers of education for their children, parents have been presented as an homogenous group by governments promoting 'parent's rights' in schools, and that this has harmed relationships between teachers and parents. Bastiani (2000) also raises doubts about the ways in which 'parent partnership' is perceived and presented, pointing out that there is a body of evidence outlining major differences between the perspectives of schools and parents and suggesting that contact between the two can lead to tension, as well as promote partnership. Despite these reservations, parent partnership is a central tenet of legislation and policy influencing the early years.

The Children Act (1989) establishes the principle that parents must be viewed as partners in all legal transactions concerning their children and, as such, must be informed, treated with respect and consulted about their wishes. To some extent, the legislative and policy framework determines the areas in which practitioners are expected to be working with parents; the reasoning behind the need for such partnerships; and how they should be approached. For example, in the Curriculum Guidance for the Foundation Stage (DfES, 2000) it is stated that 'Parents and practitioners should work together in an atmosphere of mutual respect within which children can have security and confidence.'

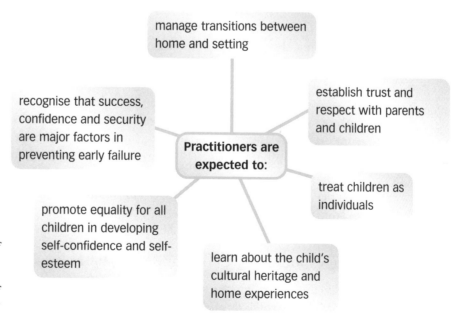

Figure 13.9
Expectations of practitioners in promoting an atmosphere of mutual respect

manage transitions between home and setting

recognise that success, confidence and security are major factors in preventing early failure

establish trust and respect with parents and children

Practitioners are expected to:

treat children as individuals

promote equality for all children in developing self-confidence and self-esteem

learn about the child's cultural heritage and home experiences

The guidance focuses on the need to understand the child's background and early experiences in order to give the child the best opportunities to achieve, through both positively acknowledging the child as an individual, and incorporating the child's early experience in learning activities. In order to achieve this understanding, practitioners are expected to develop relationships with parents through which their understanding of the child's culture, background and individual needs can be shared. In this case, the guidance clearly states both the purpose of developing partnerships with parents and the benefits that are anticipated for children when such partnerships are effective.

The SEN Code of Practice guidelines, the 'SEN Toolkit' (DfES, 2001)

The SEN Code of Practice guidelines, the 'SEN Toolkit' (DfES, 2001) emphasises the areas shown in Figure 13.10 for working with parents.

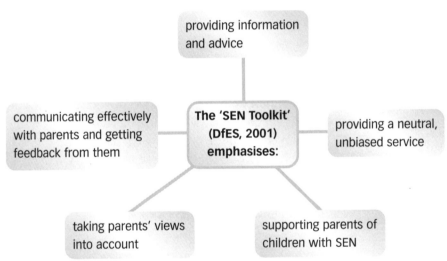

Figure 13.10
Emphasis of the 'SEN Toolkit'

In this area, the guidance emphasises that parents should be listened to and supported in dealing with the complex systems available to support children with SEN. The focus of partnership is on ensuring that parents have good quality information about their child's needs and how these can be assessed and met. Involving parents in their child's assessment and support is considered crucial to ensuring success in promoting the child's global development. Roffey (1999) argues that there has been less support for and involvement with parents at the earlier stages of the Code of Practice, but that independent support for parents and the dissemination of good practice have been introduced to address this.

The National Day Care Standards (2001)

This includes 'work in partnership with parents and carers' as one of the 14 standards on which day care providers and childminders are inspected.

Inspectors are also required to include parents in assessments. However, as Baldock (2001) points out, this can be difficult to achieve when parents are occupied with work and other activities.

Sure Start guidance (2000)

This confirms the current emphasis on the role of parents and other family members in children's learning and development. Within these projects, supporting parents in their own growth and development and their own learning is seen as central to ensuring that children receive support in their pre-school years. The projects are built on the principle that involving parents is the key issue in ensuring a better start for young children. Parent participation is, therefore, a central tenet of the Sure Start philosophy.

Focus of partnerships

These examples highlight the different areas within the legislative and policy framework in which 'partnerships with parents' need to be developed. It is clear that not all partnerships have the same focus or purpose. The type of service, the aims of the service, and the ways in which the service is delivered are all factors that influence the purposes of 'partnership with parents.' For example, in the delivery of child protection services under the Children Act (1989), the development of good relationships with parents has a number of purposes. Under the Children Act (1989), the purposes of developing good relationships with parents include:

- sharing information in order to assess the child's situation
- identifying areas of strengths and weaknesses in parenting
- gaining parental support for plans to protect the child
- gaining access to the child and information about risks to the child
- monitoring the child 'at risk'
- avoiding conflict with parents that could put the child and workers at risk.

In looking at this list, we could surmise that not all the purposes identified are necessarily seen as beneficial to the parent's position, from the parent's point of view. They also imply quite a different type of partnership to that suggested by the Curriculum Guidance for the Foundation Stage (DfES, 2000).

It is important to consider both the expectations of your relationships with parents and the purposes of these in order to understand the concept of 'partnership with parents' within your early years setting. It is also important to recognise that these expectations and purposes will differ between early years settings and agencies, and that this will have implications for multidisciplinary and inter-agency work.

1 Read through the relevant sections in the range of documents influencing or prescribing the work of your early years setting. The list could include some of the following, or other guidelines depending on your early years setting:

⊃ The Children Act (1989)

⊃ SEN Code of Practice

⊃ Curriculum Guidance for the Foundation Stage (2000)

⊃ National Curriculum (1999)

⊃ Sure Start guidance (2000)

2 Make a note of what is expected within your setting in terms of 'partnership with parents', and what the key themes are within the guidelines.

Themes on the purposes of partnership

Although 'partnership with parents' is not a single concept, there are some common themes on the purposes of partnership within the different aspects of the legislative and policy framework. These themes are given in Figure 13.11.

Common themes on purposes of partnership	
Adequate information	Ensuring that parents have adequate information to access and use educare services effectively
Communicating	Communicating with parents about the child's individual experiences and background in order to understand his or her needs
Providing a forum	Providing a forum for parents to express concerns or complaints about services to their child
Feedback	Ensuring that parents have feedback on their child's progress and attainments
Information about other services	Ensuring that parents have information about other services that will help them to support their child.

Figure 13.11
Legislative and policy framework: some common themes on the purposes of partnership

The themes illustrated in Figure 13.11 are rooted in the belief that knowledge empowers parents and can support better access to educare services and a deeper involvement in the care and education of their children. However, the extent to which parents can access and apply this knowledge varies greatly.

Types of parents and factors affecting their involvement in partnerships

In this section, we discuss the different types of parents who become involved in partnerships and consider the factors that affect their involvement.

Diverse socio-cultural contexts of parenting

One of the problematical issues with the concept of 'partnership with parents' is that parents are sometimes presented as an homogenous group, although, as all practitioners are very aware, parents vary greatly. 'Partnership with parents' is often presented as a concept relating equally to all parents, but evidence shows that there are differences in the extent to which parents become involved in partnerships with educare settings. Research findings suggest that women are much more involved in their children's care and education than men and that levels of involvement with school are also determined by race, culture and class (Vincent, 1996). These findings raise a number of questions:

- Why are some parents more likely to be involved in partnership than others?
- How does this impact on the children involved?
- What strategies can be used to involve a wider range of parents in partnership?

Different types of learning in the home

It is commonly accepted that parents have the most significant role to play in their children's early learning. Parents teach their children about the

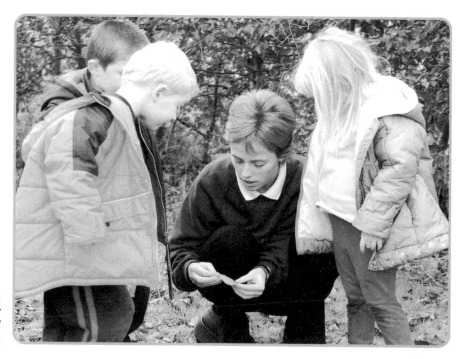

Children can learn in the home and garden

world around them, providing experiences, information and explanations as part of the day-to-day interaction between themselves and their child. The range of these experiences, the ways in which the child perceives his or her environment, and the type of cultural values and norms the child absorbs will vary significantly between families, as will the languages used within the home and the quality and quantity of communication between family members.

Social and cultural contexts

The type of learning children access within the family is linked to the social and cultural context within which the family exists. Barratt-Pugh (2000) illustrates this point in discussion of the complex and variable ways in which children develop literacy. She argues that children develop literacies according to the socio-cultural context of their family life. However, for some children, the literacies they learn in the home have less value than others when they access more formal learning situations. She states that:

> This puts some children at a disadvantage as soon as they enter formal learning contexts, where their knowledge and experiences of literacy are not recognised or built on. (Barratt-Pugh, 2000: 4)

Whilst children and families have a very wide range of understandings about what literacy is, there is evidence that 'the sorts of literacy practices carried out across educational settings appear to be quite similar' (Barratt-Pugh, 2000:20). The implications for children's learning in early years settings is determined by the ways in which some children's types of literacies are valued more than others within the setting because they more closely match the setting's own literacies, resulting in advantage to certain children over others. Drury (2000:86) also points out that we must be careful to note the discontinuities between home and setting as well as the continuities, and she gives an example about how easy it is to make assumptions about a child's home learning experiences.

In terms of partnerships with parents in developing children's early learning there are some significant considerations to be drawn from these observations. Parents who have socio-cultural roots in common with practitioners, and who support their children's learning in ways which correlate with those within the early years setting, may be more likely to enter into partnerships with the early years setting than parents who may have other socio-cultural backgrounds and different types of learning in the home.

The result may be that some parents develop close bonds with the early years setting, matching the learning styles found there and providing their children with closely connected home/setting experiences; others, however, may connect less readily with the early years setting and the children may experience dislocation between what they learn at home and in the early years setting. This may impact on the child's confidence and enthusiasm for learning, and may result in the child being less likely to take advantage of learning opportunities.

Inequalities in access to partnerships

A significant issue for those who are responsible for developing and maintaining partnerships with parents is to acknowledge and address the inequalities in access to such partnerships. Within this there are a number of issues to consider:

- ⊃ the ways in which partnerships are developed and whether they focus on and are accessible to all types of parents represented in the early years setting
- ⊃ the social, cultural, psychological and practical barriers parents face in becoming more involved
- ⊃ the power differentials between practitioners and parents, and how these may impact on access to partnership.

> **Activity 4** **Parental involvement in early years setting**

Consider your own early years setting and how parent partnership is planned and encouraged. Observe the type of parents who are closely involved with the early years setting, and those who are not.

1 Why do you think some parents are not involved?
2 Are there any links between the reasons for some parents not being involved and the ways in which parent partnership is promoted within the early years setting?
3 What could be done to encourage different types of parents into partnership with the early years setting?

Aspects of learning in the home

There are other considerations about the role of parents in partnership. It is important to recognise that the majority of parents will support their children's education and care at home and in an early years setting. For some children, however, the support may be minimal or their learning in the home may result in negative outcomes for the child. Not all of the learning that children have in the home is positive in terms of their experiences in the outside world. Some children may learn attitudes, behaviours and concepts of the world around them, which are likely to impede learning and development in an early years setting. Children who:

- ⊃ are abused and neglected
- ⊃ are in families where domestic violence dominates patterns of behaviour within the home

⊃ live in social and cultural isolation through extreme poverty

⊃ live with parents who are limited by drug or alcohol abuse

may not only receive little support at home for their learning and development, but may learn behaviours that make their access to learning in a setting problematical.

Case Study 3

Learning in the home

Sam, 4, started in nursery after his mother received a caution for assaulting him and bruising his face. The family social worker encouraged Sam's mother to take him to nursery because he had global developmental delays. His attendance was erratic, because his mother did not prioritise nursery and efforts to encourage her to become more consistent usually resulted in longer absences. Sam hardly spoke, did not get involved in activities and had occasional angry and aggressive outbursts. At home there was very little communication and day-to-day life was chaotic with no routines or plans. The children were disciplined with slaps and loud angry outbursts. They were given instructions, but there were few conversations. The family had no friends and no contact with other family members or neighbours.

Sam's mother had a fear of, and became angry with, anyone she believed to be an authority figure and Sam reflected her negative stance in his behaviour and attitude in nursery. He was at best uncommunicative with staff and other children, and at worst hostile and aggressive. In Sam's case, his learning in the home had resulted in patterns of behaviour that inhibited his development. He had learned not to talk; he had learned to treat others with suspicion, hostility and anger; he had learned to be withdrawn and to avoid involvement with others; and he had learned that, if others did things that he did not like, the response was to attack them verbally and physically.

Sam's learning in the home reflected the norms within his household, based on his mother's own negative experiences of the wider world and the ways these had shaped her beliefs, her behaviour and the development of her personality. In nursery, he was confused and unhappy because different ways of behaving were expected of him and he had little experience of these.

▶ Activity 5 Involving parents who are unwilling or hostile to partnership

Case study 3 above highlights one of the major issues in 'partnership with parents'. Despite the well-documented benefits of partnership to children, parents and practitioners, how do we engage parents in partnership where they are unwilling to be involved or are hostile to the concept of partnership?

With reference to Activity 4, consider the parents in your service or early years setting who are not involved to any great extent in partnership.

1 Can you find links between the behaviour, learning development and general progress of the child, and the parent's approach to the setting?
2 What sort of strategies could you use to work more closely with the parents and convince them of the benefits of partnership?

Remember to consider issues of confidentiality when discussing or writing about parents and sensitive issues.

Practitioners need to develop knowledge and understanding

The key issue to consider is not what 'parents' in general need in order to become more involved in partnership, but what the parents of the children you work with need in order to become involved. Practitioners must develop knowledge and understanding of the range of cultural, linguistic, economic and social contexts in which the parents they work with live and raise their children. This knowledge is crucial to developing strategies to involve more parents in partnership and it is unique to each early years setting or service. How this knowledge and understanding can be translated into positive action for developing inclusive partnerships will be explored later in the chapter. The next section analyses the various meanings of 'partnership with parents'.

What partnership means and types of partnership

The term 'partnership with parents' is somewhat glibly used to describe a whole range of ways in which parents and practitioners work together.

Equal partners?

However, 'partnership' can mean lots of different types of 'working together' arrangements depending on a number of factors. One of these factors is the extent to which parents and practitioners are equal in the partnership. Vincent (2000) developed her model of parental involvement with educational establishments with reference to what she describes as 'subject positions'. She refers to the 'parent as supporter/learner' position as the partnership between parents and teachers, but argues that:

> ... such 'partnerships', with the connotations of equality inherent in the term, are often legitimating devices used by schools to encourage parental support for their aims and objectives. (Vincent (2000:5)

The view that partnerships between schools and parents are not equal, in that the goals of the partnership are determined by the school and not the parents, is widespread. The role of parents in relationship to the early years setting can seem to be to conform to expectations of the practitioners and to perform functions suggested by the early years setting.

The ways in which partnerships with parents are developed within an early years setting and the perceptions that both parents and practitioners have about the purposes and goals of the partnership are crucial in determining the success of the partnership for all involved. As such, it is important to ensure that partnerships are based on a sense of participation by all involved, rather than dominated entirely by the perceptions of the early years setting and those who work in it. Yet to what extent does this seem practical or desirable? Parents may want very different things from partnership to those that are on offer.

The role of partnership must be based on areas of work where partnership is both possible and desirable. The key issue is how to establish genuine opportunities for communication between parents and practitioners and a clear concept of the areas in which partnership can be effectively developed.

> **Activity 6**   **Who determines what?**

1   With reference to your own work setting or service, consider the ways in which parents are involved in the work of the setting, or supporting their children's learning at home, or any other relevant function. Who determines the following?

  ⊃ The areas in which parents are involved, for example, supporting literacy at home.

  ⊃ The ways in which that involvement is expressed, for example, reading to the child.

  ⊃ The extent and level of the involvement, for example, reading with children in class.

2   Try and evaluate the extent to which parents determine what 'parent partnership' is about within the setting and discuss with a mentor or colleague to find out their views.

This poses the question about what evidence there is for partnerships with parents, within which parents have genuine power to determine the extent, goals and purposes of the partnership; and how the partnership is established, maintained and evaluated.

One of the key issues here is the extent to which parents have a sense of empowerment that will support them working in equal partnership with professionals, especially parents who have negative views of learning formed through their own experiences and family background. An example of the importance of supporting parents to choose to take a greater role in partnership is enshrined in the principles and goals of the Sure Start projects, which function partly to empower parents to sustain community based projects supporting families and children in the early years. The main goals of the Sure Start projects are shown in Figure 13.12.

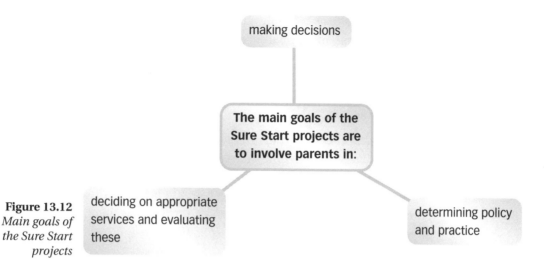

making decisions

The main goals of the Sure Start projects are to involve parents in:

deciding on appropriate services and evaluating these

determining policy and practice

Figure 13.12
Main goals of the Sure Start projects

This concept of practitioners supporting and empowering parents to participate more fully in decision-making, policy development and practice is not new. However, it is not universally applied in early years contexts, and in many 'partnerships with parents' there remains room to develop the parent's role to one that involves higher levels of responsibility and equality with practitioners.

Types of partnerships with parents

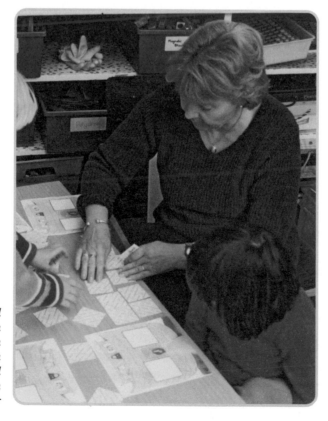

Parental involvement can be focused on helping children settle into school in the Reception year

'Partnerships with parents' appear in many different guises, many reflecting the specific purposes for which the partnership has been developed. For example, a key goal of the Sure Start projects is to improve the attainment of children at Key Stage 1. To achieve this, the projects focus on developing parent partnerships when children are very young, in order to facilitate the delivery of services to remedy what are perceived as deficits in all aspects of the children's early development. The additional goal in this situation is to help parents to become educated in community development and in sustaining community resources in order to ensure that services continue after the Sure Start funding is phased out. In the case of Sure Start, the objectives are targeted and the level of involvement is high.

In a reception class, 'partnership with parents' may focus more on helping children to settle into school, developing children's learning skills, and sharing information about a child's needs and how these can be met. The level of the parent's involvement is less intense and the parent's efforts tend to focus on their own child. The goals of partnership are general, but may become more specific if the child has any particular or special needs.

There are two dimensions on which types of 'partnerships with parents' can be explored:

- ⊃ the purposes for which 'partnership with parents' is promoted
- ⊃ the extent to which parents are involved in aspects of the service.

In other words, we can explore different aspects of the concept of 'partnership with parents' by evaluating the range of partnership types and the extent of parental involvement in the partnership. For example, Willey (2000:1) discusses the ways in which parents used to be involved in nursery education at her child's school. The children were left at the school gates and collected from the playground. Contact with teachers was restricted to assemblies and parents' evenings. A few parents were invited to help with practical tasks. The purpose of this type of 'partnership with parents' seemed to be based on the need for parents to have limited and formally presented information about their children's progress and achievements. The extent of the 'partnership' was limited.

Approaches to developing partnership with parents fall into a number of different categories as shown in Figure 13.13:

Universal approaches	Potentially involve all parents and children, for example, parents' evenings, open days.
Targeted approaches	Focus on particular parents and children, for example, parent partnership approaches within the SEN Code of Practice, literacy summer schools.
Community-based approaches	Focus on socially and economically disadvantaged geographical areas, for example, Sure Start, Education Action Zones.

Figure 13.13
Developing partnership with parents: differing approaches

Activity 7) Types of partnership with parents

Consider the types of partnership with parents in which you are involved in your service or setting.

1 What determines the type of partnership?

2 Which types of partnerships are most effective in involving a diverse range of parents?

3 What other types of partnership would benefit 'stakeholders' in your service or setting?

Factors supporting the development of effective partnerships

In this section we look at the factors that support the development of effective partnerships.

Partnership in context

The factors that may support the development of a partnership are, to some extent, contextual. The types of approaches and strategies that may work in one situation may be ineffective in another, depending on various factors, as illustrated in Figure 13.14.

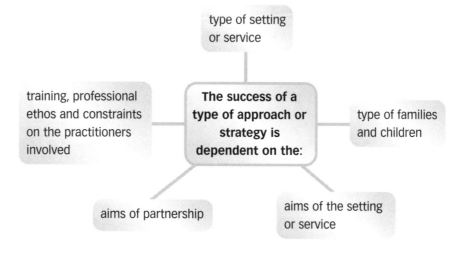

Figure 13.14
Factors determining the success of an approach or strategy in specific early years settings

Every partnership will have unique elements based on the factors shown in Figure 13.14, particularly the individuals involved in partnership.

Who is responsible?

A key question at this point could be to determine who is responsible for ensuring the development of effective partnerships? This is a complex question, relating to the power differentials between parents and practitioners and the barriers to both practitioners and parents getting involved in genuine partnership.

The legal and policy framework seems to suggest that the bulk of the motivation for partnership comes from practitioners as part of their professional responsibilities to the children in their care. This view may be supported by the fact that often the agenda for partnership is presented as one that originates from the early years setting or service and is supported by documentation outlining goals and objectives for the service and how they can be achieved more effectively through partnership. This type of approach seems to be based on an underpinning belief that parents are more passive in developing partnerships and more compliant in determining the goals of partnership than the early years setting or services. However, parents may have their own goals and motivations for involving, or not involving, themselves in partnerships, based on a number of complex and interrelated factors:

➲ the parent's own social, cultural and learning experience of education as a child and adult
➲ the family's relationship with agencies, professionals and authority
➲ the parent's views on the value and place of educare
➲ the parent's views on the deficits or problems they perceive in the educare system and how this impacts on themselves and their children
➲ the parent's own agenda for their own child
➲ the family's cultural, social, religious and linguistic background and how this shapes their approach to their children's education and care.

These factors will influence the willingness and ability of parents to involve themselves in partnership with early years settings and services, and the goals that parents may have for such partnerships.

Clearly, what needs to be acknowledged is that:

➲ parents will have their own agendas for partnership
➲ these agendas will differ between parents and may be different to the goals of the early years setting
➲ not all parents will initially have a positive view of partnership
➲ parents will have different levels of motivation, ability and skills to get involved in partnership
➲ these factors will be unique to each early years setting or situation.

Case Study 4

Three different families

Consider three different families whose children are going to nursery school for the first time. The children are all aged 3 and a half.

Shirley and Danny

Shirley is desperate for Danny to start nursery. He is extremely lively and demanding and, since his father left two years ago, Shirley has received little help with him. Sometimes she becomes very tired or angry with Danny and she feels that she never has a moment to herself. Shirley believes Danny may be bright, but she does not know much about helping him to learn, although she reads him stories sometimes. She does not play with him much, as she finds it boring and she does not see the point. Shirley did not enjoy her own school years and left with few qualifications. She had a job in a sandwich shop but has not worked since she became pregnant with Danny. It does not occur to Shirley that she will have a relationship with the reception teacher unless Danny is naughty at school.

Alex, Mary and Rose

Alex and Mary sent their other two children to nursery school and feel that it supported their early learning development and helped them to do well in school. They are very keen on learning in the home and have a wide range of educational toys and books for the children to use. They both spend time reading with Rose and helping the older children with maths and other homework. Alex and Mary have considered private schools but they believe in state education and want their children to benefit and do well in school. However, they are concerned about class sizes and the amount of individual time children receive in classes of 30. They also feel that standards in schools may be slipping and are determined that this will not affect Rose's education as they believe she is a gifted child.

Shiraz, Safina and Jamal

Shiraz works long hours and is often away from home so Safina has the main responsibility for Jamal, their only child. Safina, who came from Pakistan shortly before Jamal's birth, has little contact with English speakers in her community and does not speak much English although she would like to learn. She is worried that Jamal will be unhappy in school because of language problems. Safina is also worried that the school has no non-white teachers or Punjabi speakers. She wonders how Jamal will be supported and helped in a largely white school and whether he will be bullied.

> **Activity 8** **Differences between families**

1 With reference to each of the families outlined in Case study 4, try and think about:

- ⊃ the parent's agenda
- ⊃ strategies to meet this agenda through partnership
- ⊃ the approaches that may work to help the parent become involved in partnership
- ⊃ what issues, if any, may arise to cause tension between the school and parents.

2 Look at the differences between the families in the case study in terms of their needs, how they can be met, and the problems in achieving this. Try the exercise with reference to different types of families you are involved with.

Building partnerships

In order to build genuine and effective partnerships, practitioners need to consider the following in relation to their own early years setting or service:

- ⊃ the diverse needs of parents
- ⊃ a range of different approaches to involve parents
- ⊃ the fact that some parents will initially be more responsive than others
- ⊃ the fact that some parents may be negative about or even hostile to the concept of partnership
- ⊃ that achieving partnership requires planning, short- and long-term goals and a range of strategies to meet diverse needs

Draper and Duffy (2001:151) suggest that successful partnerships need to be based on sharing information, sharing decision-making, sharing responsibility and accountability.

Discussion Point

Building partnerships in your setting

Building partnerships with parents takes time and cannot be achieved overnight. In order to ensure partnerships have a secure basis, they need to be rooted in the day-to-day activities of the setting or services, and not a series of isolated events to involve parents on a temporary basis. They also need to involve all types of parents, not just those willing and able to join in the activities of the setting. Practitioners need to be committed to the concept and practice of partnership.

Using the list above, consider how these factors are addressed in your workplace on a day-today setting. Share your views with a mentor or colleague and discuss their views also.

Skills for building partnerships

A key factor of effective partnership is the extent to which genuine participative communication takes place between parents and practitioners. Fisher (2000) discusses the need to have 'conversations with parents' in order to learn more about the child as a learner:

A good case for home visiting is made when teachers recount what they have learnt from seeing the child in the surroundings of their own home, and how relationships change when parents meet teachers on their own territory… (Fisher, 2000:22)

It may be difficult to have conversations with some parents who may avoid engaging with you or the early years setting as a whole. Tips that may help you to hold conversations in these cases are given in Figure 13.15.

Communicate regularly	Ensure that regular communication is part of the work of the early years setting or service, for example, written communication, phone calls, informal discussion.
Actively seek out 'hard to reach' parents	Seek out 'hard to reach' parents and encourage them to share information with you about their child.
Give regular feedback about child	Give regular verbal feedback on the child's progress and achievement as well as more formal methods of conveying information to parents; for example, conversations at the beginning and end of the day, feedback on the child's work and progress.
Recognise parents' reasons for avoidance	Recognise that parents may avoid involvement for many and varied reasons.
Seek parents' views and opinions	Ask parents for views and opinions, and ask for advice about their child.
Plan	Make plans and strategies with parents for dealing with issues about their child.

Figure 13.15
Tips for participative communication with parents who may avoid engaging with practitioners or early years settings

Case Study 5

Using communication skills in building partnerships

Harriet entered reception class in a primary school when she was nearly 5 years old. Although her general development did not give cause for concern, the nursery she attended had noted that her social development was delayed and that she had difficulty relating to other children and joining in. She did not seem able to make friends easily or feel confident with others. She had some skills in dealing with other children on a one-to-one basis, but these disappeared when with a group. Harriet spent many of her breaks alone or with the lunchtime supervisor.

Harriet's teacher waited in the playground and spoke to Harriet's mother when she collected her. The teacher commented on Harriet's work and good progress with reading. She also commented on how helpful Harriet was in the class and the good standards of work she produced. She then commented that she was a little bit concerned that Harriet was shy with other children and found it hard to join in. Harriet's mother agreed that Harriet had always found it difficult to make friends. The teacher asked if Harriet's mother could come into school so they could make plans together to help Harriet gain confidence with others. She implied that the mother's knowledge and expertise on her own child would be invaluable in helping devise a successful strategy. She also suggested several different times in order to find one to suit the mother. The mother agreed and the meeting took place.

Analysis of skills used by teacher in case study 5

The teacher in Case study 5 was using her communication skills to:

- ⊃ engage the mother with the concerns she had
- ⊃ help the mother feel that she had much to offer in seeking a solution to her child's difficulties
- ⊃ help the mother feel that she was not being critical but wanted to support the child
- ⊃ develop a sense of partnership between the two of them.

Good communication is a key to effective partnership. The attributes of good communicators are shown in Figure 13.16.

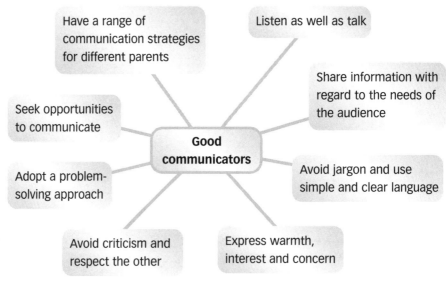

Figure 13.16
Attributes of good communicators

⊃ Factors that may inhibit the development of ⊃ effective partnerships

In this section we look at the range of factors that may inhibit the development of partnership and strategies to address these.

Parents

Parents have diverse motivations, agendas, and skills to bring to partnership with early years settings. Some will want to have a high level of involvement; others may appear to want to have no involvement at all.

Some may want to be involved but do not know how to engage; others may be hostile, even aggressive in their relationship with practitioners.

Figure 13.17 illustrates those factors that may influence parents' contributions to partnership.

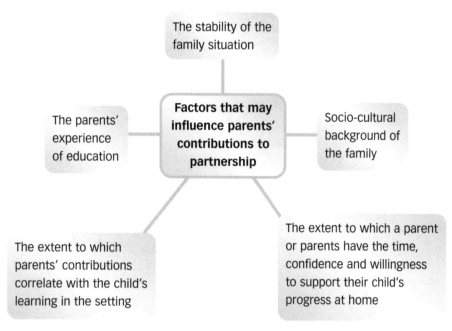

Figure 13.17 *Factors that determine parents' involvement with partnership*

Practitioners

The factors that influence the extent to which practitioners are committed to developing partnerships with parents are shown in Figure 13.18.

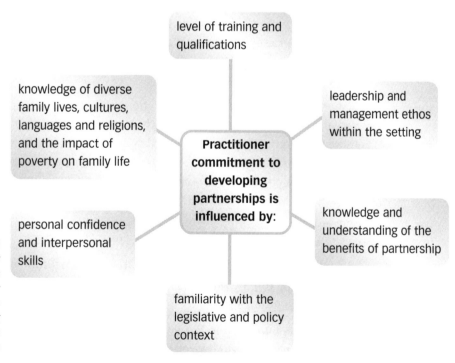

Figure 13.18 *Factors that influence practitioner commitment to developing partnerships with parents*

Early years organisations

Practitioners bring their own contributions to the development of partnership, but a key factor will be the level of commitment the work setting or organisation has to partnership and the management ethos in respect of the 'genuineness' of a partnership approach. Factors that may influence the organisational approach are shown in Figure 13.19.

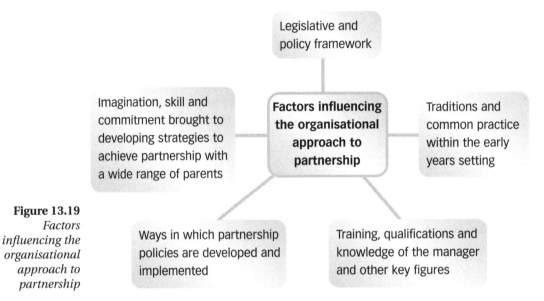

Figure 13.19
Factors influencing the organisational approach to partnership

What really works to develop partnership with parents?

In this final section we discuss strategies and approaches that work to develop partnership and ways of overcoming the inhibiting factors listed above. The strategies suggested are those that have been successful. However, Willey (2000:94) points out that 'There is no single model for working with parents that would meet the needs of every setting'.

Fisher (2002) suggests that parents should be given invitations to join in activities or use resources in the early years setting before the child starts there. She argues that such informal contacts are valuable in engaging parents as well as more formal contact. It is important to consider the extent to which parents may need support to become involved and what help they may need to access facilities. This could include:

- asking an experienced parent to 'befriend' a parent who lacks confidence
- showing parents around to familiarise them with the facilities
- checking that invitations are given in a medium that is understandable to the recipient.

Practitioners may need to befriend, encourage and support parents to cross the threshold into the setting.

Home visiting, usually prior to entry or at crucial stages, is a key determinant in establishing good relationships with parents and developing understanding of the child's needs (Fisher, 2002; Draper and Duffy, 2001). Practitioners can also gain an insight into how literacy is developed in the home so that they can build effectively on the child's previous experience (Campbell, 2000). In order to ensure that home visiting contributes to the development of partnership, practitioners need training in working with parents and families, organisations need to commit resources to home visiting and there needs to be a strong ethos supporting home visiting that is enshrined in policy within the organisation. Willey (2000:96) suggests a range of 'formal' meetings as essential contact: see Figure 13.20.

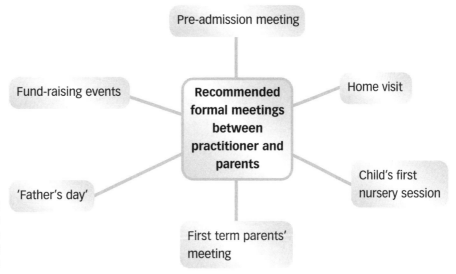

Figure 13.20
Formal meetings suggested as essential contact (Willey, 2000:96)

Settling-in period

Draper and Duffy (2001:151) emphasise the settling-in period as 'a crucial arena for the establishment of a good partnership between parents and practitioners'. Parents and children should both be given the chance to get used to the early years setting before the child stays alone. Some of the methods that may be used to achieve this are shown in Figure 13.21.

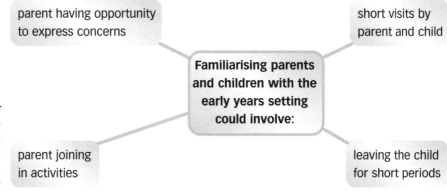

Figure 13.21
Some ways of familiarising parents and children with the early years setting

Practitioners need to be responsive to, and patient with, parents' concerns about leaving their child. They need to recognise that parents have a range of feelings at this stage and that separation can be easy or painful. They need to be sure that they listen to concerns and not assume they know what these are.

Communication between parents and practitioners

Opportunities for communication between parents and practitioners are crucial. Trying to catch busy practitioners before and after nursery or school, being told you can just have a few minutes of their time, not being able to contact key people by phone – all these barriers to communication are very frustrating for parents who may be anxious about their child. Communication should include those elements shown in Figure 13.22.

Communication between practitioners and parents should include:	
Informal and formal meetings	Opportunities for parents to meet with practitioners formally and informally to discuss aspects of their child's learning and development
Methods of conveying information about the child	Methods of ensuring information about the child is conveyed between parents and practitioners on a regular basis
Forums for parents' views	Forums for parents' views on aspects of the setting or service to be aired
Regularly updated information about the early years setting	Regular information about events, developments and items of interest to be conveyed from the early years setting to parents.

Figure 13.22
Range of communication between practitioners and parents

Practitioners need to be skilled in communication at a range of levels and audiences. They should be aware that some parents may need different communication approaches to others, and have the interpersonal skills to judge this successfully. There should be strategies within the early years setting to support communication with parents who do not have English as a first language and parents who have other communication difficulties, and there should be policy and resources to support these strategies. Written communications should be considered in terms of the audience and be appropriate to that audience.

Commitment to specific goals

Parents and practitioners need to have a common understanding of and commitment to specific goals in respect of each child's learning and development. Parents' views should be sought and incorporated in the practitioner's understanding of the child's needs. Use should be made of home-setting diaries, initial information-gathering about the child, and opportunities to meet to keep this understanding current. Willey (2000:94) describes the use of a nursery diary in which practitioners and parents record children's work, photos, observations and comments as an important tool for communication.

Practitioners should be aware of parents' aspirations for their child, their concerns and hopes. Records should be up to date, confidential and used as a working tool to aid the practitioner's work.

Parents should be made to feel part of the community of the early years setting. They should be welcomed at arrival and departure times; given verbal and written information; and involved in key events within the setting. Parents should be included in delivering the curriculum. Practitioners need to find out about parents' skills and utilise these where possible. They should pay particular attention to those parents who are not involved and communicate less with the early years setting. Stereotypes about the sort of experiences and skills parents can offer should be avoided (let the white British parents make curry with the children for a change, for example).

Parents should have access to information about the early years setting and the community. They should also have access to information about other services available, which they may want to use. Practitioners need to be knowledgeable about the range of services available to young children in their community and share this information.

Seek parents' views

Parents need to have opportunities to make suggestions; give feedback; make complaints and offer views and opinions. This entitlement should be part of policy and supported by a strong management and organisational ethos of listening and responding to feedback. Where possible, parents should be represented on the management of the service or early years setting.

Within the early years setting or service there should be policies, strategies and ongoing discussion about the best ways of reaching those parents who are less likely to get involved. Parents should be asked for their help and ideas. Schemes such as befriending, 'father's days' and other strategies targeting specific groups should be tried and assessed for their impact. There should be an ongoing and dynamic debate within the early years setting about what parents want and how best to get them involved.

Conclusion

The concept of partnership with parents is often presented simply and with the underlying assumption that developing relationships will benefit the children and the early years setting. Yet parents can gain enormously from being involved in their children's learning; developing new skills and using existing ones to support others; learning about child development; having opportunities to discuss hopes and fears and show pride in their child.

Developing partnerships is complex and messy, involving a large quantity of imagination and determination in order to reach the diverse range of parents with whom each early years setting is involved. The key elements are a strongly supportive ethos, ongoing discussion and feedback on strategies adopted and practitioners who have the knowledge, commitment and skills to work effectively in this area.

References and further reading

Baldock, P. (2001), *Regulating Early Years Services*. London: David Fulton

Barratt-Pugh, C. and Rohl, M. (2000), *Literacy Learning in the Early Years*. Maidenhead: Open University Press

Bastiani, J. (2000), 'I know it works! …Actually proving it is the problem!' examining the contribution of parents to pupil progress and school effectiveness', in Wolfendale, S. and Bastiani, J., (eds), *The Contribution of Parents to School Effectiveness*. London: David Fulton

Campbell, R. (2000), 'Literacy Learning at Home and at School', in Drury, R., Miller, L. and Campbell, R., *Looking at Early Years Education and Care*. London: David Fulton

Drury, R. (2000), 'Bilingual children in the pre-school years: different experiences of early learning', in Drury, R., Miller, L. and Campbell, R., *Looking at Early Years Education and Care*. London: David Fulton

Children Act (1989), London: HMSO

DfEE (1999), 'National Curriculum'. London: HMSO

DfES/QCA (2000), 'Curriculum Guide for the Foundation Stage'. London: HMSO

DfES (2001), 'SEN Toolkit'. London: HMSO

Draper, L. and Duffy, B. (2001), 'Working with Parents', in Pugh, G. (ed.) *Contemporary Issues in the Early Years*. London: Paul Chapman

Fisher, J. (2002), *Starting from the Child*, 2nd edition. Maidenhead: Open University Press

Plowden Report (1967), HMSO

Pugh, G. (2001), 'A Policy for Early Childhood Services?' in Pugh, G. (ed.) *Contemporary Issues in the Early Years*. London: Paul Chapman Publishing

Roffey, S. (1999), *Special Needs in the Early Years*. London: David Fulton

Shah, M (2001), *Working with Parents*. Oxford: Heinemann Educational

Vincent, C. (2000), *Including Parents? – education, citizenship and parental agency*. Maidenhead: Open University Press

Willey, C. (2000), 'Working with Parents in Early Years' Settings' in Drury, R., Miller, L. and Campbell, R. *Looking at Early Years Education and Care*. London: David Fulton

Wolfendale, S. (2000), 'Effective Schools for the future: incorporating the parental and family dimension', in Wolfendale, S. and Bastiani, J. (eds.) *The Contribution of Parents to School Effectiveness*. London: David Fulton

Useful websites

www.dfes.gov.uk
Department for Education and Skills

www.qca.gov.uk
For information provided by the Qualifications and Curriculum Authority, follow the links to the Foundation Stage section. Includes downloads and curriculum guidance.

www.surestart.gov.uk
Covers all the aims and achievements of the government's SureStart programme.

Health, nutrition and physical safety

14

Vicky Cortvriend

This chapter is designed to encourage you to extend your knowledge about various aspects of childhood health.

It addresses the following:

- ⊃ health promotion in context
- ⊃ preventing disease and promoting health
- ⊃ factors affecting children's health
- ⊃ meeting children's nutritional needs
- ⊃ common childhood illnesses
- ⊃ safety in the early years setting

After reading this chapter, you should be able to:

1 understand the role of the early years practitioner in promoting health in young children

2 recognise the various factors that can affect the health of young children, including poor nutrition, and know how to plan to minimise those factors

3 recognise signs and symptoms of childhood illnesses and be aware of when to call for medical help

4 plan and implement policies and procedures designed to ensure the safety of the children in your setting.

What defines health? Good health can mean many different things – but to the majority of people it certainly means more than just the absence of disease. One of the first published definitions of health was that formulated in 1948 by the World Health Organization (WHO), which defined health as being:

A state of complete physical, mental and social well-being and not merely the absence of disease or infirmity.

It is important for practitioners working in early years settings to have an understanding of health and related issues because children develop holistically and their health can have a positive or negative effect on their overall development.

Health promotion in context

In 1978, the WHO and the United Nations Children's fund (UNICEF) sponsored a conference at Alma-Ata in the then Soviet Union that was attended by representatives from 134 countries. A resolution was passed –

'Health for all by the year 2000'. A declaration of intent was drafted, which was designed to provide guidelines for the establishment of a primary health care service in any country. This conference was considered to be the official introduction to the concept of primary healthcare worldwide. However, even the United Kingdom, a wealthy developed country, has not achieved that resolution. In fact, the health of children in some areas of the country is declining rather than improving.

> **Activity 1** **What does feeling healthy mean to you?**

Take a moment to consider your state of health. Do you consider yourself to be healthy at the moment? Remember that health is not just a matter of physical fitness. Write down what makes you feel healthy, under the following headings: physical, emotional, psychological, social and spiritual.

For example:

I feel healthy when:

Physical: I am free from infections.
Emotional: I am free from stress.
Psychological: I don't feel miserable.
Social: I have time to go out at least once a week with my husband.
Spiritual: I feel at peace with my soul.

Now write down what makes you feel unhealthy.

For example:

I feel unhealthy when:

Physical: I have a cold, *or* I can't run for 5 miles without stopping because I have become unfit.
Emotional: I am under pressure from work, family and my pets.
Psychological: It is dark and wet outside, which makes me feel depressed.
Social: I am too busy even to chat to my husband and children.
Spiritual: I feel I have neglected my soul.

Clearly, feeling healthy or unhealthy is unique to each individual. This applies equally to the children we work with, so it is very important that we understand all the different components that influence a person's health. This will enable us to provide a balanced early years setting in which to care for the children. It is also important to be able to recognise when children are unhealthy or ill and be aware of the steps to take to help them feel better or become healthy again. This is vital for all children whatever their level of need, including those who may have a chronic illness, physical, learning or mental health needs.

Health promotion initiatives

The concept of primary health care that was introduced at Alma Ata in 1978 resulted in the governments of different countries introducing various health promotion initiatives, designed to improve the general health of their population. The initiatives differed depending upon the specific health needs of each country. In some developing countries, such as South Africa, people living in remote rural areas had little or no access to health care, so one of their first initiatives was to set up community health centres, staffed by nurses and mobile health clinics. The United Kingdom already had some health promotion programmes in place such as immunisation schedules and screening programmes for babies and young children. The present government has recognised the importance and need to provide comprehensive initiatives to promote good health in children.

Case Study

National Healthy School Standard

It is important and necessary for different national and local departments to work together to provide resources and information. The National Healthy School Standard (NHSS) is a joint initiative between the Department for Education and Skills and Department of Health. Their remit is to support the development of healthy schools in England through local education and health partnerships. Standards have been written to guide these partnerships in developing local schools programmes. A copy of this guidance can be found on the Health Development Agency website (see Useful Websites at the end of this chapter). The agency provides interactive websites aimed specifically at young people from the ages of 5 to 14. These sites cover health topics relevant for the specific age group that they are targeting; they are updated on a regular basis.

Welltown, for example, is aimed at 5 to 7-year-olds. Children are encouraged by the use of symbols and words to visit the different areas and discover ways of keeping themselves and their friends healthy and safe. There is a link for parents and practitioners in early years settings that explains the philosophy of the site and how the activities link in with the national curriculum. This site would be useful for practitioners to either download information to use with the children during health promotion activities, or for the children to have access to during free-play time.

Sure Start

The Government's £452 million Sure Start initiative, which began in 2000, aims to improve the life chances of children under 4 years of age in areas of need in England, by improving access to health, family and education services. Again this is encouraging partnerships and joint initiatives to develop projects that will build on existing good practice and link with other government initiatives. Targets included:

⊃ a 5 per cent reduction in the proportion of low birth-weight babies by 2001

⊃ a 10 per cent reduction in the number of children aged under one admitted to hospital emergency departments with severe injuries, gastroenteritis, or respiratory infections.

Local programmes work with parents and parents-to-be to improve children's life chances through better access to family support, advice on nurturing, health services and early learning.

The Sure Start initiative benefits professionals in early years settings in several ways (see Figure 14.1).

Sure Start initiative: benefits to professionals working in early years settings	
Funding	To assist in the training of unqualified staff, enabling them to become qualified. Details of funding in your area can be obtained from your local Early Years Development and Childcare partnership.
Resources	An example includes the Framework Pack, which is available to anyone working with young children. This pack consists of a booklet introducing the framework, a poster identifying the four aspects (A strong child, a skillful communicator, a competent learner and a healthy child); and the components into which each aspect is subdivided, a set of component cards, a video and CD-ROM. These resources are intended for use by practitioners in early years settings during their daily routine to support their health promotion work with the children.
Support	For good-quality play, learning and childcare experiences for children. For children and parents with special needs, including help in gaining access to specialised services. To enable services to be culturally appropriate and sensitive to particular needs.

Figure 14.1
Benefits of Sure Start initiative to practitioners

Keeping children safe

'Keeping children safe' (2003) and the Green Paper 'Every child matters' (2003) set out the government's proposals for reforming the delivery of services for children, young people and families. Children and young people, when consulted during this inquiry, considered that being healthy and staying safe were among the five outcomes that mattered most to them. Professionals in early years settings can, through planning for children's effective care and education, help them to achieve those two outcomes. This will then support children in enabling them to fulfil their potential.

Preventing disease and promoting health

There are three distinct parts to preventing disease and promoting health. These are primary prevention, secondary prevention and tertiary prevention.

Health education is part of the cycle of maintaining good health. Caring for an ill child is another part of the cycle, as is maintaining children's safety. Supporting children who have been ill or children who have a disability or chronic illness are equally important. These different parts of the health cycle have been defined as health promotion and disease prevention, and rehabilitation.

Figure 14.2 illustrates how each area, although a distinct area in its own right, interlinks with the others.

Primary prevention	Prevention of illness before it occurs	Primary health care clinics, home, early years settings
Secondary prevention	Treatment Prevention of complications	Primary health care clinics, home, hospitals
Tertiary prevention	Supporting children in their recovery Enabling children with a disability or chronic condition to maximise their potential	Primary health care clinics, home, early years settings, hospitals and outpatient specialist services

Figure 14.2
The links between primary, secondary and tertiary prevention

Disease can occur at any time during the cycle; for example, it is not uncommon for a child suffering from a common cold to then catch an ear infection at the same time. This is because the cold virus has compromised his or her immune system and enabled the bacteria to take hold, causing the ear infection. Similarly a child undergoing treatment with antibiotics for a throat infection may catch chicken pox. Chicken pox is caused by the herpes virus, which does not respond to antibiotics. This explains why the promotion of health must be ongoing whether the child is in a state of good health or not. Children who have a chronic condition such as asthma or diabetes, or children who have a special need, are also prone to catching infections. Early years practitioners should have detailed knowledge of the needs of the children in their care so they can make sure they meet their primary, secondary and tertiary health needs. An ongoing health promotion programme should ensure that this happens.

Primary prevention

Primary prevention aimed at reducing the incidence of disease in a population is an important step in disease control. The government initiatives designed to improve children's nutrition, encourage exercise and reduce poverty will all result in improving children's health and, therefore, their resistance to disease. Conditions such as rickets, anemia, gastroenteritis, malnutrition and pneumonia are all linked to poverty, poor diet and poor living conditions. Eating disorders and obesity, which are on the increase in young children, are other conditions linked to the modern lifestyle as well as peer pressure and the media.

One proven method of reducing the incidence of disease in the population is to develop an effective immunisation schedule so that babies and children are protected from some potentially dangerous diseases such as measles, diphtheria, polio, tuberculosis, meningitis, mumps and tetanus.

Immunising children against disease gives them the best chance of developing immunity against specific diseases in a safe and effective manner. Babies are not immunised until they are 2 months old because they still have antibodies in their systems from their mother prior to this, which can stop the vaccines from working. Some vaccines such as the pertussis (whooping cough) are better given at the recommended times to prevent adverse reactions (see Figure 14.3).

Age	Immunisation	Method
Sometimes shortly after birth	BCG (tuberculosis)	Skin test, then one injection if necessary
2, 3 and 4 months	Polio	By mouth on three separate occasions
2, 3 and 4 months	Diptheria, tetanus and pertussis (whooping cough) Hib (DTP – Hib)	One injection each month (total = three injections)
	MenC	One injection
13 months	MMR (measles, mumps and rubella)	One injection
3 to 5 years	Polio	By mouth
	Diptheria, Tetanus and acellular pertussis (DtaP)	One injection
	MMR	One injection
10 to 14 years	BCG	Skin test then one injection if necessary
13 to 18 years	Tetanus and low dose diptheria (Td)	One injection
	Polio	By mouth

Figure 14.3
Recommended national immunisation schedule

Note:

> ⊃ This schedule is considered the ideal.
> ⊃ The gap between the vaccinations is to ensure that each dose has time to work.
> ⊃ If a vaccine is missed it does not mean that the whole schedule has to be started from the beginning; it can continue, after a break, until all vaccinations have been given.

Activity 2 Current immunisation schedule

Research the current immunisation schedule for infants and young children in your area; it may differ slightly from the one quoted in Figure 14.3. You may consider having a copy of the schedule on the notice board in your setting, to inform parents.

Safety of vaccines

As a result of negative press coverage, many parents have become concerned about the safety of vaccines and the MMR vaccine in particular. Practitioners in early years settings should be aware of the various issues in order to be able to give parents facts rather than opinions. It is important, however, not to influence parents' decisions but to provide them with information to enable them to make an informed choice.

MMR: the facts

The following issues often give cause for concern:

> ⊃ a possible link between MMR vaccination and autism in children
> ⊃ a possible link between bowel disease and MMR vaccination
> ⊃ articles published about case histories, linking children who have developed autism after having the MMR vaccine.

The measles, mumps and rubella vaccine (MMR):

> ⊃ contains three separate vaccines in one injection.
> ⊃ is given twice, firstly at the age of 13 months, and once more while the child is aged between 3 and 5 years. The second vaccination protects any child who did not respond to the first injection.
> ⊃ was introduced into the UK in 1988, and since that time, according to Department of Health statistics, the number of children catching these diseases has dropped significantly.
> ⊃ causes some children to suffer side effects from the immunisation; these are usually mild and may include a raised temperature, swelling of the glands and a rash.
> ⊃ in about 1 in 100,000 immunisations results in a severe allergic reaction. Health professionals administering the immunisations are

trained to respond to such incidents and if treated quickly the child should recover fully.

The suggestions of MMR's risks followed research headed by Dr Andrew Wakefield at the Royal Free Hospital London. Two reports, one in March 1998, which reviewed the evidence from the Royal Free team, and one in June 1999, which evaluated over 100 children's records, concluded that the information available did not support the suggested causal associations. The first report did not find evidence to link MMR vaccination and bowel disease or autism, and the second one reported that the information available did not give cause for concern about the safety of MMR or MR (measles and rubella) vaccines. Further reports have been published by the Department of Health, reviewing the evidence on MMR safety and identified the arguments about why separate vaccines are not considered an alternative to MMR. They asserted that there is no good scientific evidence to support a link between MMR vaccine and autism or inflammatory bowel disease. They state that there is considerable evidence on the safety of the MMR vaccine and that giving separate vaccines would be a backward step in protecting children from infectious disease. They concluded by acknowledging that the final decision had to rest with the parents, but health professionals should have no hesitation in recommending its use.

In the light of this controversy, the World Health Organisation (WHO) in January 2001 issued a report that came out strongly in support of the MMR vaccine.

Various studies quoted by the Department of Health demonstrate that although there was an increase in the diagnosis of autism between 1988 to1999, there was no change in the proportion of children who had been vaccinated with MMR. In February 2004, the editor of *The Lancet*, in which Dr Wakefield's study had been published, stated that the original research had been flawed by a conflict of interest, because Dr Wakefield had been conducting research on behalf of parents hoping to take legal action.

Screening

Screening is another method of reducing the incidence of disease in children, or of reaching an early diagnosis. It helps to minimise complications and manage the disease effectively. Screening means checking babies and children for potential problems rather than waiting for symptoms to appear. Antenatal screening takes place for all pregnant women. If problems are picked up in good time, then the condition can be managed, or even prevented, depending upon the condition or illness. Screening covers a wide variety of conditions including those illustrated in Figure 14.4.

Midwives, health visitors, school nurses and medical practitioners are all skilled in screening techniques for diseases or abnormalities relevant to

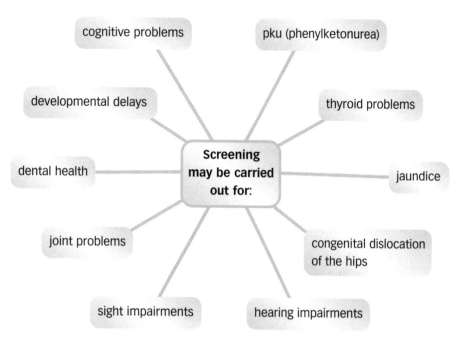

Figure 14.4
Health screening

the age of the children they work with. An example of a screening tool commonly used by health visitors, the growth chart, is described in Chapter 3.

Antenatal screening

Standards to support the screening programme in pregnancy currently in place in the UK were published in August 2003. Figure 14.5 illustrates the current antenatal screening programme in the UK.

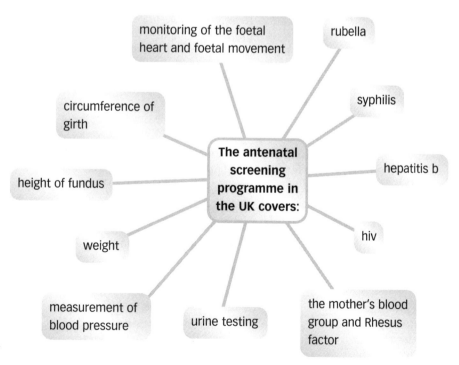

Figure 14.5
Antenatal screening in the UK

The mother may have one or more scans and possibly an amniocentesis, depending upon her individual needs.

Practitioners in early years settings should be aware of the various screening techniques used, the diseases, or conditions, that can be picked up by screening, and the age at which these procedures take place.

The National Screening Committee makes recommendations on screening that local health authorities act upon. The Child Health Screening Subgroup advises this committee on the implementation, development, review, modification and where necessary the cessation of UK childhood screening programmes.

In 1996 a report was published on the Third Joint Working Party on Child Health Surveillance. This report, by D. M. Hall, suggested that local authorities implement a programme of regular screening of children,

Timing of test	Details of screening
8 weeks	Weight Length Head circumference Heart and femoral pulses Hips Testes in males Eyes, e.g. following and fixation/red reflex Head control Behaviour, e.g.smiling Congenital abnormalities, e.g. cleft palate
7–9 months	Distraction test for hearing (currently being phased out, to be replaced by universal neonatal hearing screening) Vision, e.g. squint Hips Testes Motor development Head circumference Social behaviour
20–24 months	Parental concerns relating to: ⊃ vision, hearing or behaviour ⊃ motor development ⊃ speech ⊃ head circumference ⊃ hand/eye co-ordination.
3–4 years	Height Weight Motor development Parental concerns relating to: ⊃ vision, hearing or behaviour

Figure 14.6
Minimum assessment programme

aimed at detecting problems in children and using these opportunities to promote health. A typical programme would include a check:

- within 24 hours of birth, by a pediatrician
- at 8 weeks, by a GP and health visitor
- at 7 to 9 months, by a health visitor
- at 20 to 24 months, by a health visitor
- at 3 to 4 years, by a health visitor.

Details of the minimum assessment programme are shown in Figure 14.6.

Activity 3) Screening

Choose one of the conditions mentioned that children can be screened for.

1 Research the screening techniques used to detect any abnormalities in that area.
2 Design a chart that you could display in your setting that would inform and educate parents about that particular screening routine.

Secondary prevention

Secondary prevention of disease is concerned with early detection and prompt treatment to minimise complications and shorten the duration of the disease. Screening plays an important part in secondary prevention as well as in primary prevention. For example, in a child with suspected hearing loss, using the otoacoustic emission screening will determine the level of impairment, which can then be treated or managed. In order for the correct treatment to be prescribed it is important for infants and young children to be taken to a doctor at the first signs of illness.

Health promotion and education are also important during illness. Parents and childcare workers need to be aware of the importance of diet, rest and gentle exercise in the treatment and management of disease. A strong immune system helps to fight illness and will also help the child to recover quickly.

Tertiary prevention

This is when a diagnosis has been made and the child has a condition or impairment that is either long term or permanent. Tertiary prevention is aimed at ensuring the child continues to develop and be as healthy as his or her condition allows. The intention is to minimise the impact of an established clinical disease. It often requires specialist input and services to reduce disabilities and assist the child in living his own individual life. For practitioners working in early years settings it may mean adapting the premises in order to enable a child who uses a wheelchair to attend the setting. Specialist equipment such as walking aids, eating utensils, speaking books and sensory toys should be provided in order to include children with special needs in the daily routine of the setting. It is essential that practitioners are aware of the particular needs of each child who attends their setting in order to plan effectively for their needs. This includes knowing how to give any medication that a child may be prescribed (with parental consent); children with asthma, epilepsy and diabetes, may well require medication on a regular basis during the day.

Health promotion in early years settings

Educating children about their own body and how to take care of it is part of both the Foundation Stage Curriculum and the National Curriculum. The 'Keep Children Safe' (2003) document is concerned with all aspects of child safety, not only abuse. Practitioners in early years settings, therefore, have a responsibility towards the children in their care. Health promotion topics and activities should be a routine and regular part of the daily curriculum.

Practitioners in early years settings are in a unique position because there are a number of ways in which they can practise health promotion in their setting. Some examples are shown in Figure 14.7.

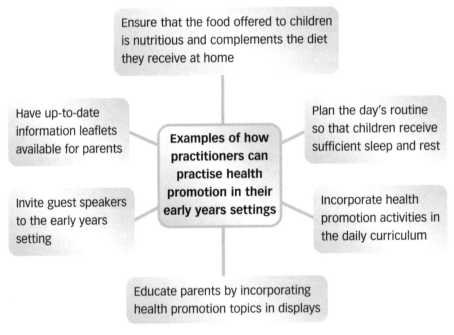

Figure 14.7
How practitioners can practise health promotion

> **Activity 4** **Health promotion**

1 What health promotion topics would you choose as being suitable for a group of 4-year-old children? What sort of activities would you do?

2 Use the curriculum guidance/standards for Foundation Stage/Key Stage 1 or 2 to devise a short-term and medium-term plan that would be appropriate for the children in your setting.

3 Explain how you would adapt any activities to ensure that all children could take part.

4 How would you involve parents in the programme?

Comment on Activity 4

Examples could include:

⊃ healthy eating: introducing different fruits to the children, or different vegetables. Include foods from other countries, for example, guavas, yams, okra, Sharon fruit

⊃ hygiene, for example, why we need to wash our hands. Introduce the idea of germs

⊃ keeping teeth clean, inviting a dental hygienist to visit the nursery

⊃ exercise is fun. Plan an indoor and outdoor sports day with games and sports that everyone can join in with

⊃ road safety. Invite your local traffic officers, or road safety team to pay you a visit.

Involve parents by giving them a complete programme of the activities you have planned. Invite comments and suggestions. Invite any who may be able, to join you and their children in taking part in the activities.

⊃ Factors affecting children's health

If we accept that good health is not just the absence of illness, then it follows that there are many factors that can influence health. Hubley (1994) subdivides these factors into three main areas, as shown in Figure 14.8.

Factors influencing health:	
Lifestyle and behaviour	Including health knowledge, customs, cultural beliefs, and the influence of people in society (for example, peer groups).
Environment	Including housing, water supply, sanitation, hazardous waste, pollution, food production and climate.
Primary health care services	

Figure 14.8
Factors influencing health (Hubley, 1994)

Other factors, cited in the Black report (1980) but not mentioned by Hubley are **education**, **unemployment** and **poverty**. This report published the results of a research project that considered the health status of the different social classes found in Britain. The results demonstrated that social class and, by association, wealth had a definite impact on health. People in social class 1 had the best health status and those in class 5 the worst. There was a gradual decline of good health from class 1 through to class 5. A further disturbing point, which was highlighted, was that in cases of illness or disability those in the higher classes were significantly better off in terms of health than those in the lower classes. See Figure 14.9 for an explanation of social classes 1 to 5. The Registrar General's scale is an occupational scale ranking social class according to employment status and occupational skill.

Social classes 1–5	Occupations
Class 1: Professional	Doctors , lawyers, architects
Class 2: Intermediate	Nurses, teachers, farmers, managers
Class 3: Skilled non-manual	Clerical, receptionists, sales assistants
Class 3: Skilled manual	Bus drivers, bricklayers, electricians
Class 4: Semi-skilled manual	Postal workers, bar workers, agricultural workers
Class 5: Unskilled manual	Road sweepers, refuse collectors, labourers

Figure 14.9
The Registrar General's scale of social class

This scale, although quoted in the Black report, was largely replaced in the 1990s by the Standard Occupational Classification, which contains a wider range of occupational groups. There are nine major groups as shown in Figure 14.10.

Class	Occupations
Class 1	Managers and administrators
Class 2	Professional
Class 3	Associate professional and technical
Class 4	Clerical and secretarial
Class 5	Craft and related
Class 6	Personal and protective services
Class 7	Sales
Class 8	Plant and machine operatives
Class 9	Other occupations

Figure 14.10
The Standard Occupational Classification (Browne, 1998)

In 1998, Sir Donald Acheson published a report commissioned by the government on health inequalities. This demonstrated that the health gap is in fact widening between the professional or rich people and the unskilled or poor. The report highlighted a range of areas where these inequalities could be targeted. These included increasing benefits for women of childbearing age, expectant mothers, young children and older people, as well as providing more funding for schools in deprived areas, better nutrition and health promotion in schools. Another proposal was to restrict smoking in public places, ban tobacco advertising, increase the price of tobacco and prescribing nicotine replacement therapy on the NHS.

Lifestyle and behaviour

Ignorance about the causative factors of some health problems is a very real threat to good health. This ignorance is reflected in the way that we live our lives. Children learn by example and cannot be expected to always know what constitutes a healthy lifestyle or what might be dangerous.

Examples of harmful situations could include:

- eating or drinking poisonous substances, for example, berries, medicines, cleaning fluids
- crossing the road dangerously
- not being aware of 'stranger danger'.

Examples of ways in which children may maintain and improve their health include:

- knowing how to clean their teeth correctly
- understanding the need to wash their hands after using the toilet
- taking sufficient exercise
- eating healthily.

Practitioners in early years settings have a responsibility to the children in their care to educate them in age-appropriate ways about how to protect themselves and to teach healthy living practices. They have a further responsibility to protect children while they are in their care. This means meeting their individual health needs and ensuring their safety while in the setting.

Our customs and cultural beliefs prescribe the way in which we live our lives; they influence our diet, our social habits, our dress, the way we exercise and our belief in medical practices. In turn, the adults of any culture influence the children. For example, many Jehovah's Witnesses do not accept any form of human tissue as a medical treatment. This includes blood transfusions. As a practitioner in an early years settings, you should have an awareness and understanding of the cultural background of the children in your care, again, so that you can plan how best to meet their individual needs.

Environment

This discussion of how the environment affects health looks at the impact of poverty, poor housing and pollution.

Poverty

Childhood is a critical and vulnerable stage when health inequalities can have lasting effects throughout life and into other generations. Poverty is generally regarded as the most important determinant of health and also one of the most difficult areas in which to achieve change. The worst health is found amongst social groups with the lowest income or in areas with the highest deprivation. Causes of poverty are manifold and include:

- ⊃ unemployment
- ⊃ poor qualifications or lack of them
- ⊃ ill health (mental, or physical)
- ⊃ disability and reliance on the state
- ⊃ addictions
- ⊃ crime.

Lone parent families are most at risk of living in or falling into poverty.

The possible outcomes for children born into poverty are shown in Figure 14.11.

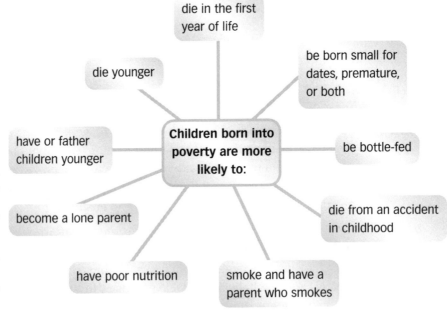

Figure 14.11
Possible outcomes for children born into poverty (source: www.esbhhealth. nhs.uk/publicati ons/public- health/inequaliti es.asp)

die in the first year of life

be born small for dates, premature, or both

die younger

Children born into poverty are more likely to:

be bottle-fed

have or father children younger

die from an accident in childhood

become a lone parent

smoke and have a parent who smokes

have poor nutrition

The NHS plans to reduce inequalities in health, recognising that one-third of children under the age of four live in poverty in Britain today. A children's fund was initiated in 2001, to be implemented over three years to address some of these inequalities.

Housing

Access to affordable and good quality housing is an important factor in determining health status. Poor housing conditions include overcrowding, damp, cold and infestations of pests. These all have a negative effect on children's health, leading to recurrent or chronic illness and in some cases hospitalisation. Conditions identified by the Health of Londoners Project 1998 that were directly linked to the quality of housing are shown in Figure 14.12.

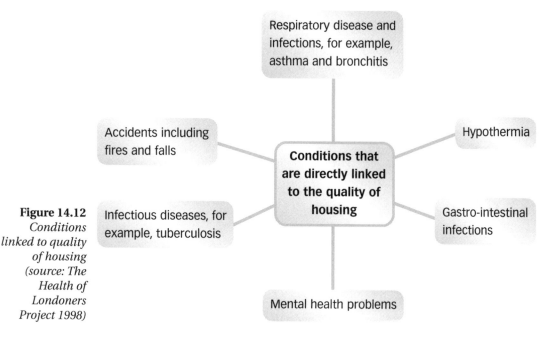

Figure 14.12
Conditions linked to quality of housing (source: The Health of Londoners Project 1998)

Poor housing is often associated with poverty and a variety of other social factors, including poor educational qualifications and unemployment.

Primary health care services

Access to primary health care services should be the right of every person and child in Britain today, particularly in the light of the NHS plan to reduce health inequalities for people living in Britain. If everyone had equal access, all children would be able to take part in screening programmes, which would reduce the incidence of childhood morbidity and mortality (the incidence of childhood disease and death). Unfortunately, there are many groups of children who do not have easy access to primary health care clinics. These include children of travelling families, illegal immigrants and itinerants (children whose parents do not have any fixed abode). These children may not attend any childcare setting (where they would have their basic health care needs met), despite the fact that the government provides five free childcare sessions per week in a recognised setting for children between 3 and 5 years of age. At age 5 they are eligible for school.

Meeting children's nutritional needs

As a practitioner in an early years setting you need to have an understanding about what the components of a healthy diet are, and you need to work in partnership with the parents/carers to provide a healthy diet for the children in your care.

Healthy eating is absolutely vital for all-round development and physical growth. Individual children grow and develop at different rates. There are charts designed to provide standardised norms of development to help guide parents, carers and health professionals (see Chapter 3).

By carrying out detailed observations on children and comparing the results with the expected norms you can decide if a child falls within the expected norms for his or her height and age.

Food classification

Food is classified by organising it into groups according to type. There are five separate groups, as shown in Figure 14.13.

Classification	Foods
Group 1	Cereals, potatoes, yams, couscous, rice, polenta and pasta
Group 2	Vegetables and fruit
Group 3	Milk (cow, goat, ewe and buffalo) and dairy products such as cheese, yogurt and fromage frais
Group 4	Meat and alternatives, for example, soya, some beans and pulses
Group 5	Sugars/fats

Figure 14.13 *Food groups*

All food contains some nutrients (nutrients are collections of the components that occur in food). The important point is to get the balance right, to provide the required mixture of essential nutrients that will enable the body to grow, repair damage and fight infections. We need to take in sufficient nutrients to support a healthy energetic lifestyle. The seven essential nutrients:

- carbohydrates
- protein
- fats
- fibre
- water
- vitamins
- minerals.

Carbohydrates

These are found in Group 1. They are our single most important source of energy.

Carbohydrates	Foods
Simple carbohydrates (for example, sugars, monosaccharides and disaccharides)	Found in fruits, milk, vegetables and honey.
Complex carbohydrates, or polysaccharides (for example, starches and glycogen)	Found in potatoes, root vegetables, cereals, rice, pastas, yams and sweet corn. Glycogen is found in animal muscle and liver.

Figure 14.14
Carbohydrates

A deficiency in carbohydrates results in thinness, failure to thrive and an inability to maintain body temperature.

Protein

This is found in Groups 2, 3 and 4. It is required for growth and to build and repair all the cells that make up the human body.

Proteins do not all have the same nutritional value so it is important that childcare workers know which foods provide the best quality protein. These are known as complete proteins or high biological value (HBV).

Proteins	Foods
Complete proteins or high biological value (HBV)	Found in animal products, fish and seafood and also in soya beans.
Incomplete proteins or low biological value (LBV)	Found in vegetable products such as nuts, seeds, beans, peas, lentils, chickpeas and cereals, pasta, chapattis and other breads.

Figure 14.15
Proteins

Protein deficiency results in a condition known as kwashiorkor. Children with kwashiorkor do not initially always appear undernourished, because they are not thin. They have swollen bellies and a distinctive orange tint to their hair.

Fats

These are found in Group 5. Fats provide more concentrated energy than either carbohydrates or proteins. The body requires energy for all its functions including organ functioning, growth, repair and movement. The body also uses fat to protect internal organs; it cushions delicate structures and forms a layer of insulation beneath the skin. Excess fat is stored in the body as adipose or fatty tissue.

Fatty acids play a part in regulating blood pressure and assists in the maintenance of the body's immune system. Recent research also indicates that they may help to reduce the incidence of strokes/heart attacks due to blood clots.

Fats	Foods
Essential fatty acids	Found in foods high in polyunsaturates such as oily fish, soya beans, sunflower oils, seeds and nuts.
Saturates and monounsaturates	Found in dairy products, meat products and other oils.

Figure 14.16
Fats

Fats containing a majority of saturated fatty acids tend to be solid at room temperature, while unsaturated are liquid. The exceptions are margarine spreads that can be up to 75 per cent unsaturated, and palm and coconut oils, which are liquid, but contain a high proportion of saturated fat.

Fibre (cellulose or roughage)

This is found in Groups 1 and 2 and is a form of carbohydrate. There are two types of fibre: Type 1 and Type 2 as shown in Figure 14.17.

Fibre (cellulose or roughage)	Foods
Type 1 Insoluble Dietary Fibre (IDF)	For example, bran, found in some breakfast cereals. IDF is indigestible by humans but is necessary to provide bulk to help the digestive system in the formation of stools to remove waste products from the body. It also helps us to chew our food properly and gives us a full, satisfied feeling following a meal. However, it provides little or no energy, nor any other nutrients for the body to use. Raw bran should never be given to children under 5 as it can cause bloating and wind, and can affect the absorption of other important nutrients.
Type 2 Soluble Dietary Fibre (SDF)	This is digested and absorbed in the intestine or gut. As well as providing similar functions to ID, it also helps to control blood sugar levels and lower cholesterol levels. Soluble fibre is found in fresh fruit and vegetables, pulses and cereals. It is also found in some dried fruit such as raisins, sultanas, dates apricots and prunes. It is a source of energy and provides other nutrients, particularly vitamins and minerals.

Figure 14.17
Fibre

Minerals

These are found mainly in Groups 3 and 4.

Minerals	Importance
Magnesium	Vital for the conversion of food into energy
Calcium, phosphorus, zinc and fluoride	Developing bones and teeth
Sodium and potassium	Functioning of the nervous system
Iron	Functioning of the circulatory system
Iodine	Functioning of the endocrine system
Selenium	Functioning of the immune system

Figure 14.18
Minerals

A calcium deficiency can result in rickets and fluoride deficiency in tooth decay (but too much fluoride results in mottling of the tooth enamel). Iron deficiency causes anemia.

Vitamins

These are found mainly in Group 2. But yeast, meat and fish are important sources of the B group vitamins, whereas vitamins D and A are found in oily fish.

Thirteen vitamins have been identified as essential to health and for fighting infections caused by bacteria and other microorganisms. They are required in very small quantities compared with some other. Vitamins are either soluble in water or in fat.

Vitamins		
Fat-soluble vitamins	A D E and K	These are stored in fatty tissue until needed by the body. Note: because the body can store these vitamins, if too many are ingested then they can reach toxic levels. The body requires sunlight in order to manufacture and absorb vitamin D.
Water-soluble vitamins	C and the B group	These dissolve in water, the body does not store them and excess amounts are excreted in the urine.

Figure 14.19
Vitamins

A deficiency in vitamin A will result in skin problems and problems with vision. Vitamins B2, B6 and B12 are necessary for the circulatory system and a deficiency can result in anaemia. A deficiency of vitamin C can result in a depleted immune system, leading to slow healing of wounds and infections.

Water

This is found in Groups 1 and 2. Water makes up about two-thirds of our body weight.

Water is required for:

- the formation of cells and tissues, lymph, blood and all body fluids
- transport of oxygen, carbon dioxide, nutrients and enzymes around the body
- the excretion of waste products
- helping to regulate the temperature.

Children who are ill and running a fever can become dehydrated very quickly and will require extra water and other fluids.

The body cannot store water and is constantly losing it through respiration, sweat, urine and stools. Therefore, it needs to be replaced regularly. Adults need at least 2 litres of water daily and children's requirements vary according to their age and weight. Should the children be very active or the weather hot then they will need to increase their intake.

Water is found in many foods, for example, juicy fruit and vegetables, but the best source is water from the tap or bottled water.

Special requirements

Practitioners in early years settings need to take into account the particular needs of the children in their care when planning how best to cater for their daily nutritional requirements. Some examples of children who may have particular dietary requirements are children:

- following vegetarian or vegan diets
- following coeliac diets
- with food intolerances or allergies
- with a disability
- whose culture or religion determines what foods they may eat.

Vegetarian and vegan diets

A strict vegetarian will not eat any fish, meat products or poultry. A vegan does not eat any animal, dairy, fish or fowl products at all. Some people are part-vegetarian in that they don't eat red meat, but are happy to eat fish and sometimes poultry. It is important to determine exactly what the children in your care are allowed to eat and ensure this is recorded. It is possible that without careful planning a child who is following a vegetarian or vegan diet could become deficient in one or more nutrients, particularly iron and protein. A balanced nutritional diet can be provided that will ensure that the full range of amino acids is eaten, by including foods from each of the four main food groups on a daily basis – and always combining foods from Group 1 (grains: carbohydrates) and Group 2 (pulses, nuts and seeds: proteins) in a single meal. Figure 14.20 shows an example of a day's menu suitable for a three-year-old vegetarian child.

Figure 14.20
An example of a day's menu for a three-year-old vegetarian child

Meal	Suggested menu
Breakfast	Fresh orange juice diluted with water Cornflakes and milk Brown toast, with some low fat spread and honey or jam
Mid-morning snack	Milk to drink Oatcake with low fat spread
Lunch	Water to drink Potato curry with rice, dhal, chapatti and an orange
Mid-afternoon snack	Milk to drink Apple Breadsticks and cheese
Tea	Orange juice diluted with water Pizza with tomato, apple and fruit yogurt to follow

Food intolerances and allergies

The distinction between food intolerances and allergies is highlighted in Figure 14.21.

Figure 14.21
Food intolerances and food allergies

Distinction between food intolerances and allergies:		
Food intolerance	Causes an unpleasant reaction to the ingestion of a particular food. Intolerances can cause diarrhea, vomiting and skin rashes.	It is not life threatening and may disappear or appear at different times of life. Because the reaction does not involve the immune system it is not considered an allergy.
Food allergy	The ingestion of a particular food causes an immune reaction and can result in anaphylactic shock.	Can be life threatening.

True food allergies only affect about 5–8 per cent of young children under the age of 3 and about 2 per cent of older children. Most children will grow out of their allergy by the time they are 3 years old. However, if a child has had a severe allergic reaction under the age of 3 it is very important to refer to the doctor before reintroducing the same food later on. Among adults, about 1 per cent suffer from an allergy to a particular food. Symptoms of a food allergy can include those identified in Figure 14.22.

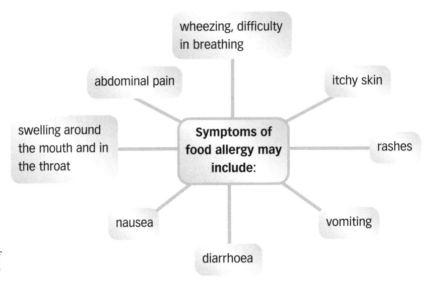

Figure 14.22
Symptoms of food allergy

Symptoms of food allergy can occur within minutes of ingesting the food but may take a few hours to appear.

The most common foods that cause food allergies in children are peanuts, tree nuts (for example, walnuts or pecans), fish, shellfish, eggs (particularly egg whites), milk, soy and wheat.

It is important to remember that just because a child has eaten a food and not had a reaction it is not true that he or she is definitely not allergic to that food. Children can develop allergic reactions to foods that they have happily eaten in the past. This is because it may take some time for the immune system to build up a reaction to a food.

A doctor can carry out skin tests or blood tests if you suspect a food allergy. If the child is found to be allergic to a particular food then he or she may be issued with an EpiPen (epinephrine auto injection device) and should wear a medic alert bracelet to warn people of his or her allergy.

It is vital that there is always a member of staff on duty who is capable of giving an EpiPen injection.

A food diary is a good method of recording what the child eats over a period of time and may assist in making a diagnosis of food allergy. Practitioners and parents should record whatever the child eats, the symptoms he or she develops and when they develop, to enable them to share this with the child's GP or pediatrician.

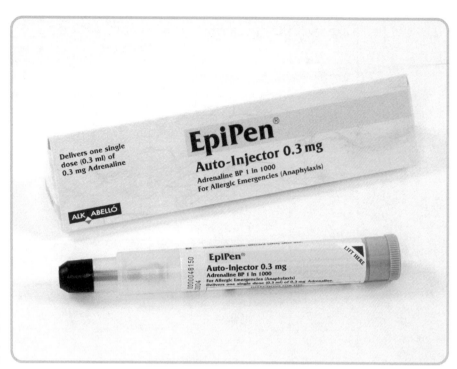

An EpiPen may be carried by some children with allergies

Children who have physical or learning difficulties

Eating independently requires physical coordination, social skills and cognitive ability. Where one or more of these areas is challenged then the child may have difficulty in eating and, therefore, requires help in order to have a balanced diet. This cannot be achieved in isolation so the practitioner in an early years setting needs to work in conjunction with the child's parents and other professionals such as a dietician, pediatrician and health visitor.

A portage programme may be planned to suit the child's individual needs. Portage originated in America in the 1960s and consists of developmental tasks and skills put together in an individual programme worked out to meet the needs of the child. It aims to support the children in a way that builds upon the child's strengths. The specially trained portage worker works with the child, parents and other helpers in the home and the setting to support the child in achieving the tasks. A recent study in Egypt investigating the role of antioxidant nutritional support in conjunction with an early intervention portage programme for children with Down's syndrome reported, 'The most striking finding was the marked improvement in the group of children attending the programme in conjunction with the antioxidant treatment.'

Figure 14.23 illustrates a portage record chart.

Several local authorities support a portage programme. For example, Tameside has a successful programme up and running and the Isle of Wight is running a pilot scheme involving nine families at present.

Age level	Card	Skill/behaviour	Entry skill/ behaviour	Date achieved	Comments
0 to 1	1	Sucks and swallows liquid			
	2	Eats liquified food when fed			
	3	Eats strained food when fed			
	4	Eats mashed food when fed			
	5	Eats semi-solid food when fed			
	6	Feeds self with finger foods			
	7	With help, takes spoon filled with food to mouth			
1 to 2	8	Uses spoon independently			
2 to 3	9	Feeds self from spoon and cup			
	10	Begins to use fork to feed self			
	11	Uses fork and spoon independently			

Figure 14.23
Example of portage record chart

4 Devise a portage programme for a child in your setting who you consider would benefit from such input.

Note: The portage programme you design does not necessarily have to do with nutrition per se. It could be for developmental delay, either physical or cognitive. However, whatever the need, it will have an effect on the child's ability to receive a balanced diet, which is why a portage programme should meet the child's nutritional needs.

Multicultural and religious aspects

Practitioners in early years settings must respect the culture and beliefs of the children in their care. The following recommendations and menus give the key points and ideas for meals, in relation to the main cultures found in society. This is a very broad outline; there is a wide range of diverse cultures and beliefs in society and it is of the utmost importance that each child's beliefs are upheld and that the early years setting provides a balanced diet in accordance with what the child is allowed to eat. Practitioners have a responsibility to liaise with the child's parents to ensure that they are fully aware of any dietary restrictions and that the setting complies with the parents' wishes. This information should be shared with the rest of the team and the cook so that no mistakes are made. The information should also be recorded on the child's records. Examples of the dietary requirements of some religious faiths are shown in Figure 14.24. Obviously, these may vary from person to person.

Religion	Dietary requirements of adherents
Hinduism and Sikhism	Strict followers do not eat eggs, meat, fish and some fats.
Islam	Do eat meat, except for pork, but it must be Halal.
Rastafarianism	Some are vegan.
Jainism	Do have restrictions on some vegetable dishes
Buddhism	Do not eat meat or poultry, but some eat fish except for shellfish. Also do not eat butter, ghee, or lard.
Judaism	Do not eat meat with milk or cheese products. The meat eaten must be Kosher. Only fish with fins and scales is eaten; pork, shellfish and lard are not eaten. Separate utensils are used for meat and dairy products.

Figure 14.24
Religion and diet

An example of a suitable menu for children with special dietary requirements is shown in Figure 14.25.

Menu for a four-year-old child in a day-care setting	
Mid-morning snack	Milk, scone and margarine
Lunch	Baked sweet potato, rice and peas, spinach Pineapple to follow
Mid-afternoon snack	Milk, banana, plain popcorn
Tea	Orange juice diluted with water Pasta, cheese sauce and sweet corn Mandarin orange to follow
Drinks offered with meals or when thirsty could be water, milk, goat or soya-milk, diluted fresh fruit juice.	

Figure 14.25
A menu for children with special dietary requirements

Menu for a three-year-old who attends nursery mornings only	
Mid-morning snack	Milk, muffin and margarine
Lunch	Fried tofu, stir fried vegetables, noodles Fruit yogurt to follow
Drinks offered with meals or when thirsty could be water, milk, goat or soya-milk, diluted fresh fruit juice.	

Figure 14.26
A menu for children attending nursery only in the mornings

Children have different nutritional requirements according to their age, gender and also differing needs. The Caroline Walker Trust, (dedicated to the improvement of public health through good food) in 1998 commissioned an expert working group to research nutritional guidelines for practitioners in early years settings working with children under the age of five years. This report, 'Eating well for under-fives in child care', explains why nutritional guidelines are required and describes how practitioners can ensure the children in their care have a healthy diet.

Offer alternative lunchtime options such as vegetable and chicken curry, shepherd's pie, lamb stew, fish fingers and other home cooked main meals. Puddings such as fresh fruit crumbles and pies, rice pudding and fresh fruit jellies are all nutritious options.

A useful reminder that provides a nutritional daily guide for early years practitioners, and which can be adapted for educating children of appropriate age, is the Food is Fun pyramid pictured opposite.

Activity 6) Meeting all children's dietary needs

Imagine that you are the manager of a busy private day nursery. Children arrive from 7am and some don't leave until 6pm. An important part of your role is to ensure that the nutritional needs of all the children in your care are met. You have

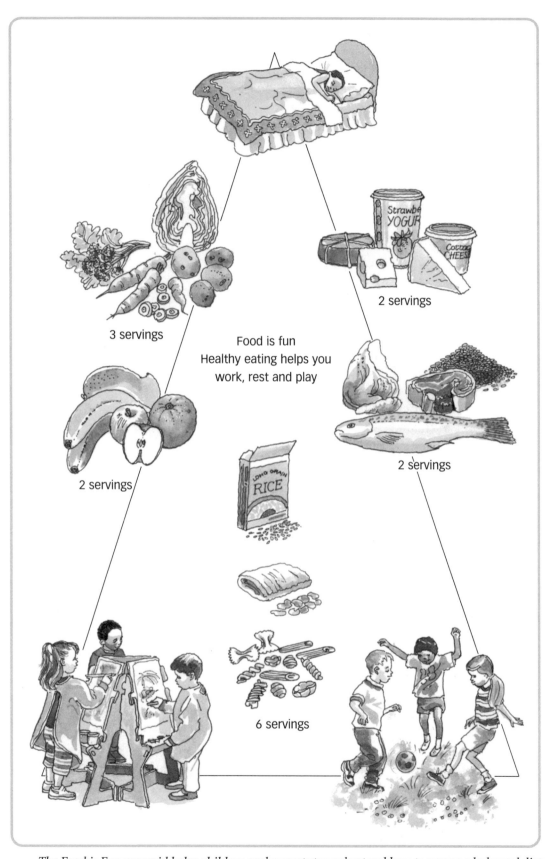

3 servings

2 servings

Food is fun
Healthy eating helps you
work, rest and play

2 servings

RICE

2 servings

6 servings

The Food is Fun pyramid helps children and parents to understand how to ensure a balanced diet

received application forms from four new families requesting full day care for their children. Their ages range from 1 year to 4 years. The 1-year-old has a diagnosed milk and egg allergy, while the other three are all members of the Hindu faith, one being a strict Hindu. Their parents have requested a meeting to discuss their individual dietary needs.

1 How will you ensure you meet these children's needs as well as the other children in the setting?

2 What precautions should you take for the child with allergies?

3 Plan a menu for a week that will meet all their nutritional needs and that you could share with the parents to allay any fears they may have.

Common childhood illnesses

Illness in infants and young children is inevitable. There is a school of thought that we are becoming overprotective and 'over hygienic' so that our babies and young children are not being allowed to come into contact with dirt and germs that would help them to build up a strong immune system. There may be some merit in this argument and apart from helping to build a strong and effective immune system, playing in dirt and mud is good fun! See Figure 14.27 for some details of chronic and acute illnesses in children.

Childhood illnesses		
Chronic	juvenile arthritis, asthma, epilepsy, progeria, cystic fibrosis	Long-term illnesses or conditions that can be terminal
Acute	measles, mumps, chickenpox, flu, gastroenteritis	Last for only a short time. While the child is incubating the illness, he or she may be lethargic, fractious, clingy and have little appetite. During this period, the parent may remark that the child is 'off colour' or 'sickening for something'

Figure 14.27
Chronic and acute illnesses in children

Children should not be in an early years setting if they are unwell, but sometimes a child may run a slight temperature when teething, or when suffering from a slight cold. If after 3 days there is no improvement then the child should be cared for at home and medical attention sought. In the majority of cases there will be no lasting after effects.

General signs and symptoms of illness

Practitioners in early years settings need to know the general signs and symptoms of illness in children and, in particular, any danger signs that would require immediate medical attention. The practitioner needs to use common sense when dealing with sick children in his or her care.

⊃ There should be a set of policies and procedures in place to cover such issues as a child being taken ill while at the setting, the giving of medicine and first aid.

⊃ There should be regular in-service training for staff to update them on any changes to the policies.

⊃ There should be a room, or quiet place, where children can rest until a parent or carer can collect them.

⊃ It is important to keep children warm (not hot) and dry, and give plenty of fluids, especially if they have sickness and diarrhoea.

⊃ They should be kept amused and distracted with stories and quiet activities.

⊃ They should not be left on their own.

⊃ A record should be kept of when the child began to feel ill, or when the early years practitioner first became worried. Any signs and symptoms, (including behavioural changes), what food or fluid was taken by the child and whether the child vomited, had diarrhoea or urinated, should be carefully recorded. These notes should be entered in the child's records and shared with the parent or doctor. Medical attention is required if a baby or child has any of the symptoms shown in Figure 14.28.

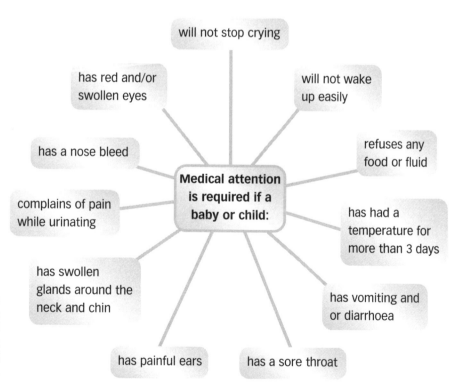

Figure 14.28
Symptoms in a baby or child that require you to seek medical attention

Should the child have any of the symptoms shown in Figure 14.29 (on the next page) then a doctor should be called immediately.

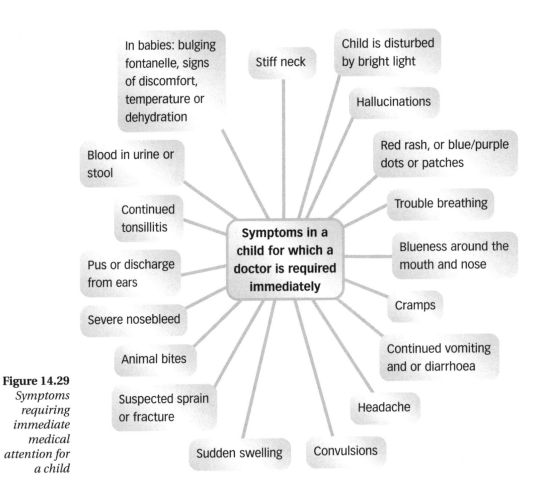

Figure 14.29
Symptoms requiring immediate medical attention for a child

Symptoms in a child for which a doctor is required immediately:

- In babies: bulging fontanelle, signs of discomfort, temperature or dehydration
- Stiff neck
- Child is disturbed by bright light
- Hallucinations
- Red rash, or blue/purple dots or patches
- Blood in urine or stool
- Trouble breathing
- Continued tonsillitis
- Blueness around the mouth and nose
- Pus or discharge from ears
- Cramps
- Severe nosebleed
- Continued vomiting and or diarrhoea
- Animal bites
- Headache
- Suspected sprain or fracture
- Sudden swelling
- Convulsions

In addition if you are at all worried about the health of a child or baby in your care then you need to seek medical advice and inform the parents or carer.

Some common childhood illnesses are shown in Figure 14.30 below.

Illness	Incubation period	Signs and symptoms	Treatment	Complications
Common cold	1 to 3 days	Sneezing Sore throat Runny nose Headache Irritability		Pneumonia Tonsillitis Laryngitis Sinisitis Otitis media
Chicken pox	10 to 14 days	Rash of itchy red spots with a white centre that starts on trunk and spreads to limbs The rash blisters, then scabs over Slight fever	Fluids Rest Calamine lotion on rash to stop itching	Impetigo Scarring Encephalitis

Illness	Incubation period	Signs and symptoms	Treatment	Complications
Diarrhoea/ Gastroenteritis	7 to 14 days (if bacterial)	Loose, runny stools Stomach cramps Dehydration	Replacement fluids, e.g. Dioralyte No food Medical attention	Dehydration can be fatal
Food poisoning	Half an hour to 36 hours	As above, plus vomiting	As above	As above
Hand, foot and mouth	3 to 10 days	Blisters on hands, soles of feet and in mouth Feeling unwell Mild fever	Plenty of fluids Soft food, e.g. soup, fruit	Ulcers in mouth may last for 3 to 4 weeks
Measles	7 to 14 days	Feeling fluish Sore, red eyes Day 1: koplick (white) spots on inside of cheeks Day 4: blotchy red rash starts behind ears, back of neck and on fact, then spreads to rest of body. Dislike of bright light (photophobia)	Rest Fluids Keep cool Shady room Medical attention	Otitis media Pneumonia Encephalitis
Meningitis: viral bacterial meningococcal	2 to 14 days	Fever Drowsiness Temperature Headache Nausea Vomiting Stiff neck Photophobia Bruise-like rash with flat, purple spots that do not fade if pressed	Call for medical help immediately	Deafness Epilepsy Brain damage Can be fatal
Mumps	14 to 24 days	Fever Swelling of jaw on both sides Pain when eating or drinking	Fluids	Orchitis (swelling of the testicles) in males Meningitis Encephalitis

Illness	Incubation period	Signs and symptoms	Treatment	Complications
Roseala Infantum	5 to 15 days	High temperature Mild diarrhoea Cough Ear ache Enlarged glands in neck After 4 days: temperature recedes and rash appears: tiny pink spots on head and neck	Treat temperature Fluids	Rare
Rubella (German measles)	14 to 21 days	Slight fever with cold-like symptoms Swollen glands behind ears Rash: mild, flat, pink and not itchy	Rest Fluids	Encephalitis Serious damage to the foetus if contracted in the first 12 to 16 weeks of pregnancy
Slapface (erythema infectiosum)	4 to 14 days	Bright red cheeks with pale mouth High temperature After 1 to 4 days, a lace-effect rash may appear on arms, legs and (occasionally) trunk	Fluids Reduce temperature	Serious if child has an inherited blood disorder, e.g. sickle cell anaemia or thalassanaemia
Scarlet fever	2 to 4 days	Bright red pinpoint rash over face and body Fever Sore throat Pale mouth Red 'strawberry' tongue	Rest Fluids Reduce temperature	Kidney infection Otitis media Rheumatic fever
Tonsillitis		Sore throat Pain on swallowing Fever General aches and pains	Rest Fluids Control temperature	Abcess on tonsils Otitis media Kidney infection

Illness	Incubation period	Signs and symptoms	Treatment	Complications
Whooping cough (pertussis)	7 to 10 days	Cold-like symptoms Dry cough followed by a whoop (deep intake of breath) Vomiting Cough may last for months	Fluids Rest Feed after whoop to try to avoid vomiting	Convulsions Hernia Pneumonia Encephalitis Dehydration Weight loss

Figure 14.30
Common childhood illnesses

Some of these illnesses are notifiable (see below). Medical help should be sought for clarification of diagnosis, possible antibiotic treatment and prevention of complications.

Fevers, febrile convulsions/fits

The normal body temperature is between 36°C and 36.8°C. (97.7°F and 99.1°F). A fever or high temperature is the body's defence mechanism against infection. The body tries to kill the organism causing the infection or illness by creating heat. Children's temperatures can rise and fall very quickly because their temperature control in the brain is not yet fully developed. They can also suffer from convulsions or fits caused by this sudden change in temperature. One in 20 children can be affected between the ages of 1 and 4 years of age. But children as young as 6 months can suffer from febrile convulsions, as can children as old as 5 years.

If a child has a high temperature they need more fluid than usual, rest and sleep. Parents should seek advice from a doctor or pharmacist regarding the best medication to use and the correct dosage. Practitioners in early years settings should follow the policy regarding the giving of medicines in their setting. This should explain the procedure to be followed when a child requires medication.

Notifiable diseases

There are some diseases that are designated as notifiable. This means that it is a statutory requirement under the Public Health (Control of Disease) Act 1984 and in the Public Health (Infectious Diseases) Regulations 1988 for doctors to notify a 'Proper Officer' of the local authority, usually the Consultant in Communicable Disease Control of cases of certain infectious diseases. Should any of the children in your care develop symptoms of any of these diseases then you must inform a doctor and the parents immediately. Practitioners in early years settings should develop a procedure to explain how to manage this eventuality. The procedure should cover exclusion from the nursery and state how long the child should be excluded for. The procedure could be included in a general illness procedure, covering all instances when a child should be sent home, seen by a doctor, or excluded until the infection is clear. Alternatively there could be a separate procedure or appendix to cover notifiable disease. These procedures should be part of the setting's health and safety policy.

Notifiable diseases in England and Wales

- Acute encephalitis
- Acute poliomyelitis
- Anthrax
- Cholera
- Diphtheria
- Dysentery (amoebic or bacillary)
- Food poisoning
- Leprosy
- Leptospirosis
- Malaria
- Measles
- Meningitis
- Meningococcal septicemia (without meningitis)
- Mumps
- Ophthalmia neonatorum
- Paratyphoid fever
- Plague
- Rabies
- Relapsing fever
- Rubella
- Scarlet fever
- Smallpox
- Tetanus
- Tuberculosis
- Typhoid fever
- Typhus
- Viral haemorrhagic fever
- Viral hepatitis
- Whooping cough
- Yellow fever

Although AIDS is not a notifiable disease, certain powers can be applied to people with AIDS under regulations issued in 1985. Doctors are urged to report HIV infections and AIDS cases to the voluntary confidential surveillance schemes at CDSC (Communicable Disease Surveillance Centre).

Infection from animals

Playing with and owning pets is, on the whole, a positive experience for children. Hamsters, mice, chipmunks and chinchillas are small and easy to care for within an early years setting. Looking after them is a good way of teaching children about responsibility for animals. Maintaining hygiene and preventing infection is largely a matter of good sense and may be achieved by observing the following:

- ensure that the children do not go near the animals on their own
- ensure children wash their hands after touching animals
- ensure that a child with an allergy to pet fur does not go too near to the cage
- don't allow pets to lick the children

- ensure faeces are cleared away immediately
- as cats and dogs could foul the outside areas of the setting, take care not to allow children to play outside until the area has been thoroughly checked and cleaned
- always act in accordance with parents' wishes in all matters including playing with animals.

Figure 14.31 shows some illnesses that can be caught from animals.

Illness	Cause	Symptoms	Prevention
Toxocariasis	Roundworm in dog and cat faeces	Allergic symptoms (Rarely) blindness	Ensure play areas are clean Ensure children wash their hands after touching dogs or cats
Ringworm	A fungal infection of the skin caught from infected children, cats or dogs	Round, red itchy area	Treat with prescribed cream Do not allow child to touch infected area
Fleabites	Fleas are usually found on cats or dogs	Small, round, red lumps	Cream, prescribed by GP or pharmacist

Figure 14.31
Some illnesses that can be caught from animals

Safety in the early years setting

The Health and Safety at Work Act 1974 is still the main piece of legislation giving general guidance about health and safety. Several regulations have been passed since the introduction of the Act, designed to bring the United Kingdom into line with European laws. These are:

- The Control of Substances Hazardous to Health Regulations1994 (COSHH)
- The Health and Safety (First Aid) Regulations 1981
- Reporting of Injuries, Disease and Dangerous Occurrences Regulations 1995 (RIDDOR)
- Fire Precautions (Workplace) Regulations 1997
- The Food Handling Regulations 1995

National Standards for Child Care

These explain in detail what early years settings need to do in order to comply with the above regulations, and to ensure good practice and quality care.

The Office For Standards in Education (Ofsted) and the Department for Education and Skills (DfES) have produced publications that explain the National Standards that providers of childcare and education should aim to achieve. There are different publications for different childcare settings; they include full day care, out-of-school care, sessional care, crèches and child minders.

Ofsted expects providers to demonstrate how they achieve each of the standards and the guides have been produced in order to help them do this.

These standards refer to the Children Act 1989 and explain what the setting should be providing to meet the needs of the children in its care. The Children Act 1989 called for policies to be in place in early years settings in order to protect the children. The four main policies demanded by the act are:

⊃ Equal opportunities

⊃ Parents as Partners

⊃ Health and Safety

⊃ Child Protection (see Chapter 15).

A health and safety policy should include the various procedures necessary to ensure that the health and safety needs of all children in the setting are met. The relevant standards in relation to health and safety in the setting, which can be used to help formulate some policies and procedures, are discussed below.

Safety

The standards suggest carrying out a risk assessment in order to identify hazards inside and outside the early years setting. Security is an important factor today, not just ensuring that the children remain on the premises, but also keeping unwanted people out. Are outside areas secure? What is the general security of the building like? Other points to consider under safety include questions about potentially hazardous areas. Are there any:

⊃ poisonous plants or bulbs on the premises

⊃ hazardous shrubs or trees

⊃ water features

⊃ outdoor play areas?

Fire safety

A statement of the procedures to be followed in the event of fire must be kept. It would also be a good idea to have an evacuation procedure that could be followed in the event of a terrorist attack or other disaster.

Health

This standard covers hygiene practices, aimed at reducing the spread of infection and maintaining the cleanliness of the premises. Smoking, animals in the setting, sandpits, food handling and medicine are all included. Procedures should be in place to inform staff on how to manage and work with those issues. The Children Act 1989 states that a record must be kept of all medicines administered to children. The standards state that non-prescription medication may be administered to children in day care, but only with the prior written consent of the parent and only when there is a health reason to do so. Blanket consent should not be given by the parent to cover all non-prescription medicine.

This Standard also covers First Aid in the setting, and sick children. In this section it mentions the care of the sick child while awaiting collection and contingency arrangements that should be in place if the parents cannot be contacted, or cannot collect a sick child. The setting's procedures should state when to seek medical advice and what to do in the case of infectious, notifiable and communicable diseases. The Children Act regulations state that you must notify Ofsted of any infectious disease that a qualified medical person considers notifiable.

Activity 6) Risk assessment

1 With regard to the above information relating to illness and safety, carry out a risk assessment of your setting. Then design a set of procedures to minimise or remove those risks.

2 Describe how you would ensure the safety of the children and staff once they were in the setting.

Comment on Activity 6

1 Did you include procedures to cover both the sick child and excluding a child from the setting: when ill, or if suffering from a notifiable disease? Did you cover accident procedure, giving of medicine, animal care, evacuation procedures, record of visitors, procedures for the safe collection and arrival of children and outings?

2 The following are all effective methods of improving security and ensuring the safety of children and staff: monitoring access to the early years setting, use of a visitor's book, seeking advice from a crime prevention officer, making arrangements for answering the door, the use of security systems (including locks, alarms, intercoms and cameras), up-to-date CRB checks on all people who work in the early years setting (including parents and students).

Accidents

Childhood injury has overtaken infectious disease as the main source of death in young children in the United Kingdom. Road accidents, or transport-related deaths, are the commonest cause of accidental death at all ages, including babies less than one year old. As with infectious disease, poverty is a major contributing factor in childhood injury. The cost of childhood injury is high: road accidents and accidents in the home are estimated to cost the community in Britain alone over £10, 000 million each year.

Practitioners in early years settings have a responsibility to the children in their care, as part of the ongoing health promotion programme, to educate them in all aspects of safety, including road safety.

Road safety

Educating children about road safety should begin at an early age. Every local authority employs a Road Safety Officer who is always happy to visit childcare settings with new ideas about teaching children about road safety.

> **Activity 7** **Road safety**
>
> Contact your local Road Safety Officer to find out what is on offer in your area. Invite him or her to your setting to share new ideas with you.

The Green Cross Code is still an effective way of teaching young children about road safety. You should ensure everyone practises it when they take children out of the early years setting for walks or outings.

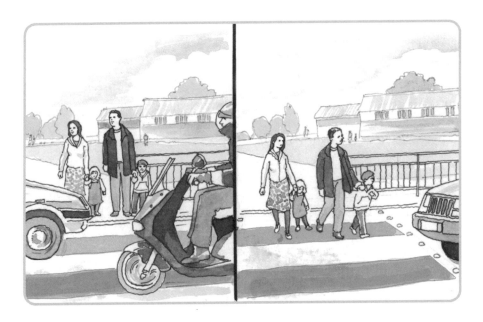

1 Find a safe place to cross with a clear view in both directions.

2 Stand on the pavement facing the road.

3 Look right, then left, then right again.

4 Listen carefully.

5 Wait until you cannot see or hear any traffic coming.

6 Walk swiftly across the road. Do not run.

7 Keep looking and listening while crossing the road.

Accidents in the setting

Accidents in the home and early years settings happen very easily and are often directly linked to the child's stage of development. Accidents, however, do happen despite your best efforts.

Activity 8 Assessing children's safety

1 Refer back to the chapters on development. Make developmental notes on three different ages of children, linking these to the age range found in your setting or place of work.

2 Carry out a situational analysis of your workplace and perhaps your home, (particularly if you are a childminder). Highlight any areas of concern in relation to children's safety, in the light of your knowledge about their holistic development.

3 Using your analysis, design new procedures to ensure the children's safety when playing with toys and equipment inside and outside the setting. You may need to design a different set of procedures for the different age groups of children who attend the setting.

Comment on Activity 8

For example, if you research the holistic development of 2 year olds you will find that they are curious and impulsive; they want to explore independently and easily become frustrated. At this age they can run and enjoy climbing. They can easily walk up and down the stairs. Therefore, when you carry out your situational analysis you will be checking for such things as safety gates on stairs, space to run safely, soft and safe surfaces under playground equipment and large equipment that allows them to climb in safety. You will also check that the equipment is in good condition and carries the British Kite mark for safety.

Making your early years setting and home as safe as possible is an important factor in reducing the possibility of an accident, but it cannot be stressed strongly enough that the most important factor in reducing the incidence of accidents is adult supervision. This is one reason why the Government, in the Children Act 1989, set down minimum requirements for the ratio of adults to children in childcare settings. The standard recommended ratio is 1 approved adult to 8 children between the ages of 3 and 7 years. This ratio is increased with younger children; for 0 to 2 years it is 1:3, and for 2 to 3 years it is 1:4.

First Aid

Accidents will happen however vigilant you are and however safe you make your early years setting. It is the responsibility of the manager of early years settings to ensure that there is a qualified first aider, skilled in resuscitation techniques, on every shift. However, it is advisable for all practitioners to obtain a recognised qualification in first aid. This should be updated every three years. The following advice is a general guideline only, covering a very small example of common accidents and is not intended to replace professional instruction. There should be an accident and emergency procedure to be followed that states:

- what to do in accidents or emergencies
- who the first aiders are
- where the first aid box is (which needs checking weekly)
- who to contact in the case of an accident or emergency
- how to record the incident.

See Figure 14.32 (opposite) for details of some of the treatments for common injuries and accidents.

Should any accident occur in your setting, no matter how minor, then it should be recorded and the child's parents notified.

Sudden Infant Death Syndrome

Sudden Infant Death Syndrome (SIDS) is a term is used to describe the unexpected and unexplained death of babies up to the age of two. It may be referred to as cot death because the infant is often found dead in his or her cot. There is currently a lot of research being carried out into the causes and incidence of cot death, particularly in the light of two recent cases of suspected infanticide when the mothers were accused of killing their babies only to have the ruling overturned on appeal when the judge found there was evidence of unexplained infant deaths in the mother's family history. Research has shown that the risk of cot death is greatly reduced if the baby is put to sleep on its back. Other factors that may have an influence on sudden infant death syndrome are overheating, smoking and infections.

SIDS is more common in boys, premature babies and low birth-weight babies, and during the winter months. (Continued on page 493)

Injury/ Accident	Treatment	Call medical help
Burns and scalds	Limit the extent of the damage and prevent the burn from becoming worse by: cooling the area quickly by running under cold (not freezing) water. It should be kept under running water until the pain has stopped. If necessary use clean wet towels to keep the area wet and cold while taking the child to the doctor, if the burn is severe.Do not lance any blisters, do not remove anything sticking to the area and do not apply any creams	Notify parents and, if severe, take the child to the doctor as soon as possible.
Sunburn	Remove child out of the sun. Give sips of water frequently. Use an after sun cream only with parental consent.	Should the sunburn be extensive, or blister seek medical help
Nosebleeds	A nosebleed can be very distressing for a child. They may feel something is seriously wrong with them, so it is important that the practitioner in an early years setting remains calm. The child should not tilt his or her head back or lie on his or her back. Sit the child down and pinch the lower soft part of the nose between the thumb and forefinger, keep the grip firm and steady. Hold the nose for ten minutes before letting go. Once the bleeding has stopped the child should play quietly for a couple of hours to prevent a further attack. The child should be discouraged from picking, rubbing or blowing his nose. The nosebleed should be recorded and reported to the child's parents/carers.	If you suspect the child of putting a foreign body up his or her nose then take the child to the doctor immediately. If, after ten minutes the bleeding still has not stopped, **or** if you are at all concerned, at any, time, call a doctor, or an ambulance.
Poisoning	Write down exactly what the child has had to eat or drink. Keep any bottles you suspect the child might have got hold of. The doctor will need to know the child's weight. Do not give the child anything to drink or make him vomit unless you are acting on the express orders from the doctor.	If you think that one of the children in your care has eaten something that is poisonous then you must call a doctor immediately and notify the child's parents/ carer. Take a sample of what the child ate or drank to Accident and Emergency with you.

Injury/ Accident	Treatment	Call medical help
Choking	First open the child or baby's mouth; if the obstruction is visible, try to hook it out. Do not use your fingers to feel blindly down the throat. **Babies**. Lie the baby face down along your forearm and give five sharp slaps on the back. Look in the mouth and if the object is visible hook it out. Repeat for two cycles; if the object does not appear, call an ambulance. (Continue until the ambulance appears.) **Young children**. Lie the child head down across your lap. Give five sharp slaps between the shoulders. Look in the mouth and if the object is visible hook it out. Repeat for two cycles, if the object does not appear, call an ambulance (continue until the ambulance arrives). The Heimlich manoeuvre is the method of choice for older children (do not use on a baby). 1. Kneel behind the child, place your arms around their waist and bend them well forward. 2. Clench your fist and place it right above the child's navel. 3. Place your other hand on top of your fist and thrust both hands back and up, into the child's tummy. Repeat this, for two cycles; if the object does not appear call for an ambulance (continue until the ambulance arrives).	Seek medical help if the child or baby continues to choke or, if the baby or child becomes unconscious, begin resuscitation and send someone to call an ambulance. Notify the parents.
Falls	Assess the damage; if the child has an obvious injury such as a cut or scrape to a limb; then take inside, wash the area with sterile water and, if necessary, cover with a sterile non-stick dressing. (Do not use cream or antiseptic in case of allergic reactions.) If there is any sign of head injury this needs to be carefully assessed. If the head injury is mild then a headache may be the only sign.	If the child shows signs of: concussion (loses consciousness, vomits, is drowsy and/or disorientated, eyes not focusing, or pupils enlarged or pinpoints), call an ambulance immediately. Call an ambulance also, in the case of suspected fracture, or if there is any discharge from eyes, ears, nose.

Figure 14.32
Examples of common injuries and accidents

In order to minimise the chance of cot death, parents and carers are advised to:

➲ put babies to sleep on their backs with their feet touching the foot of the bed

➲ keep the room temperature at 18°C

➲ use sheets and blankets rather than a duvet because these can be adjusted to suit the temperature of the room

➲ do not smoke near the baby, and keep babies out of smoky atmospheres (parents should stop smoking during pregnancy)

➲ always take the baby to a doctor if it is at all unwell

➲ parents should consider keeping the baby in the same bedroom as themselves, in a separate cot, for at least six months

➲ ensure that the room is supervised at all times.

Alternative therapies

Today more people are becoming aware that there are alternatives to conventional medicine, not only for themselves but also for their children. It is important as a practitioner in an early years setting for you to have some knowledge if not about the efficacy of various therapies then at least where to obtain relevant information, as you may well be asked for an opinion on such matters. Alternative therapies most often used effectively with children include homeopathy, massage (in particular baby massage), cranial head massage and aromatherapy.

> **Activity 9** **Alternative therapies**

Choose a common childhood condition, for example, asthma, or one perhaps that a child in your early years setting suffers from. Research the alternative therapies that could possibly be used for this condition and describe the rationale behind them.

If each member of your group chooses a different condition then you could share your findings and increase your knowledge.

Note: it is important you do not try to influence the parents or carers in their choice of treatment. Rather, you should increase your own knowledge so you can give objective factual information, if asked.

➲ Conclusion

The purpose of this chapter has been to encourage you to think about different aspects relating to the health of children and also your own health. Some areas have been covered very briefly and you are urged to do your own more in-depth research into those areas that interest you. There are many texts covering health and illnesses that you can refer to and the Internet is a useful source of valuable information. Health promotion activities and initiatives are constantly being updated as research continues to grow and develop. As a practitioner in an early years setting you have a duty to stay informed about new research related to health, and review your own practice and the policies and procedures of your early years setting accordingly.

References and further reading

Acheson, D. (1998), 'The Acheson Report: Independent Inquiry into Inequalities in Health'. London: HMSO

Caroline Walker Trust (1998), *Eating well for under-5s in child care*. London: The Caroline Walker Trust

Childs, C. (2001), *Food and Nutrition in the Early Years*. London: Hodder Arnold.

Department of Health (1989a), 'The Children Act 1989 Guidance and Regulations'. London: HMSO

Department of Health (2003), 'Every Child Matters'. London: HMSO

Department of Health (2003), 'Keeping Children Safe'. London: HMSO

DfES/DfWP (2003), 'Birth to Three Matters'. London: Sure Start/DfES

DfES (2001), 'Full Day Care: National Standards for Under 8s Day Care and Childminding'. Nottingham: Sure Start/DfES

DHSS (1980), 'Inequalities in health. Report of a research-working group to the DHSS (the Black report)'. London: HMSO

Disability Information Trust (2001), 'Children with Disabilities'. Oxford: Disability Information Trust

Fullick, A. (1998), *Human Health and Disease*. Oxford: Heinemann

Hall, D. and Elliman, D. (2003), *Health for All Children* (4th edition). Oxford: Oxford University Press

Hubley, J. (1993), *Communicating Health*. Oxford: Macmillan Education Ltd

Keene, A. (1999), *Child Health: Care of the Child in Health and Illness*. Cheltenham: Stanley Thornes.

McCormick, A. (1993), 'Communicable disease Report'. Volume 3, Review Number 2.

Meggitt, C. (2001), *Baby and Child Health*. Oxford: Heineman

Meguid, N.A. and Ismail, S. (2002), 'Early Intervention in Down's Syndrome: The Effect of Antioxidants'.

Paterson, G. (1999), *First Aid for Children Fast*. London: Dorling Kindersley

Roberts, I., Norton, R., Taua, B. (1996), 'Child pedestrian injury rates: The importance of exposure to risk relating to socio-economic and ethnic differences in Auckland, New Zealand', in *Journal of Epidemiology and Community Health* 50: pp162–165

Stordy, B.J. (1994), 'Is It Appropriate to Apply Adult Healthy Eating Guidelines to Babies And Young Children in the Growing Cycle?'. London: National Dairy Council Conference

Thompson, J. (1997), *Nutritional Requirements of Infants and Young Children*. Oxford: Blackwell Science

Varma, V. (ed) (1992), *The Secret life of Vulnerable Children*. London: Routledge

World Health Organization (1978), 'Report on the International Conference on Primary Health Care, Alma Ata, USSR, 6–12 Sept 1978'. Health for all series (1). Geneva: WHO

World Health Organization (1999), 'International Consultation on Environmental Tobacco Smoke (ETS) and Child Health'. Geneva: WHO

Useful websites

http://society.guardian.co.uk/publichealth/story/0,11098,941030,00.html
Report from the Guardian newspaper's website about the rise in children's consumption of ready meals.

www.keepkidshealthy.com
This website has useful tips and up-to-date information relating to children's health.

www.netdoctor.co.uk
Net Doctor is a constantly updated website produced by doctors in the UK to answer queries relating to health, including treatment of illnesses. Follow the links to find information specific to children.

www.sids.org.uk
Contains the latest research findings on Sudden Infant Death Syndrome.

www.welltown.gov.uk
Welltown is an excellent website produced by the government, which contains health promotion activities for adults to carry out with children. It can also be accessed by children, who can try the interactive activities.

www.hda-online.org.uk
The Health Development Agency website, which contains details of the National Healthy Schools Standard, for reducing health inequalities and promoting social inclusion.

www.tameside.gov.uk
Local authority that runs a successful portage scheme.

http://eduwight.iow.gov.uk
The Isle of Wight council's education site. The council is running a pilot portage scheme involving nine families at present.

Child protection and children's rights

15

Janet Kay

This chapter explores issues relating to child protection work in the early years, in relation to the concerns and problems that working within the child protection system presents to many practitioners. The role of practitioners in early years settings in child protection is discussed in terms of the rights of young children and our responsibilities towards them. The role of the legislative framework and procedural guidelines in shaping these responsibilities is critically examined in the context of a multi-agency response to child abuse. Ways in which child protection work can be integrated into the role of the practitioner or organisation are discussed, as are supporting children's rights to protection through implementing strategies to raise standards in this area within early years settings.

This chapter addresses the following areas:

- ⊃ concepts of child abuse
- ⊃ defining child abuse
- ⊃ responding to suspected child abuse
- ⊃ the child protection enquiry process
- ⊃ the legal and procedural framework for the child protection process
- ⊃ raising standards in child protection work

The discussion on procedure and legislation relates to England and Wales. Legislation and the structure of the court system are different in Scotland.

Introduction

Child protection is one of the key roles of any practitioner working with children whatever their professional status, discipline or job. It is also one of the most closely regulated systems within which practitioners in early years settings operate, with a raft of legislative and policy requirements, procedures and guidelines to know, understand and implement. Or, as Baldwin (2000:5) states:

> *Extreme cases, where children have died, where gross abuse and neglect have not been recognised early enough, or responses have been inadequate, have led to a child protection system which has been procedurally and legalistically driven*

Yet levels of child protection training remain a problem within many organisations, and many practitioners do not feel equipped for the demands of the child protection role. Widespread media coverage of key cases in the last 20 years has supported the notion that it is both easy to 'get it wrong' and disastrous when this happens. The sheer level of responsibility the child protection system places on individual practitioners is daunting to many, and fears about making errors of judgement in this area of work are rife.

It is common to find that child protection work is considered a 'bolt on' within early years settings, rather than an integral part of the work of the organisation. As such, child protection issues may only be considered when the relevant policy is due for review or when abuse of an individual child is suspected.

The notion of children's rights has been enshrined for some years in the 1989 UN Convention on the Rights of the Child which supports the concept, amongst others, of children having the right to be protected from abuse (Article 19). The ideas inherent in the concept of children's rights have become part of theory and practice in the early years, and the principles of the Children Act 1989 and other significant legislation and policy reflect these ideas. The theory behind the concept of children's rights within child protection is that by upholding this notion, the child does not become forgotten within the child protection process. As Howitt's research (1992) established:

> *once started, the child protection process can acquire such powerful momentum of its own that it can sometimes operate against the child's best interests (Pettican, 1998:194).*

Exploring child protection work through the concept of children's rights allows us an alternative view of the child protection system and the role of the practitioner in early years settings within this. In this view, child protection work is part of the practitioner's and organisation's roles in supporting the development of children's rights. Rather than regarding child protection work as a rare (hopefully) and unwanted part of the job, building the concept of a 'child protecting setting' into the day-to-day work of the setting, and the regular duties of practitioners, can improve standards in this area and support a clearer understanding of how children can best be protected from abuse.

One of the key issues to consider when discussing professional roles in child protection is the conflict between private and public aspects of child abuse, between the role of the state and the role of the family (Pettican, 1998). Inherent in British culture is the belief that the family is a private entity with rights to conduct family life without state intervention and to raise children in accordance with the parent's beliefs and wishes. Child protection work often involves a breach of this privacy, invading the lives of adults and children alike. The notion that children's rights may only be protected at the expense of the family's rights to privacy can be a difficult concept for practitioners and organisations to negotiate (Hodgson, 1999). Often making a decision about whether to refer a child protection case onwards feels like a Catch-22 situation. If you do refer the case, the child and family's rights to privacy may be destroyed and they may suffer considerably through a child abuse enquiry. If you do not refer the case, the child may continue to suffer abuse.

Another key issue to consider is the complex nature of the influences in every child's life. Child protection procedures emphasise standard responses to suspected child abuse incidents, focusing on key issues, such as the quality of parenting, identified as making a difference to the child's welfare. However, as Baldwin (2000) points out, every child is uniquely influenced by (at the very least):

⊃ his or her own personal characteristics

⊃ family relationships

⊃ environment

⊃ socio-economic circumstances

⊃ local and wider cultural context.

As such, responding to child abuse issues with simple, one-dimensional views of the causes of abuse, how to respond to it, and how to best protect the child will impinge on the rights of the child to be viewed and treated as an individual. Instead, practitioners need to be acutely aware of the range of factors and influences in every child's life and the complex interrelations between these, or as Baldwin (2000:2) states 'the feelings, thoughts, lived experience of individual children'. As such, a number of issues relating to children's rights need to be at the forefront of child protection work within the early years.

It is important to remember the rights of children in the child protection process. These are shown in Figure 15.1.

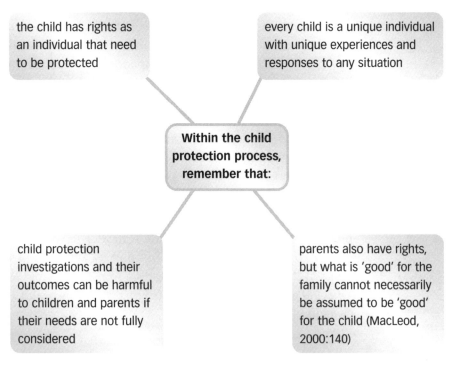

Figure 15.1 *Children's rights in the child protection process*

the child has rights as an individual that need to be protected

every child is a unique individual with unique experiences and responses to any situation

Within the child protection process, remember that:

child protection investigations and their outcomes can be harmful to children and parents if their needs are not fully considered

parents also have rights, but what is 'good' for the family cannot necessarily be assumed to be 'good' for the child (MacLeod, 2000:140)

Concepts of child abuse

In order to analyse child abuse it is important to recognise what would and would not be considered abusive within the boundaries of the child protection system. Practitioners are sometimes concerned that there is no action taken in respect of children who appear to be poorly cared for and where parenting is of a low quality.

Significant harm

The Children Act 1989 makes it clear that to be legally considered as abuse, behaviour must result in 'significant harm' to the child's health and development. Therefore, child abuse may appear to be quite a narrow concept, excluding many cases where there is genuine concern for the child's welfare. However, one of the key tenets of children's rights is that children should be raised in their own families where possible. To achieve this, it is important to ensure that the law does not allow professionals to intervene because of poor standards of parenting alone. The Children Act 1989 introduced a demarcation between children who are abused and those who are 'in need' to support this right.

The abuse of children is a not a static concept

Gibbons et al (1995) argue that child abuse 'is a socially constructed phenomenon which reflects values and opinions of a particular culture at a particular time.' The sorts of behaviours that are deemed to be abusive to children have changed over time and differ between cultures. This does not mean that the behaviours are different, but that our view of whether they are abusive or not abusive has changed (Munro, 2002:58). For example, it would now be generally considered to be emotionally abusive to a child to lock him in a dark cupboard for any period of time, but in the past this was a common punishment. In addition, certain behaviours towards children that can be or are harmful to their welfare and development may not be defined as abusive. For example, regularly smoking in the same room as a child may be strongly disapproved of by many but would not at this moment in time be described as abusive (although this may change in the future as smoking becomes less acceptable as a social habit).

Developments in the parameters of what is considered abusive are ongoing. In a widely reported case in the US a few years ago, a parent was prosecuted for child abuse after her teenage daughter died in an appalling physical condition related to extreme obesity. However, in terms of the rights of children to safety and freedom from harm, child abuse is only one aspect of a wide range of issues affecting children's health and development.

Child abuse is measured by Department of Health statistics based on data drawn from social services across England and Wales. These statistics reflect the number of children who are registered on Child Protection Registers across the country. Registration takes place when there has been a child protection enquiry leading to a child protection case conference. Therefore, the figures reflect only the cases which have drawn official attention and been drawn into the child protection system. It is widely understood that these figures do not represent anywhere near all of the children who suffer 'significant harm' from the actions or omissions of their parents or carers. Currently, there are about 56,000 children's names on Child Protection Registers in England and Wales. In March 2001, 46 per cent of children were registered in the category for neglect; 30 per cent for physical injury; 16 per cent – sexual abuse; 17 per cent – emotional abuse.

Perhaps the most significant gap in our understanding of child abuse is the child's view of what is abusive. MacLeod (2000:131) in discussion on the influential compilation of research findings in the field of child abuse, *Child Protection: Messages from Research* (DoH, 1995) points out that 'there was no discussion about how children might define abuse. The question was not even posed'. There is very little research to help us understand the child's view of what is abusive or how children assimilate the experience of being categorised as abused. This is particularly true of children in their early years.

Defining child abuse

There have been many definitions of child abuse over time, but the definitions currently used are those set out within the *Working Together to Safeguard Children* (1999, DoH) guidelines. These definitions are used as a guideline to remind practitioners of what may be the full range of abusive behaviours and to clarify some particular questions about what is and is not abusive. However, definitions may only cover certain specific behaviours and it is important to recognise that they have limitations.

Child abuse is currently defined within four categories: physical, sexual, emotional and neglect. These categories are useful tools for analysis, but do not reflect the real lives of children who may experience a range of different abuses over time. Definitions can also fail to clarify the extent to which an event has to take place in order to be abusive or whether the age of the child makes a difference to the nature of the behaviour. For example, shaking a baby to only a moderate degree may result in serious and possibly fatal injuries. Shaking an 8 year old to the same degree may be undesirable but not injurious or abusive.

Recognising abuse

Recognising abuse is not usually about identifying single indicators against a checklist of possible signs and symptoms. Evidence of abuse is often gathered over time and from different sources. This evidence may include observations of the appearance and behaviour of the child, linked to knowledge of the family situation, and observations of the interactions between the child and parent. It may include records of conversations and the concerns of other practitioners or parents, or professionals from other agencies. Evidence should relate to aspects of the child's welfare and development that are being affected by the suspected abuse and any indicators of abuse that have been identified. Some points to consider when gathering evidence are shown in Figure 15.2.

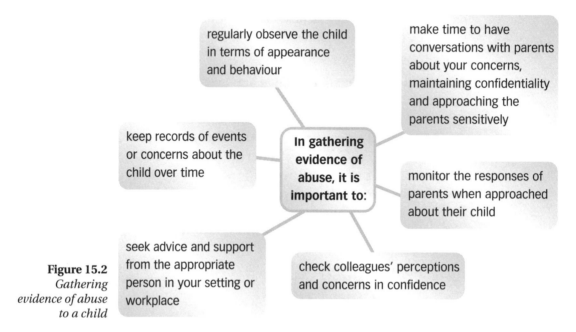

regularly observe the child in terms of appearance and behaviour

make time to have conversations with parents about your concerns, maintaining confidentiality and approaching the parents sensitively

keep records of events or concerns about the child over time

In gathering evidence of abuse, it is important to:

monitor the responses of parents when approached about their child

seek advice and support from the appropriate person in your setting or workplace

check colleagues' perceptions and concerns in confidence

Figure 15.2
Gathering evidence of abuse to a child

Effective recognition of child abuse depends on your ability:

- ⊃ to believe abuse takes place
- ⊃ to believe that many different types of parents are involved in abuse
- ⊃ to accept that it is your responsibility to respond to evidence of any such abuse
- ⊃ to observe and accurately record events, conversations and behaviour.

The need for practitioners working in the child protection system to develop child observation skills and knowledge of child development has been highlighted by Rouse and Vincenti (1994:68). They argue that recognition of child abuse should be factually based, drawing conclusions from observations of children's appearance and behaviour. In this way, recognition of abuse should be more clearly based on 'hard evidence' and the problems of opinion, hearsay, prejudicial judgments and skewed perceptions can be avoided.

The use of observation to identify indicators of abuse means that judgments are soundly based and robust. It is significant that of all professionals working with children, practitioners in early years settings are probably the best trained and most able to use observation effectively in this way.

It is particularly important when discussing the recognition of indicators of abuse to consider the needs of children with disabilities, children with communication difficulties, and children who do not have English as a first language. The indicators may be more difficult to recognise and confirm with some children and there may be barriers to believing that all types of children can be abused (Kennedy, 2000).

There are a number of factors which can make it difficult to develop and exercise skills in observation and identification of indicators of abuse:

- ⊃ lack of time with individual children in large groups or classes
- ⊃ the demands of the curriculum
- ⊃ recording and other paperwork
- ⊃ rising numbers of children with special needs
- ⊃ poor standards of training in child protection
- ⊃ lack of clear policy guidelines within some early years settings or workplaces.

These factors may act as real deterrents to practitioners involving themselves in child protection work. However, as discussed above, children have a right to be protected from abuse and the Children Act 1989 and the guidelines in *Working Together to Safeguard Children* (DoH, 1999) place the responsibility for upholding this right firmly on the shoulders of early years practitioners.

Physical abuse

Physical abuse may involve hitting, shaking, throwing, poisoning, burning or scalding, drowning, suffocating or otherwise causing physical harm to a child. Physical harm may also be caused when a parent or carer feigns the symptoms of, or deliberately causes, ill health to a child whom they are looking after. This situation is commonly described using terms such as factitious illness by proxy or Munchausen syndrome by proxy. (DoH, 1999:2.4)

Physical abuse may be one of the better-understood types of abuse of children, but recognising physical abuse and defining it are complex. One of the main issues is the relationship between corporal punishment and physical abuse in some cultures. Debates about physical abuse are dominated by what is or is not 'normal and lawful' chastisement of a child (Pettican, 1998). In Britain there is a long-held cultural belief in the use of smacking to punish children or control their behaviour, supported by the existence of a strong pro-smacking lobby. Recent attempts to introduce anti-smacking legislation in Scotland, and to consider such a move in England and Wales, have been strongly opposed. Smacking remains a common experience for young children in this society, although national organisations such as the NSPCC are campaigning for legislation to outlaw harsh physical punishment of children.

Practitioners often report problems of assessing the extent to which children have to be harmed by their parent or carer in order to be deemed abused. There is no doubt that a significant proportion of physical abuse arises from over-chastisement and that this can escalate to dangerous levels of assault in some cases. The commonly held view that physical abuse must result in a bruise, mark or other injury in order to be seen as abusive gives practitioners some guidelines as to the 'benchmark' between punishment and abuse.

Another problem with recognising physical abuse is the difficulty in determining the difference between accidental and inflicted injuries. Guidelines can give some help with this, but there are a number of pitfalls in following these faithfully. Children do have injuries that may be unlikely to have been caused accidentally, but in fact are. They may have other injuries where the explanation is likely and the story acceptable. Recent cases such as Victoria Climbie and Lauren Wright have highlighted the plausibility of some physically abusive carers. In both cases, injuries were not identified as abuse because the carer asserted that they had been caused accidentally, and this was believed.

How can we recognise physical abuse?

Practitioners have a responsibility to ensure that their assessments of whether a child has been abused or not are made in the context of their knowledge and understanding of the child and family. One of the difficulties that arises when child protection work is not a regular part of the work of the practitioner or early years setting is that judgements can be made out of context. For example, the appearance of a bruise on a child may result in a referral where there have been no other concerns or injuries to the child. Guidelines have to be followed in the light of what is already known and understood about the child and family.

One of the major pitfalls practitioners face when assessing whether abuse has taken place or not is the belief system they have about particular types of families or individuals. These stereotypes about the likely behaviour of particular types of people can predispose practitioners to assume that certain parents could abuse or others will not. Stereotypes of parents often arise from the degree of social and cultural congruence between the parent and the practitioner. In other words, we are less likely to believe that individuals who are socially and culturally similar to us would abuse. Practitioners have a responsibility to ensure that they are aware of how such stereotypes may affect their work.

In considering whether an abuse referral should be made for physical abuse, it is important to ensure that the points shown in Figure 15.3 have been addressed.

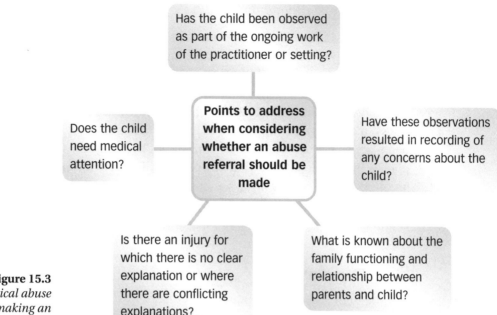

Figure 15.3
Physical abuse and making an abuse referral

The diagram shows "Points to address when considering whether an abuse referral should be made" connected to:
- Has the child been observed as part of the ongoing work of the practitioner or setting?
- Does the child need medical attention?
- Have these observations resulted in recording of any concerns about the child?
- Is there an injury for which there is no clear explanation or where there are conflicting explanations?
- What is known about the family functioning and relationship between parents and child?

Case Study 1

Deciding whether an abuse referral is appropriate

Ben, aged 4 years, attended a family centre day nursery as part of a family support package; this had been designed to help his single parent mother, Brenda, to improve her parenting skills and to support Ben's delayed speech and learning development. Brenda attended parenting classes but often went out to have a cigarette or chatted to other mothers in the centre instead. She sometimes smelled of alcohol when she arrived in the mornings and slurred her words, talked very loudly or became verbally abusive with staff and other parents. Sam, Ben's key worker, noticed that on several occasions over a period of time Ben was very distressed on entry to nursery and that he would remain withdrawn and easily upset all day. Sam recorded these observations and the fact that Ben's mother was often abrupt with him, handled him roughly and made disparaging remarks about him to the staff.

One day, Sam noticed bruises on Ben's thigh and buttocks when helping him in the toilet. He asked Brenda how Ben might have got the bruises. She became angry and told him to mind his own business and that she did not know how the bruises had happened. However, later she came back and gave a long explanation about how Ben had fallen off his skateboard and bumped his bottom. Brenda kept telling Ben that he must tell the truth about what had happened, insisting that her version was the truth. When Ben looked bewildered and said he had not got a skateboard, Brenda shouted at him.

1 Using the list in Figure 15.3, write down the points you believe should be considered within this case study.

2 Do you think a referral should be made? Give your reasons.

The impact of physical abuse on the child

For some children, physical abuse results in death or permanent injury. Every year about 80 children die at the hands of their parents or carers. The most common causes of death are head injuries and internal injuries. For example, Lauren Wright died when her digestive system collapsed after a beating. For other children, the long-term impact of physical abuse is less to do with injuries and more to do with the emotional impact of being abused. The long-term outcomes for physically abused children may be linked more to the 'harshly punitive, less reliable and less warmly involved style of parenting' associated with physical abuse, than with the direct impact of the physical abuse on the child's development (Gibbons et al, 1995).

Emotional abuse

Emotional abuse is the persistent emotional ill-treatment of a child such as to cause severe and persistent adverse effects on the child's emotional development. It may involve conveying to children that they are worthless or unloved, inadequate or valued only insofar as they meet the needs of another person. It may feature age or developmentally inappropriate expectations being imposed on children. It may involve causing children frequently to feel frightened or in danger or the exploitation or corruption of children. Some level of emotional abuse is involved in all types of ill-treatment of a child, though it may occur alone. (DoH, 1999:2.5)

Emotional abuse of young children can be analysed in two categories: active emotional abuse and emotional neglect. It is important to remember that, although active emotional abuse involves active behaviour on the part of the parent and emotional neglect involves passive behaviour, the child must be deemed to have suffered 'significant harm' in order to be considered abused. Emotional abuse is usually ongoing over a period of time, tending to involve a range of behaviours from the parents that are 'low on warmth and high on criticism' (Pettican, 1998; DoH, 1995; Kay, 2003). Parental behaviour may include indifference to the child's needs; rejection of the child; verbal assaults on the child's self-esteem (scapegoating, blaming or constant criticism); or a refusal to accept the child as he or she is. The parent may be unattached to the child and/or hostile and rejecting. Emotional abuse may appear alone or as part of other types of abuse.

Emotional neglect

Emotional neglect is sometimes used to describe the passive process of ignoring or failing to respond to the child's needs, and is linked to parenting by those who have severe unmet needs of their own (Iwaniec, 1995). Emotional neglect involves the failure of parents to meet the child's need for love, security, positive regard, warmth, praise and a sense of 'belonging' in their family and the wider world. Emotional neglect may be associated with a failure to respond to even the child's most basic needs or with a parent who is 'psychologically unavailable' to the child; in other words, a parent who is unresponsive to the child's needs because he or she does not recognise these. An emotionally neglected child may have insecure attachments within the family, and as a result may suffer from poor self-esteem, delays in development and difficulties in social relationships. Emotional neglect may be accompanied by other sorts of neglect, such as failure to meet the child's basic physical needs on a consistent basis, and failure to ensure the child is safe and secure through proper supervision.

Active emotional abuse

Emotional abuse is a more active assault on the child's emotional and psychological welfare. It may involve:

- ⊃ targeting the child for ridicule and verbal abuse
- ⊃ shaming the child
- ⊃ treating the child as unwanted and unloved
- ⊃ forcing the child to perform tasks for food and comfort
- ⊃ locking the child in a room alone.

For example, in one case, a 5-year-old boy was forced to sleep on the floor, told every day that he wasn't wanted or loved, refused food if he misbehaved, and never touched or picked up by his mother. His two sisters were treated as loved and cherished children. The boy became very distressed, wetting and soiling himself at school and ripping wallpaper and setting it on fire at home.

How do we recognise emotional abuse?

Recognising emotional abuse and neglect involves observing and monitoring the child's behaviour. Emotionally neglected and abused children are usually very low in self-esteem. They may lack confidence to tackle their tasks in the early years setting and may respond emotionally under pressure. They may seek inappropriately close relationships with staff or draw attention to themselves through unwanted behaviour. Alternatively, the child may be withdrawn and sad, unable to join in and be socially isolated. Emotionally abused children may demonstrate neurotic behaviour at times, such as pulling out their own hair or self-harming. They may have bursts of anger or distress or complete withdrawal. On the other hand, the child may be over-compliant and try too hard to please.

Emotional abuse and neglect of a child need to be monitored over time in order to demonstrate that there is 'significant harm' to the child's health and development. The effects of emotional abuse and neglect are found in the child's developmental rates, including physical growth, speech and cognitive development and social skills development. Close observation and careful recording are needed to ensure that there is an ongoing record of concerns about the child's development. Measures to ensure that the child is properly monitored should include a multi-agency response involving health professionals who can monitor growth and weight, and the child's attainment of developmental milestones. Factors to consider when monitoring a child to check for emotional abuse are shown in Figure 15.4.

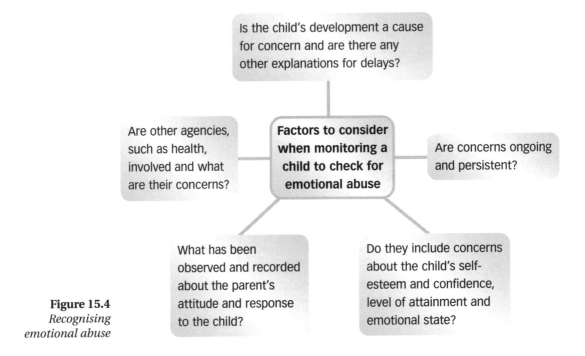

Figure 15.4
Recognising emotional abuse

Is the child's development a cause for concern and are there any other explanations for delays?

Are other agencies, such as health, involved and what are their concerns?

Factors to consider when monitoring a child to check for emotional abuse

Are concerns ongoing and persistent?

What has been observed and recorded about the parent's attitude and response to the child?

Do they include concerns about the child's self-esteem and confidence, level of attainment and emotional state?

Case Study 2

Emotional abuse

Adam, aged 3 years, has just started at nursery school. He has very limited speech and a chronic inability to concentrate. He tends to sit in a slumped position, staring into space unless directly addressed by a staff member. He does not make eye contact and has not attempted to join in activities with either adults or other children. Adam is thin and small and unkempt in appearance. When his mother collects him from nursery she likes to talk to the staff. She does not speak directly to Adam and she tends to put him into his coat hurriedly, without looking at him or responding to his struggles. She does not make eye contact with him and is apparently unresponsive to him at all levels.

The school nurse has contacted the health visitor with the mother's permission and the health visitor reports delays in Adam's speech, weight, height and cognitive development that have no explanation in terms of illness or disability.

1 What steps might you take in response to any concerns about Adam?
2 Who might be involved?

The impact of emotional abuse on the child

Emotional abuse and neglect may occur alone or as part of a more complex abusive situation. For example, the relationship between sexual and emotional abuse is well-documented. Emotional abuse is present in most cases of abuse and can have the most significant effects on the child. Long-term outcomes of emotional neglect can be amongst the most significant (Parton, 1996). They may include:

- ⊃ lack of achievement in school
- ⊃ failure to develop supportive relationships
- ⊃ drug and alcohol abuse
- ⊃ chronic low self-esteem and lack of confidence
- ⊃ self-harming and possibly even suicide.

Sexual abuse

Sexual abuse involves forcing or enticing a child or young person to take part in sexual activities, whether or not the child is aware of what is happening. The activities may involve physical contact, including penetrative (for example, rape or buggery) or non-penetrative acts. They may include non-contact activities, such as involving children in looking at, or in the production of, pornographic material or watching sexual activities, or encouraging children to behave in sexually inappropriate ways. (DoH, 1999:2.6)

The extent and nature of the sexual abuse of children was little understood before the 1980s, when it became apparent through the work of a range of professionals in the field that sexual abuse of children was much more common and widespread than previously believed. The secret and taboo nature of child sexual abuse within the family meant that many cases never came to light prior to this, and worse still many others were dismissed or not responded to by the professionals involved. Many sexually abused children never received the support and help they needed to help them with the trauma they suffered, and grew to adulthood without sharing their secret.

Sexual abuse within the family is more common than stranger abuse

Now it is widely recognised that sexual abuse within the family is common in comparison with stranger abuse, with the majority of children, both boys and girls, abused by close male relatives. The debate about child sexual abuse over the last two decades has erased some of the taboos surrounding this type of abuse and raised awareness among professionals and public alike. However, child sexual abuse remains a secret act, often only known to the child and the abuser. Successful prosecutions of perpetrators continue at a low rate, and many cases are suspected but not proven. A number of widely reported cases in the 1990s highlighted the dangers of child sexual abuse within institutional settings, particularly those which were meant to provide a safe and secure environment for children who have already suffered from abuse.

Sexual abuse of children can take many forms, including using pornography to stimulate children sexually, abuse by groups of adults, and involving children in the making of pornographic material for distribution to others. Sexual abuse can involve coercion, violent attack, threats and intimidation. It can also occur within an apparently loving relationship where the child is gradually introduced to sexual activity through a series of small steps, progressing towards penetrative sex. This is sometimes described as 'grooming'.

Recent developments include an increased recognition of the role of children in abusing other children, particularly within the family. An NSPCC survey (NSPCC, November 2000) found a much greater prevalence of sibling abuse than has been previously recognised. The child abused was usually a sister or stepsister, the abuser usually a brother or stepbrother. Brothers were found to be responsible for more than one-third of sexual abuse committed by relatives (reported in the *Independent on Sunday*, 19/11/2000).

How do we recognise child sexual abuse?

Recognising child sexual abuse can be difficult unless the child 'discloses' the abuse by telling an adult about it. Although this can and does happen, the child may find it difficult to talk to others about the sexual abuse if it has been accompanied by threats of violence or separation from non-abusing family members, or if the child has developed a sense of shame about the abuse.

Many children who are sexually abused will show signs of emotional abuse. The child may perceive himself or herself as worthless and unlovable, valuable only in terms of the extent to which he or she can satisfy adult sexual needs. The impact of the emotionally abusive aspects of the sexual abuse may last longer and have more negative implications for the child than any physical consequences.

Depending on the type and severity of the sexual abuse, not all children will show physical symptoms. However, for some children the physical consequence can be very severe, in terms of diseases such as hepatitis, HIV, gonorrhoea and syphilis, and physical damage to the reproductive organs. One of the common indicators of child sexual abuse is inappropriate sexual knowledge and behaviour in the child. This goes far beyond the normal curiosity and experimentation that every child involves himself or herself in during different stages of sexual development. It may involve persistently:

- ⊃ introducing sexual themes into conversation, play and art work
- ⊃ sexual attacks or sexually coercive play with other children
- ⊃ sexualised behaviour with adults.

Other indicators that should not be ignored are related to the child's sense of self and self-esteem, any self-harming behaviour and social isolation. Sexually abused children often carry a burden of secrets that make the day-to-day sharing of friendship difficult to sustain. These children are emotionally distressed, isolated, feel different to other children and often blame themselves for the abuse.

Case Study 3

Sexual abuse

James, 6, had developed some problems in school over a period of several months. These involved aggressive behaviour with peers, sexually explicit comments to adults and children, poor performance, lack of concentration and weeping fits if tackled about his behaviour. His teacher was deeply concerned that James had made comments about her breasts, and, as she put it, 'leered at me'.

Attempts to discuss these issues with the parents had met with complete denial and a fear that James had been severely punished at home for attracting attention by his behaviour in school. James began to linger in the classroom at breaks and avoid other children. Social services contacted the school to ask for information about James when an older sister who had just left home came to the social services office and alleged that an uncle was abusing all the children in the family.

1 Discuss with a mentor or colleague how James could be supported through the ensuing investigation.

2 What sort of issues may arise for James' teacher in offering this support and how could they be dealt with?

The impact of sexual abuse on the child

Sexual abuse of young children may lead to physical harm including disease and physical damage. However, often (but not always) this type of harm is short term. The long-term effects can be severe and relate to the emotional damage that is common in sexual abuse. These effects can include low self-esteem, failure in education, difficulties in making relationships, abusive relationships, self-harming, drug and alcohol abuse and even suicide.

Neglect

Neglect is the persistent failure to meet a child's basic physical and/or psychological needs, likely to result in the serious impairment of the child's health or development. It may involve a parent or carer failing to provide adequate food, shelter and clothing, failing to protect a child from physical harm or danger, or the failure to ensure access to appropriate medical care or treatment. It may also include neglect of, or unresponsiveness to, a child's basic emotional needs. (DoH, 1999: 2.7)

The debate about neglect used to relate to the dividing line between low standards of care related to poverty and social deprivation and the wilful neglect of children by their carers. However, this debate has moved on in response to the development of clearer legislative and procedural foundations for our understanding of abuse. To be categorised as abusive, neglect must result in 'significant harm' to the child's welfare and development and must involve a substantial failure to meet the child's basic needs.

Maccoby and Martin (1983) included neglect as a category in their classification of parenting styles, arguing that neglect occurs where the child's needs have low priority within the family and, therefore, there is little or no attempt to meet them to any acceptable extent. Their model of neglecting parents suggested that they are both low on warmth towards the child and poor on communication within the family, and also that they have low expectations of the child and poor controls over the child's behaviour. Neglect is not, therefore, just about food, warmth and shelter. It is also about the failure to give children appropriate guidance and support, discipline and controls. Children who are neglected may receive little instruction about behaviour and social presentation and, as such, may be socially isolated not only because they are poorly dressed or smelly, but also because they do not know how to behave in ways that are acceptable to others. Similarly, they may have little support for their educational progress or for their efforts to develop friendships.

How do we recognise neglect?

The impact of neglect is not instantaneous, but develops over time and is evident in a range of aspects of the child's growth and development. Neglect can be identified through indicators such as the child's appearance and behaviour, and also observation of the parent's behaviour and attitude towards the child. Neglecting parents tend to be disinterested in or unconcerned about their children's physical and psychological state. The cues that tend to elicit a response in a non-neglecting parent may have little impact on a neglecting parent. For example, crying, screaming, evidence of illness or distress in the child may not seem to gain the expected response. In a recent child abuse case in which a young child died after drinking his mother's methadone, it was reported that she took him on a shopping trip to town despite the fact that he was showing serious symptoms of illness. The mother then left the child with a friend so she could smoke heroin, although by this time he was dying.

Other indicators of neglect are found in the results of assessments of the child's developmental and educational progress. A neglected child may fail to thrive in terms of physical development and this will be reflected in height and weight charts for children under the age of 5 years, where no other cause of delays in physical development are identified. Neglected children often struggle educationally, lacking a strong basis of early learning and home support for education on which to build. Parents are unlikely to engage significantly with practitioners unless it is to access support for themselves.

With reference to the discussion above, the child's social relationships may be poor, and the child may be socially rejected. This may be a due to a lack of appropriate social knowledge, lack of self-control or disturbances in the child's behaviour.

Recognising neglect involves careful observation and recording of incidents, events about the child, the child's appearance and behaviour and the parent/child relationship over time. The issues shown in Figure 15.5 need to be considered.

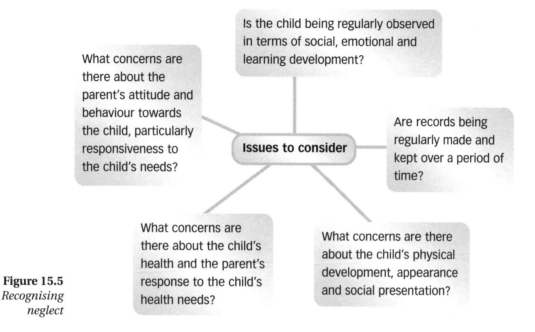

Figure 15.5
Recognising neglect

Issues to consider:

- Is the child being regularly observed in terms of social, emotional and learning development?
- What concerns are there about the parent's attitude and behaviour towards the child, particularly responsiveness to the child's needs?
- Are records being regularly made and kept over a period of time?
- What concerns are there about the child's health and the parent's response to the child's health needs?
- What concerns are there about the child's physical development, appearance and social presentation?

Case Study 4

Neglect

Jessica, aged 5, entered school after a short period in a family centre day care unit. She was extremely shy, saying very little to anyone and avoiding eye contact when spoken to by adults. Jessica was a thin child, poorly dressed in ill-fitting clothes that were not suitable for the weather conditions. She had difficulty sitting still in class and often got up and wandered around. Some of the other children started to avoid sitting near Jessica in the classroom and she was usually alone at breaks. The teacher suggested that some children could try and get Jessica to join in, but they complained that she smelled and that she did not know how to play their games.

The teacher asked Jessica a few questions, as she often smelled strongly of urine. It became clear that Jessica did not use toilet paper after urinating and that as a result she was extremely sore in the genital area. The teacher spoke to the mother about this, suggesting a visit to the doctor was required, but received little response. The mother took no action, although Jessica was obviously in discomfort, and she began to avoid the teacher at the end of school, waiting outside the playground. Jessica's attendance became erratic and she was often absent without explanation. It also became obvious that she did not read or play at home, and the contents of her reading folder grew as unread letters from school to home gathered in it.

1 Plan a strategy that the teacher could use to engage this parent with the school and within which concerns could be raised effectively.

2 Discuss the proposed strategy with a colleague or mentor.

The impact of neglect on the child

There is evidence that the long-term effects of severe neglect may be extremely serious. See Figure 15.6.

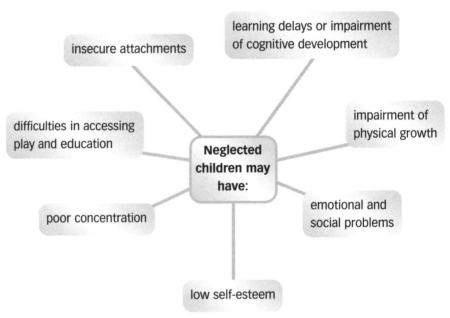

Figure 15.6
Long-term effects of neglect

The life chances of the child may be permanently impaired if the neglect is serious and long term.

Disclosure

Some child abuse is made apparent or is confirmed by a disclosure from the child. Disclosure simply means that the child tells an adult or another child what has been happening to him and this includes evidence of abuse or neglect. For example, a child, when asked about a nasty bruise, may tell a teacher or practitioner in an early years setting that a parent has inflicted it. Disclosure is most common where there is physical or sexual abuse. Children may disclose in a range of contexts including public settings. Young children's disclosures may be unclear if they do not have the language skills to explain what is happening to them and it is possible not to recognise such a disclosure for what it is. The question of whether a disclosure is genuine or not has long been considered a difficult area of judgment. However, evidence shows that younger children are unlikely to fabricate disclosures and that all such events should be taken seriously. Other factors to consider are whether the child's story remains consistent through retelling, and whether there are other concerns that support suspicions of abuse. However in a small number of cases, particularly those of sexual abuse, disclosure can come 'out of the blue' with no forewarning.

Responding to disclosure

Responding to a child who discloses requires patience, sensitivity and a calm and structured approach. Children may be significantly affected if a disclosure is handled poorly. Children are most likely to disclose to those adults they like and have warm relationships and regular contact with. The child has placed trust in the individual to whom she discloses and it is important that this trust is not broken, as discussed below.

Disclosure may have a different meaning to the child than to the adults involved. For the adults, disclosure often heralds the start of a child protection enquiry within the framework of procedures. The child is often unaware of what may happen after disclosure. He or she may simply want to tell a trusted adult about what is happening to make him or her so unhappy and for that adult to stop the events that are causing the unhappiness.

As a practitioner you need to consider the following if a disclosure is made to you:

- ⊃ privacy and a quiet place for the child to talk
- ⊃ using active listening skills to promote the disclosure without asking questions
- ⊃ the role of the person who comforts and supports the child and the limitations of this role, for example, not being able to keep this to yourself; knowing the enquiry will be painful for the child
- ⊃ accurate and objective recording of the conversation, i.e. facts only and no speculation, opinion or assumptions
- ⊃ evidence of other indicators of abuse that may support the child's disclosure, for example, previous enquiries, observations of the child's relationship with parents, behaviour, attitude and ability to engage with the setting
- ⊃ the setting's policy on how to handle a disclosure from the practical point of view.

Case Study 5

Disclosure

Karen, age 6 years, asked her teacher if she could stay in at break, as she wanted to help clear up after art. The teacher had been concerned about how quiet Karen had been in the last few weeks and agreed to the plan. Karen said nothing for 15 minutes, and as the other children started to flock back through the door, she urgently whispered 'Dave touches me on my front bottom and I don't like it…'. The teacher turned the first child round and told her to go to the office and ask another adult to come immediately. She took Karen into the corridor, explaining that she wanted to listen to what she had to say but she needed to sort the other children out first. She then asked the returning children to sit down quietly. When the head teacher arrived she explained that she needed to talk to Karen urgently and asked him to cover the class for 10 minutes. The teacher took Karen into the cooking room and listened to what she had to say. A teaching assistant stayed with Karen doing quiet reading while the teacher and head discussed the situation and contacted social services for advice.

1 What would you do in the same situation and how would you deal with the practicalities in your setting?

2 What are Karen's needs in this situation and how can they best be met?

Responding to suspected child abuse

Responses to suspected child abuse need to take place within the procedural framework supporting the child protection process. The Area Child Protection Committee (ACPC), a multi-agency body in every local authority, has the responsibility for producing child protection procedures, based on the *Working Together to Safeguard Children* (DoH, 1999) guidelines.

ACPC procedures outline the roles of all professionals involved with children, based on the principles of the Children Act 1989. Each setting or workplace should have its own procedures as well.

Practitioners involved with children are encouraged to recognise that their role in child protection is not voluntary, but part of their more general professional roles and responsibilities. Within the procedural guidelines there is a strong theme of supporting parents and children through the child protection process and ensuring that they are kept informed and consulted at all stages.

Referring suspected abuse

The decision to refer suspected abuse to the police or social services is never taken lightly. For many practitioners, such referrals involve a weighty responsibility and a number of concerns. Some common fears, which you may experience, are shown in Figure 15.7.

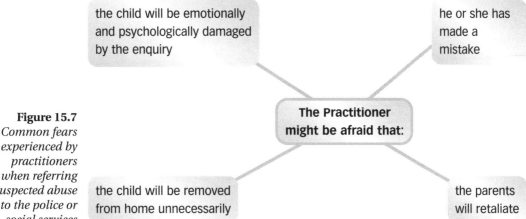

Figure 15.7
Common fears experienced by practitioners when referring suspected abuse to the police or social services

Why refer?

Referring suspected abuse is not an individual choice in theory. Practitioners are encouraged to consider their role in relation to that of colleagues and professionals from other agencies, and to act within prescriptive guidelines, particularly ACPC Child Protection Procedures. Perceptions that practitioners may hold about making a referral to child protection agencies are shown in Figure 15.8.

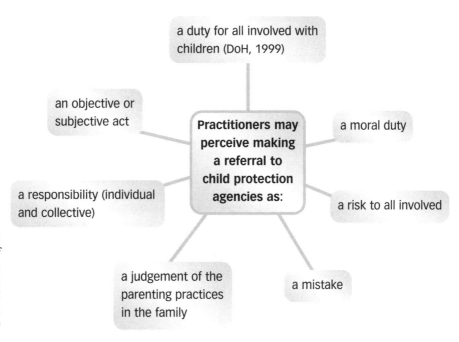

Figure 15.8
Perceptions of practitioners when making a referral to a child protection agency

The decision to refer abuse to a child protection agency needs to be objective and with the child's best interests in mind. Factors influencing this decision must be weighed and considered in the light of the primary goal, which is to promote the child's welfare. In order to ensure this goal remains primary, other factors need to be evaluated in terms of their validity, and perceptions need to be considered in terms of their objectivity.

For example, a belief that particular parents could not be involved in abuse of their children needs to be considered objectively. Why do we believe this? What evidence do we base this belief on?

> **Activity 2) Why not report abuse?**
>
> 1 List any reasons why a practitioner may not wish to refer suspected abuse of a child.
> 2 Note down the possible consequences of not referring suspected child abuse.

Making a child protection referral

The practitioner should first discuss concerns about the child with the appropriate person. In schools, this will be the child protection liaison teacher. In other early years settings, this could be a designated member of staff or the manager. In some cases, it is appropriate to contact social services and ask for advice on how to proceed. It is possible that after taking advice:

⊃ you make referral to social services, or

⊃ social services decide to act on the information you have given them.

Not all types of abuse require the same response. See Figure 15.9 for information about the options available.

Responding to abuse:	
Child protection referral	If there is evidence of physical or sexual abuse then a referral to social services should be made promptly
Single-agency response	If there are concerns about neglect or emotional abuse you may agree to monitor the situation and work with the parents on your concerns
Multi-agency response	You may agree to work with other agencies or professionals working with the family to provide support, for example, health visitors, social services

Figure 15.9
Making an appropriate response to abuse

The circumstances in which a referral to social services should always be made are where:

⊃ the child makes an allegation of abuse

⊃ there are physical injuries which are cause for concern

⊃ there are concerns about sexual abuse

⊃ there are concerns about emotional abuse or neglect and the situation has deteriorated to the extent that the child may be suffering significant harm

⊃ a child is being refused vital medical treatment

⊃ there is a credible allegation from a member of the public

⊃ the child is in contact with an individual who may put them at risk

⊃ there are further concerns about a child who is already on the Child Protection Register.

Referrals can be made in one of two ways, as shown in Figure 15.10. Either way it is important to record your concerns as soon as possible.

A child protection referral	
Make the referral:	Either By completing an inter-agency referral form for reporting suspected child abuse to social services *or* By making a telephone referral first in situations where there appears to be some urgency
The report should include:	Basic details about the child, for example, name, age, address, class, any special needs or particular issues affecting the child including any communication difficulties the child may have Details of your concerns, including dates, and any discussion you have had with the child and parents about these concerns Details of any discussions you have had with other staff about your concerns The level of your concern and extent of risk you believe the child to be in.

Figure 15.10
Making a child protection referral

It is important to ensure that reporting is factual, based on observation and evidence, rather than opinion, hearsay or speculation. This means that practitioners need to attend closely to the language used in their reports and to ensure that they are objective and not subjective in tone and content.

Working with parents

In order to ensure that parents' rights are maintained in this situation, in line with the requirements of the Children Act 1989, and 'Working Together to Safeguard Children', parents need to be:

⊃ informed that a referral to social services is to be made and why (unless informing the parents could put the child at risk of acute physical harm)

⊃ kept informed of the progress of the child protection process

⊃ supported to remain as involved as possible in the process and any decision-making within that

⊃ supported to continue to care for their child wherever possible.

Parents differ in their responses to child protection enquiries, but many will feel angry, threatened, frightened or distressed by the process. This may mean that they behave in ways that are hard to manage and may feel very disturbing to practitioners. Factors that may help to support parents and reduce the possibility of conflict are shown in Figure 15.11.

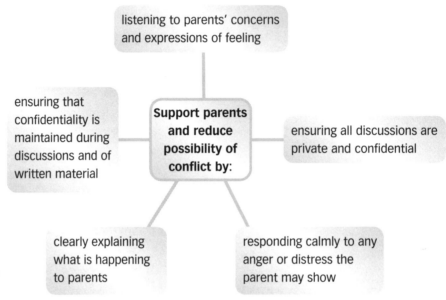

Figure 15.11
Factors that may help to support parents and reduce the possibility of conflict

Working with the child

Referring a child, whether the child has disclosed or you have collected information about indicators of abuse, can feel like a betrayal of the relationship you have. Part of this feeling can come from the knowledge that you have about the possible consequences of a child protection enquiry, and the recognition that the child's wishes in the situation may not be complied with. Evidence shows that many abused children do not want separation from their abusing parent, but that they want the abuse stopped. Young children in particular many have difficulty in understanding that this may not be possible in all cases.

Case Study 6

The rights of children

Hayley, aged 4 years, has been in nursery for about 3 months and you are her key worker. Today your manager was contacted by social services, who want information about Hayley, and to interview her with her mother's permission about allegations of sexual abuse made by Hayley's older sister to a teacher in school. The social worker intends to see Hayley after nursery finishes and asks if she can speak to her at the nursery as the alleged abuser, a friend of the mother's, is a lodger in the home. The mother arrives at the end of nursery absolutely distraught, crying and incoherent.

Referring back to Figure 15.1 on page 499 ('Children's Rights in the Child Protection Process') discuss what could be done to support both Hayley and her mother in this situation and what issues need to be born in mind.

The skills and abilities required for working with children in a child protection enquiry include:

➲ good listening skills – the child's concerns may not be what you assume they are

➲ ability to offer emotional and practical support

➲ trustworthiness

➲ time and energy

➲ ability to focus on the child when under pressure to ensure procedures are being followed correctly

➲ ability to recognise and focus on the child's needs where others' needs and wishes are strongly competing.

Staff development and training issues

There are a number of issues arising from the role of the practitioner in an early years setting in child protection in terms of staff development and training that, as a practitioner, you may wish to consider. They are:

➲ the need for practitioners to develop child observation skills and knowledge of child development (Rouse and Vincenti, 1994:68 Fig. 5.1)

➲ developing skills in providing emotional support for children

➲ anti-discriminatory practice

➲ training to support multidisciplinary and inter-agency approaches. (Kay, 2003; DoH, 1999: Rouse and Vincenti, 1994)

❯ The child protection enquiry

The majority of reports of child abuse go to social services child protection services. However, in situations where it is clear that the child has been harmed by someone outside the family it may be appropriate to refer to the police, who have specialist Child Protection Units to deal with such cases.

Local authorities have a duty to investigate any allegations of child abuse under Section 47 of the Children Act 1989. The main purposes of any such investigation are to:

- establish the facts and make a record of them
- assess the risk to the child as a basis for taking action to protect him or her
- assess the extent to which the child's needs are being met within the family.

Since 2000, assessment of the child and family, which is a central part of any investigation, is achieved through the *Framework for Assessment of Children in Need and their Families* (DoH, 2000), which is a detailed assessment tool used to establish what the child's needs are and the extent to which they are being met within the family and wider environment (see page 533 for a full discussion).

Action following a child protection referral

The child and family are initially assessed within the 'Framework for Assessment' by an experienced child protection social worker, within seven days from referral. This assessment covers the needs of the child, the extent to which parents can meet these needs, and the family and environmental factors that support or hinder this process. The initial assessment will conclude whether:

- immediate action, possibly legal measures, should be taken to protect the child
- a child protection enquiry should be instigated under section 47 of the Children Act 1989
- the child and his or her family should be referred for family support services under section 17 of the Children Act 1989, as a 'child in need'
- no further action should be taken.

A section 47 enquiry will be instigated if there is evidence that the child is suffering or likely to suffer significant harm related to the care he or she is receiving. This involves a core assessment within the 'Framework for Assessment'. This establishes a range of factors, as shown in Figure 15.12.

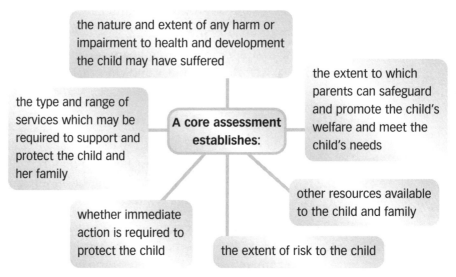

Figure 15.12
A core assessment

the nature and extent of any harm or impairment to health and development the child may have suffered

the extent to which parents can safeguard and promote the child's welfare and meet child's needs

the type and range of services which may be required to support and protect the child and her family

A core assessment establishes:

other resources available to the child and family

whether immediate action is required to protect the child

the extent of risk to the child

Assessment is achieved through interviews with family members and key professionals mainly, and examination of any relevant records. However, if it is considered that there is a high level of risk of 'acute physical harm' to the child, the social worker may:

➲ try and persuade the suspected abuser to leave the household or make other arrangements to safeguard the child in the short-term

➲ apply for an Emergency Protection Order (EPO)

➲ apply for a Child Assessment Order, if the parents refuse access to the child for medical or other assessment

(see section on the 'Legislative and Procedural Framework' page 527, below).

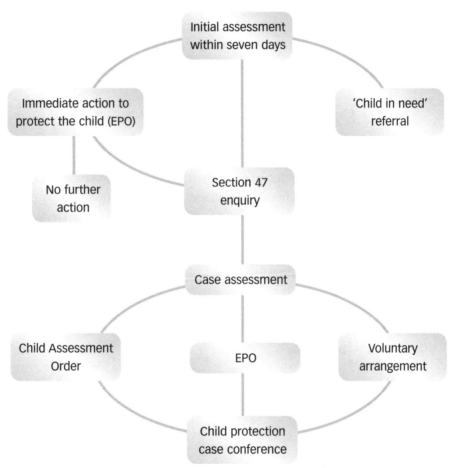

Figure 15.13
Action following a Child Protection Referral (within the 'Framework for Assessment')

The role of the practitioner in child protection enquiries

The roles of all professionals are outlined in the *Working Together to Safeguard Children* (DoH, 1999) guidelines and it is important that you are fully aware of your responsibilities. Knowing what is expected of you as a practitioner in an early years setting is a significant step in working towards supporting the child in this situation. Perhaps one of the child's most essential rights is to have competent and well-prepared adults working with him or her within the child protection process. You, as a practitioner in an early years setting in child protection enquiries should have the knowledge and ability to:

- ⊃ recognise indicators of possible abuse
- ⊃ make considered decisions about referring children to social services where abuse is suspected
- ⊃ ensure all communication with children and parents is sensitive and involves active listening
- ⊃ report accurately, based on observation
- ⊃ inform the investigating social worker of any special needs or communication difficulties the child may have
- ⊃ give information to any social worker involved in a section 47 enquiry
- ⊃ support the child in the setting and be aware of the stress the enquiry may place on the child and his family
- ⊃ maintain confidentiality of speech and written record.

The child protection case conference

The child protection case conference is a meeting with social services and other professionals, also involving parents, in order to pool information about the child and family in relation to child protection concerns. The meeting may include professionals from health, education and voluntary organisations. Parents may be invited to all or part of the child protection case conference depending on the ACPC guidelines for the local authority. The purpose of the child protection conference and details of decisions made are given in Figure 15.14.

The child protection case conference	
Its purpose	Pool information about the child and any concerns about him or her Discuss factors which affect the family functioning Assess the risk of further abuse and the extent of concern about the child Make plans to safeguard the child and support the family
It makes two decisions	Who is to be the key worker for the child (usually a social worker) and who will be in the 'core group' Whether the child's name should be added to the Child Protection Register

Figure 15.14
Purpose of the child protection case conference

The child protection register

The child protection register is a centrally held record of children who are considered to have been abused. A child is only registered when he or she has been the subject of a child protection case conference and the decision to register has been taken by the conference. Registration usually takes place where there are ongoing concerns about the child's safety and welfare. It is used to ensure that professionals can find out if a child has suffered previous abuse and there are ongoing concerns. Registration also triggers the commitment of resources to a child and family to safeguard the child and help the family to cope better, or remove the child to alternative carers. Whilst a child's name is on the register, there will be ongoing review case conferences to monitor the child's welfare and situation, usually at 3- or 6-monthly intervals.

Child protection case conference recommendations

The child protection case conference also makes a series of recommendations designed to support and promote the child's welfare and the parents' ability to parent safely and effectively. These recommendations are incorporated in a child protection plan, which sets out goals for involved agencies on how they can contribute to safeguarding and promoting the child's welfare. The plan may include legal action to protect the child, such as Care Proceedings to make the child the subject of a Care Order or Supervision Order. This may involve, in a small number of cases, removal of the child into local authority care on a short- or long-term basis. The child protection plan is subject to regular review, usually 6-monthly or more frequently, and is monitored by the key worker.

Core groups

The 'core group' is made up of professionals with direct responsibility for the child and family. They monitor and discuss the progress of the child protection plan in-between case conferences. You may be involved in the 'core group' for a particular child in your care. However, research evidence shows that 'core groups' often fade away after the initial case conference, leaving the social services to monitor and implement the child protection plan alone. Clearly, this is not in line with current guidelines and policy and continuing efforts to strengthen multi-agency approaches to child protection are taking place, with more initiatives in the pipeline since the Victoria Climbie enquiry (January 2003).

The role of practitioners in the child protection case conference

Early years practitioners involved in child abuse cases may be asked to attend the case conference and contribute their knowledge of the child and family to the proceedings. Normally, a report is written based on the records kept within the early years setting or workplace. Your knowledge and experience of the child and family is crucial to ensuring that a clear picture of the child's welfare and situation is established. You may also be asked to be part of the core group, as discussed above, and to take on responsibilities within the child protection plan. In order to support the child and parents within this process, the following needs to be considered:

- ⊃ factual verbal and written reporting based on observations
- ⊃ objective, not subjective, views and opinions
- ⊃ consideration of what your early years setting or organisation can offer to support the child and family in order to meet the child's needs.

Objective views and opinions are factual and based on observation and actual knowledge rather than speculation, hearsay or assumptions. For example, we could describe a child as 'really battered, covered in bruises and obviously been beaten' or we could say ' the child had a number of bruises on her upper arms and shoulders that appeared to be of different ages: some purple, some green and yellow'.

The child protection plan

The core group develops the child protection plan in response to recommendations made by the case conference. Targets are set to ensure the child's safety, to promote the child's welfare and to support the family to parent more safely and effectively. The plan will also determine the roles and responsibilities of different professionals and agencies in meeting these targets.

In early years settings the practitioner's roles and responsibilities may include those identified in Figure 15.15.

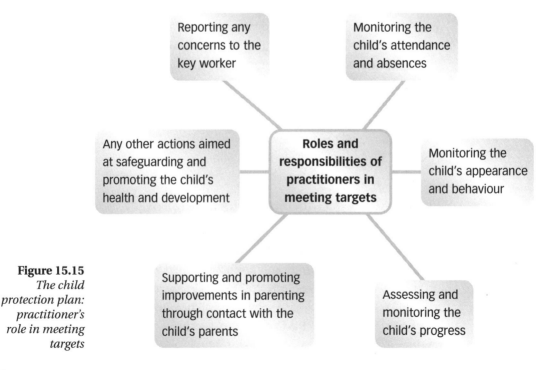

Figure 15.15
The child protection plan: practitioner's role in meeting targets

Reporting any concerns to the key worker

Monitoring the child's attendance and absences

Any other actions aimed at safeguarding and promoting the child's health and development

Roles and responsibilities of practitioners in meeting targets

Monitoring the child's appearance and behaviour

Supporting and promoting improvements in parenting through contact with the child's parents

Assessing and monitoring the child's progress

Case Study 7

Monitoring development

Harry, aged 4 years, has been placed by social services for part of the day with a childminder after he was found to be neglected by his parents. The childminder is expected to monitor Harry's health and welfare as part of the child protection plan.

1 Describe which aspects of Harry's development the childminder could be expected to monitor.

2 How she might go about this?

3 Which areas of Harry's development would the childminder not be monitoring?

The legal and procedural framework

The legal and procedural framework for child protection processes in England and Wales determines the responses that are available to professionals when faced with suspected child abuse. Knowledge and understanding of the legal and procedural process can help practitioners in early years settings to perform their roles more effectively. This knowledge includes:

- the rights of the child and parents within the legislative and policy framework
- the roles and responsibilities of different professionals involved in protecting children
- the role of legal intervention in protecting children
- the limits and boundaries of legal intervention.

The Children Act 1989

The Children Act 1989 is based on a number of key principles that underpin the ethos in which child protection work should take place. The key principles of the Children Act 1989 are:

- the child's welfare is paramount
- delay in legal processes is prejudicial to the child's welfare and should be avoided
- courts should only make orders where it is better for the child to do so than not (the non-interventionist principle)
- decisions should be made in partnership between professionals from different agencies, and families
- the child's views and opinions should be considered (but cannot override the need for the child's welfare to be paramount)
- 'parental responsibility' is retained by parents throughout, even if the child is in care (it is transferred only through the making of an adoption order).

Essentially these principles support a child-centred approach, based on partnership between parents and professionals, and between professionals. They underline the belief that legislative action is a last resort when acting to protect children.

Under section 47 of the Act, local authorities have a duty to:

- investigate suspected child abuse cases
- take steps to ensure the child's welfare is safeguarded.

Although many cases are investigated under section 47, only a small proportion of these result in legal action. Procedural guidelines support the non-interventionist principle, in that steps have to be taken to try and safeguard the child without resorting to the law. Legal action can be traumatic for the child and family and may result in the child being separated from her caregivers. It is in the child's best interests to avoid legal intervention unless this is the only way to protect the child. For example, if the child can remain with a non-abusive parent within his or her own home, with siblings, school and friends, then the impact of abuse will be lessened. If the child is removed from home through the legal process, this means disruption to family and other relationships, education and care arrangements, and loss of familiar environments, routines and people.

'Significant harm'

In order for legal steps to be taken, the child must be deemed to be suffering or likely to suffer significant harm for such intervention to take place. 'Harm' is defined as:

> *ill-treatment or the impairment of health and development (section 31, Children Act 1989)*

'Development' refers to all aspects of the child's physical, emotional and social development and learning development. There must be evidence that the quality of care the child is receiving will result in or has resulted in 'significant harm' to the child. Evidence of 'significant harm' will be gathered in a child protection investigation from the observations of practitioners, medical evidence, educational and psychological assessments and the child's story. Such evidence may include charting of physical injuries or impairments to growth and development.

Court orders

Court orders will only be granted if it is in a child's best interests for the court to make the order. Normally court orders are applied for by local authority social services, but the police and NSPCC have authority to apply for orders also. The evidence that is presented to the court can be drawn from a range of sources, so it is important to ensure that all relevant records are kept.

Emergency Protection Order

An EPO is used to remove the child to, or keep the child in, a safe place in cases where the child is considered to be in 'acute physical danger.' It is used where:

- ⊃ delay could be extremely harmful to the child, and immediate action to protect the child needs to be taken
- ⊃ when a child protection investigation is taking place and access to the child is being 'unreasonably refused'; for example, the parents consistently refuse to allow the social worker to see or speak to the child.

The person applying for the EPO must ensure that no alternative arrangements can be made to safeguard the child, such as:

- ⊃ parents agree for the child to be accommodated (cared for by the local authority on a voluntary basis)
- ⊃ parents agree that the child can placed with a suitable relative or other person
- ⊃ the person suspected of abuse agrees to leave the household for the time being.

EPOs are short term, lasting 8 days initially, with provision for a 7-day extension. The options available to the child after this time are shown in Figure 15.16.

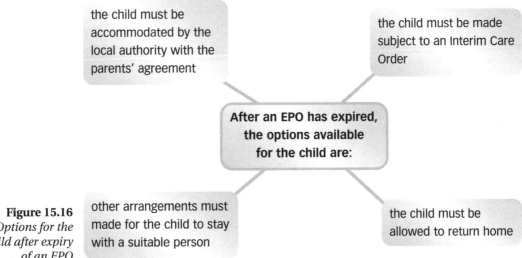

the child must be accommodated by the local authority with the parents' agreement

the child must be made subject to an Interim Care Order

After an EPO has expired, the options available for the child are:

other arrangements must made for the child to stay with a suitable person

the child must be allowed to return home

Figure 15.16
Options for the child after expiry of an EPO

Child Assessment Order

The CAO allows the local authority social services to gain access to a child for medical or other types of assessments. Criteria for successfully applying for a CAO include proving:

- ⊃ that the child may suffer or be likely to suffer from significant harm, and
- ⊃ that an assessment is necessary to determine this, and
- ⊃ that an assessment is unlikely to take place without the CAO.

A CAO lasts for 7 days and requires the parents to make the child available for specific assessments, which could include stays away from home. Assessment is interpreted very broadly and can include physical and mental health assessments; psychological assessments; and educational assessments.

In order to ensure that children have some control in this situation, children who have 'sufficient understanding to make an informed decision' can refuse an assessment. However, this tends to apply to children over the age of 10 years at least.

Care Orders

A Care Order made in respect of any child results in that child being placed in the care of the local authority, although the parents continue to share parental responsibility. The conditions under which a Care Order is made are shown in Figure 15.17.

Figure 15.17
Requirements for a Care Order

For a Care Order to be made:	
a child must be shown to be suffering from or likely to suffer from significant harm	due to the standard of care he or she receives *or* because the child is beyond parental control

The child is 'looked after' by the local authority until the Care Order expires (when the child is 18) or is revoked, usually through application by the parents.

The court can make an Interim Care Order for 8 weeks to give the local authority time to make a full case; for example, where an EPO has previously been made and it is not considered safe for the child to go back to his parents' care. Care Orders are not made lightly, as they involve the long-term removal of the child from the parent's care. As such, alternative solutions to protecting the child are sought, such as the removal of the abuser from the home or for the child to live with other caretakers. While the Care Order is in place, the local authority has to promote contact between the child and her significant others, except where there is considerable risk, in which case an application can be made to deny contact with named individuals.

The majority of children under 12 years old in local authority care are placed with foster carers, but chronic shortages of the full range of foster placements in many areas means that policies supporting placements which reflect the child's religious, linguistic and cultural background cannot always be complied with. Children may be placed in short-term or inappropriate placements, and many children experience multiple placements. A small number of children under the age of 12 may still spend periods of time in residential care, although local authorities usually have policies to place children under 12 years in foster care.

Supervision Orders

Supervision Orders can be made for a period of from 1 to 3 years. The local authority monitors and supports the child and family where a Supervision Order is in place. The usual reason for a Supervision Order is when there are concerns about the child's welfare and regular monitoring needs to be enforced. The child is usually supervised by a social worker, who is charged with advising, assisting and befriending him or her and ensuring the parents cooperate with the supervisory process.

Accommodated children

Accommodated children are 'looked after' by the local authority with their parent's agreement. The majority of children under 12 years of age will be accommodated with foster carers. The parents can reclaim their child at any time, as there is no legal transfer of parental responsibility. Accommodation can be a long- or short-term arrangement and can sometimes be arranged as an alternative to a Care Order.

The role of the practitioner in legal proceedings

The role of the practitioner in an early years setting is often limited in terms of direct involvement in legal proceedings. Giving information during investigations and at child protection case conferences; monitoring and supporting the child and family; and providing support services to the family may be the extent of your involvement. However, perhaps the most significant role you can take is that of providing continuity of care and support for the child during what is often a very difficult time. Parents need to be supported also, and their needs considered within the process. Practitioners in early years settings need to recognise that their role in supporting the child can be central in helping the child come to terms with some difficult changes in his or her life.

'Working Together to Safeguard Children' (DoH, 1999)

These Government guidelines provide every relevant professional with information about their role in child protection. The guidelines also include definitions of abuse and information about the indicators of abuse. They are based on research that has been carried out to establish 'best practice' in protecting children and supporting children and families in the child protection process. The role of the Area Child Protection Committee is outlined in terms of producing area child protection procedures and supporting and monitoring a multi-agency approach to child protection within the local authority. The guidelines can be found at www.doh.gov.uk.

The key principle of the guidelines is that the best way of protecting children is through cooperation between different agencies and professionals involved with the child and family. *Working Together to*

Safeguard Children is seen as a key feature of successful child protection. The string of child death enquiry reports that dominated professional views of child protection from the 1980s into the 1990s all identified lack of collaboration between agencies as a major contributory factor in the failure to protect the child in question. Multi-agency cooperation is now perceived as central to the child protection process.

Why do professionals need to work together in child protection?

Some of the reasons why professionals need to work together in child protection are:

- ⊃ lessons from child death inquiry reports about failures in inter-agency communication (Reder et al, 1993)
- ⊃ to prevent social disadvantage and exclusion through support for children and families
- ⊃ to reduce incidents of abuse and the costs of these
- ⊃ to maximise resource use by avoiding duplication of services. (DoH, 1999; DoH, 1995)

Working together in conjunction with other agencies is clearly an important principle of successful child protection work. Agencies and professionals need to share information, work together to protect children and support families, in order to improve parenting to a safe standard. While social services take a lead in child protection work, the legislation and guidelines emphasise that health and education need to provide support by providing information and services, as required. All practitioners involved with children have a role. However, inter-agency cooperation is not always easy to achieve. There are a number of problems in developing a multi-agency approach, as shown in Figure 15.18.

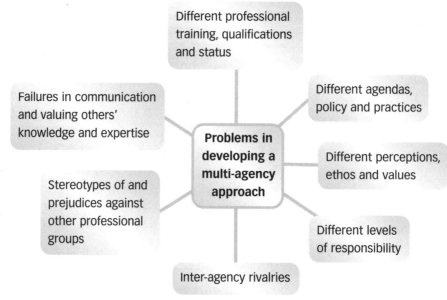

Figure 15.18
Factors that contribute to problems with a multi-agency approach (Hallett and Birchall, 1995 in DoH, 1995; Kay, 2000; DoH, 1999)

Different professional training, qualifications and status

Failures in communication and valuing others' knowledge and expertise

Different agendas, policy and practices

Problems in developing a multi-agency approach

Different perceptions, ethos and values

Stereotypes of and prejudices against other professional groups

Different levels of responsibility

Inter-agency rivalries

Those factors shown in Figure 15.18 need to be considered and addressed by agencies and professionals in order to ensure that inter-agency work is successful. Initiatives such as joint child protection training are in place to try and improve relationships, but not all practitioners have access to this.

> **Activity 3** **Dealing with professionals from other agencies**
>
> 1 Think of an example of your dealings with professionals from other agencies recently. What was the value of these? What were the problems, if any, and the cause of these? How could working together have been improved?
> 2 Write a short summary and discuss your notes with a colleague or mentor.

The 'Framework for Assessment of Children in Need and their Families'

The 'Framework for Assessment' is a tool for assessing all 'children in need' including cases where abuse is suspected. An initial assessment within the framework will establish if there are child protection issues to consider or if children and families only need to receive services for 'children in need' under Section 17 of the Children Act, 1989. Figure 15.19 identifies key areas of assessment and reasons for the development of the assessment framework.

The 'Framework for Assessment of Children in Need and their Families'	
3 key areas of assessment:	The child's developmental needs The parent's capacity to meet these needs Wider family and environmental factors
'Framework for Assessment' has been developed to:	Provide a more comprehensive approach to assessment of 'children in need' and their families Ensure family strengths and supports are acknowledged as well as failures or weaknesses in parenting Target services more accurately on identified need

Figure 15.19 *Key areas of assessment and reasons for development of Framework for assessment*

Social services are responsible for undertaking assessments, but other agencies are required to offer information, expertise and support towards the assessment of and provision of services to the child and family. Early years settings and organisations may be involved in assessment of:

- ⊃ the child's educational achievements and ability
- ⊃ the child's behaviour, and any difficulties in the setting
- ⊃ the child's ability to access the curriculum
- ⊃ the parent/child relationship
- ⊃ the parent's ability and willingness to support the child.

These contributions can be significant in ensuring that children and families are comprehensively assessed and a clear picture of the full range of their needs and areas of strength is gathered.

Failures in child protection

Failures in child protection tend to only be widely discussed when there are tragedies associated with a breakdown in the child protection system, such as the death of children like Victoria Climbie. However, failure in child protection can lead to misery for the child and family through lack of provision of services to prevent abuse and support the family. Failures in child protection are complex and involve many interrelated factors. These can include:

- ⊃ failure to recognise the indicators of abuse or respond to disclosure
- ⊃ failure to refer suspected abuse
- ⊃ incomplete investigation/no investigation/poor assessment of risk
- ⊃ lack of necessary information at the child protection case conference
- ⊃ poor or incomplete recommendations
- ⊃ inadequate child protection plan
- ⊃ the child protection plan is not implemented or is only partially implemented
- ⊃ liaison between key professionals fails or is unclear.

There are a number of reasons for failures in child protection; these are shown in Figure 15.20.

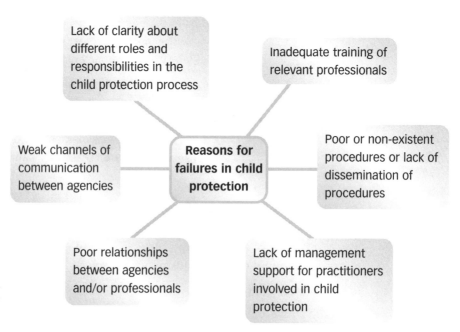

Figure 15.20
Some reasons for failures in child protection

The investigation of abuse and action taken by professionals can result in damage to the child and family. This may be due to:

- ⊃ failure to keep parents and children informed
- ⊃ separation of the child from significant others
- ⊃ failure to focus on the child and family's needs within the enquiry
- ⊃ disruptions to the child's routines, care and education.

Case Study 8

Coping with loss

Annie, 6 years, and her younger brother and sister lived with both their parents, who have severely neglected them from birth. Yesterday, social services removed Annie and her siblings from their parents care and placed them in foster homes on the other side of the city. Unfortunately, Annie's baby brother has gone to a different foster home because Annie's foster carer could only cope with two children. Annie has looked after her brother from birth and she loves him very much.

1 Consider how Annie must be feeling today.

2 What losses has she suffered? How do you think an adult could help Annie to understand what has happened? What steps need to be taken to help her cope?

In the next section the role of early years settings and organisations in developing high standards in child protection will be discussed, and the requirements of a supportive environment to promote the welfare and safety of all children will be outlined.

Raising standards of child protection in the early years

The role of early years settings and organisations, including education settings, within child protection procedures is outlined in *Working Together to Safeguard Children* (DoH, 1999). Early years settings should also be supporting children and families through the child protection process and in the aftermath of an enquiry. Their role is outlined in Figure 15.21.

Child protection training in the early years

Child protection training has improved in many early years settings, partly through the work of Early Years Development and Childcare Partnerships, which have promoted and supported training and policy development in many areas. Child protection is part of the OFSTED inspection requirements within the National Standards for Day Care. However, training varies in quality and availability and multi-disciplinary training is still much less available than single disciplinary training.

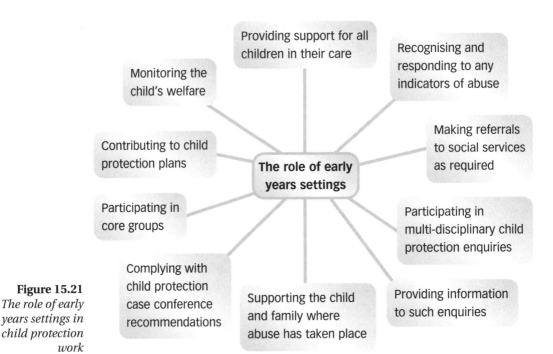

Figure 15.21
The role of early years settings in child protection work

There is a lack of adequate training in child protection on many initial teacher training courses, a fact which has been highlighted by the Victoria Climbie inquiry. Not all teaching staff have access to training after qualification, and joint training with other professionals may only be available to a few. This is despite findings by Baginsky (2000) that 94 per cent of schools have a child protection policy in place.

Working together in child protection

The development of a multidisciplinary approach to child protection has gone a long way towards improving professional relationships in child protection work. However, inherent differences in professional approaches to working with children and families are still a cause for concern. These differences and consequences if they are not resolved are identified in Figure 15.22.

Figure 15.22
Professional differences apparent in a multidisciplinary approach to child protection

Inherent differences in professional approaches to working with children and families and their consequences	
Professional differences include:	Organisational aims and objectives Professional approaches to work Training and professional qualifications Pay and status Use of language and different jargon
If professional differences are not resolved, they may lead to:	Poor communication and information relay Poorly planned and implemented efforts to protect the child and support the family Higher risk to the child Failure to support the family

A multidisciplinary approach needs to be supported through the development of joint protocols between agencies around working together; joint training; regular contact with other professionals; and the recognition of others' roles in the child protection process.

Developing a safe environment for all children

A 'child protecting' setting does not just react to individual cases of abuse that may arise, but creates an environment in which children's needs come first and where children are supported to develop confidence and high self-esteem. It is an environment in which children's security is promoted and this is achieved through working with children directly and also though developing supportive relationships with parents. It is also an environment in which observation is used to monitor the welfare of children as well as their educational progress.

In a 'child protecting' setting the care of children is seen in terms of emotional and psychological care as well as meeting children's physical needs. In a safe environment children are:

- valued in all aspects of their selves and their achievements, including their religious, cultural and linguistic background
- given genuine and considered praise and rewards for achievement
- supported to behave appropriately
- encouraged to respect themselves and others
- protected from all forms of bullying including verbal assaults
- encouraged to try new activities, make mistakes and experiment.

Activity 4 **Promoting a 'child protecting' environment in your early years setting**

In discussion with a colleague or mentor, make some suggestions for your early years setting about how a 'child protecting' environment could be promoted further.

These could include how children from diverse backgrounds are best supported; how the self-esteem of all children can be supported; how mutual respect is developed. Remember the role of practitioners as models of behaviour and ways in which all staff can be involved.

Supporting children who have been abused

Abused children may feel angry and bewildered, confused and scared, guilty about the impact of their abuse on the family, sad and unloved. Those who are separated from their parents may be in despair and unable to understand the outcomes of the abuse enquiry. Stopping the abuse may seem a simple solution to the child's problems, but the process of doing this may result in further pain. Butler and Williamson (1999:12) conclude that to work effectively with children who have been abused 'it is vitally necessary to establish what children themselves see as the primary causes of pain, distress and fear.'

Some children may receive therapeutic support, such as play therapy or counselling, in the aftermath of abuse, but this is not always available or relevant for all children. A child's response to abuse will depend on:

⊃ the extent, severity and type of abuse

⊃ the child's relationships with the abuser and other carers

⊃ the support the child has

⊃ the child's personality and personal characteristics.

Other factors may affect the child's response to abuse differently. Children who are disabled may 'have to work through the dual oppression of disablism and abuse' (Kennedy, 2000). Lees (1999:79) suggests that 'the inability of disabled children to communicate experiences is one of the factors that make them, as a group, more vulnerable to abuse.'

It is characteristic of abused children that they will suffer learning delays, social withdrawal or isolation, behavioural problems and low self-esteem.

Practitioners have a responsibility to support children during the aftermath of abuse on a number of fronts. These include:

⊃ maintaining a supportive and caring relationship with the child

⊃ using routine, daily activities and familiar events to 'normalise' the child's days

⊃ helping the child with difficult and painful feelings

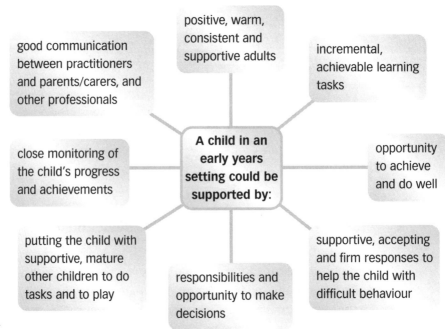

good communication between practitioners and parents/carers, and other professionals

positive, warm, consistent and supportive adults

incremental, achievable learning tasks

close monitoring of the child's progress and achievements

A child in an early years setting could be supported by:

opportunity to achieve and do well

putting the child with supportive, mature other children to do tasks and to play

responsibilities and opportunity to make decisions

supportive, accepting and firm responses to help the child with difficult behaviour

Figure 15.23
Examples of how a child could be supported in an early years setting

- supporting the child's behaviour
- helping the child to maintain friendships and other social relationships
- supporting the child's self-esteem and confidence
- helping the child to continue learning
- getting specialist support for children with disabilities/communication difficulties.

In order to support the child, there needs to be a clear understanding between practitioners, parents or carers and other professionals involved as to what the child's needs are and how best to meet them. Some of the ways in which the child could be supported in an early years setting are shown in Figure 15.23.

> **Activity 5** **Supporting an abused child**

Refer back to the case study of James on page 511 and answer the following questions:

1 How would you respond to James' behaviour?
2 What strategies would you use to help him behave more acceptably?
3 What other needs does James have and how else could you support him?

Supporting children who have been abused requires a range of interpersonal skills in order to ensure that the child is benefited by the relationship with the adults who care for him or her. Shemmings (1999) suggests that in order to make effective helping relationships with children, the six qualities and skills identified in Figure 15.24 are required.

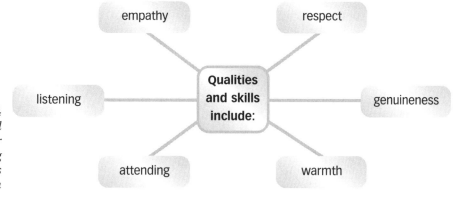

Figure 15.24
Qualities and skills required for effective helping relationships with children

empathy · respect · listening · **Qualities and skills include:** · genuineness · attending · warmth

Improving skills to work with emotionally damaged children is a crucial part of an early years practitioner's own self-development and learning.

Conclusion

The role of practitioners in early years settings in supporting children within the child protection process is extremely important in terms of the outcomes for the child and family. Children particularly need to know that familiar adults are going to be able to cope with what has happened and continue to meet their needs. Upholding the rights of the child through good practice, positive relationships with other professionals, and strategies to support the child and family is part of the development of a 'child protecting' setting. Recognising that child protection work is ongoing within the setting and not just related to individual cases is an important part of this process. Knowledge of legislation and procedures can give practitioners confidence to work well in this area and to apply their understanding of the child and family within the child protection process. Keeping the child and his or her needs at the centre of the process at all times ensures that good practice is developed and the child is protected within the child abuse investigation as well as within the family situation.

References and further reading

Baginsky, M. (2000), *Child Protection and Education.* London: NSPCC

Baldwin, N. (2000), 'Protecting Children: Protecting their Rights?', Chapter 1 in Baldwin, N. (ed), *Protecting Children: Promoting their Rights.* London: Whiting and Birch Ltd

Butler, I. and Williamson, H., 'Children's views of their involvement', Chapter 2 in Shemmings, D. (ed), *Involving Children in Family Support and Child Protection.* London: HMSO

Children Act 1989. London: HMSO

DoH (1995), *Child Protection: Messages from Research.* London: HMSO

DoH (1999), 'Working Together to Safeguard Children'. London: HMSO

DoH (2000), 'Framework for Assessment of Children in Need and their Families'. London: HMSO

DoH (2001), 'Children and Young People on Child Protection Registers – Year End 31st March 2001, England'. London: HMSO

Gibbons, J. et al (1995), 'Development after Physical Abuse in Early Childhood: a follow-up study of children on Child Protection Registers'. London: HMSO

Hobbs, C. (1994), 'Key Issues in diagnosis and response in child abuse' Chapter 1 in Pugh, G. and Hollows, A. (eds), *Child Protection in Early Childhood Services.* London: National Children's Bureau

Hodgson, D. (1999), 'Children's rights', Chapter 3 in Shemmings, D. (ed.), *Involving Children in Family Support and Child Protection.* London: HMSO.

Howitt, D. (1992), *Child Abuse Errors – When Good Intentions Go Wrong*. Hemel Hempstead: Harvester Wheatsheaf

Iwaniec, D. (1995), *The Emotionally Abused and Neglected Child*. Chichester: Wiley

Kay, J. (2003), *Protecting Children*. 2nd ed. London: Continuum Publishing Group

Kay, J. (2000), 'Working Together: the role of schools in child protection', in *ChildRight*, October 2000

Kennedy, M. (2000), 'The abuse of disabled children', Chapter 7 in Baldwin, N. (ed), *Protecting Children: Promoting their Rights*. London: Whiting and Birch Ltd

Lees, J. (1999), 'Children with communication difficulties', Chapter 12 in Shemmings, D. (ed), *Involving Children in Family Support and Child Protection*. London: HMSO

MacLeod, M. (2000), 'What do children need by way of child protection? Who is to decide?', Chapter 10 in Baldwin, N. (ed), *Protecting Children: Promoting their Rights*. London: Whiting and Birch Ltd

Munro, E. (2002), *Effective Child Protection*. London: Sage Publications

NSPCC (November 2000), 'Child Maltreatment in the United Kingdom', reported in the *Independent on Sunday* 19/11/2000.

Parton, N. (1996), 'Child Protection, Family Support and Social Work', *Child and Family Social Work*, 1, pp3–11.

Pettican, K. (1998), 'Child Protection, Welfare and the Law', Chapter 10 in Taylor, J. and Woods, M. (eds), *Early Childhood Studies*. London: Arnold

Reder, P., Duncan, S. and Gray, M. (1993), *Beyond Blame – Child Abuse Tragedies Revisited*. London: Routledge

Rouse, D. and Vincenti, O. (1994), 'Observation assessment and support: the contribution of early years workers', Chapter 5 in Pugh, G. and Hollows, A. (eds) *Child Protection in Early Childhood Services*. London: National Children's Bureau

Shemmings, D. (1999), 'The importance of relationships', Chapter 13 in Shemmings, D., (ed) *Involving Children in Family Support and Child Protection*. London: HMSO

Victoria Climbie Inquiry – Report of an Inquiry by Lord Laming, (January 2003)

Waterhouse, L. (ed.) (1993), *Child Abuse and Child Abusers*. London: Jessica Kingsley

Useful websites

www.doh.gov.uk
Department of Health website. Contains 'Working Together to Safeguard Children' and the 'Assessment Framework'.

www.victoria-climbie-inquiry.org
Report on the inquiry into the death of Victoria Climbie.

www.nspcc.org.uk
NSPCC website containing information and advice about child protection.

www.dfes.gov.uk/everychildmatters
Introduction to the 2003 DFES Green Paper, 'Every Child Matters'.

Index

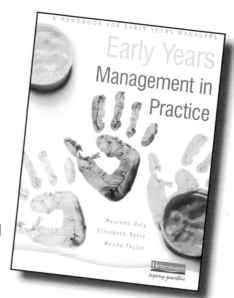
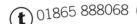 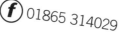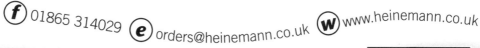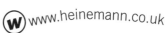
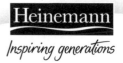